'Jess Glenny has produced an invaluable guidebook for the Hypermobile community. Her uniquely intersectional and thorough research offers useful tips, validating information and a wealth of resources for use – on and off the mat! Highly recommended for hypermobile yoga practitioners, teachers and bodyworkers.'

– Georgina Obaye Evans, Yoga Teacher and
Art Psychotherapist

'This is a book I will recommend to all my yoga and dance students and fellow teachers, whether hypermobile or not; Jess's approach combines insightful somatic perspectives with rigorous yet easy to understand scientific knowledge and methodology. Traditions in yoga are respected, whilst individual solutions to a healthy and enjoyable practice are presented in a way that is sustainable, enabling and forward moving.

Jess's knowledge of hypermobility and yoga is second to none, her book needs to be in every yoga and dance teacher's library.'

– Susanne Lahusen, Teacher Trainer, Lecturer at Yoga
Campus and London Contemporary Dance School

'*Hypermobility on the Yoga Mat* is a wonderful resource for yoga teachers and students alike. Jess uses her lived experience of hypermobility and her expertise as a yoga teacher in order to shed light on this fascinating and under-researched area. Written in both a scholarly and accessible way, I would recommend this be on every teacher training's book list.'

– Dr Abby Hoffmann, Dance and Yoga Specialist, Director
of Embodied Dancer Teacher Training, Freelance Tutor,
Rambert School of Ballet and Contemporary Dance

'Another useful book from Jess, not just for yoga teachers, but for anyone working with or living with hypermobility. The book carefully lays out both the science and the anecdotal experiences of a hypermobile body, and links this to a number of key related conditions, from POTS to autism. An important read, especially in conjunction with her previous book, *The Yoga Teacher Mentor.*'

– Theo Wildcroft, PhD

'As someone with Ehlers-Danlos, I found the information in Jess's book invaluable. If you are a person who is hypermobile and starting to explore yoga as tool for better health, I would strongly suggest you read Jess's book first. I only wish this book had been available when I started my yoga journey.'

– *Mick Lawton, Musician and Community Musician, Hypermobile Yoga Practitioner*

'A tremendously useful book for both teachers and students. Jess has brought together a wealth of information in a clear and accessible way. A must-read for anyone wanting to improve their knowledge and teaching skills relating to the important topic of hypermobility within a yoga setting.'

– *Stuart Girling, Founder of Loveyogaanatomy.com*

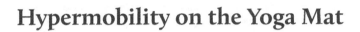

Hypermobility on the Yoga Mat

by the same author

The Yoga Teacher Mentor
A Reflective Guide to Holding Spaces, Maintaining
Boundaries, and Creating Inclusive Classes
Jess Glenny
Foreword by Norman Blair
ISBN 978 1 78775 126 2
eISBN 978 1 78775 127 9

of related interest

A Guide to Living with Ehlers-Danlos Syndrome (Hypermobility Type)
Bending without Breaking (2nd edition)
Isobel Knight
ISBN 978 1 84819 231 7
eISBN 978 0 85701 180 0

A Multidisciplinary Approach to Managing Ehlers-
Danlos (Type III) – Hypermobility Syndrome
Working with the Chronic Complex Patient
Isobel Knight
With contributions from Professor Howard Bird, Dr Alan Hakim, Rosemary
Keer, Dr Andrew Lucas, Dr Jane Simmonds and John Wilks
ISBN 978 1 84819 080 1
eISBN 978 0 85701 055 1

Yoga for a Happy Back
A Teacher's Guide to Spinal Health through Yoga Therapy
Rachel Krentzman, PT, E-RYT
Foreword by Aadil Palkhivala
ISBN 978 1 84819 271 3
eISBN 978 0 85701 253 1

Yoga Teaching Handbook
A Practical Guide for Yoga Teachers and Trainees
Edited by Sian O'Neill
ISBN 978 1 84819 355 0
eISBN 978 0 85701 313 2

Hypermobility
on the YOGA Mat

*A Guide to Hypermobility-Aware
Yoga Teaching and Practice*

JESS GLENNY

Foreword by Jules Mitchell

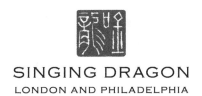

SINGING DRAGON
LONDON AND PHILADELPHIA

First published in Great Britain in 2021 by Singing Dragon, an imprint of Jessica Kingsley Publishers
An Hachette Company

3

Copyright © Jess Glenny 2021

The right of Jess Glenny to be identified as the Author of the Work has been asserted
by her in accordance with the Copyright, Designs and Patents Act 1988.

Foreword copyright © Jules Mitchell 2021

A CIP catalogue record for this title is available from the British Library and the Library of Congress

ISBN 978 1 78775 465 2
eISBN 978 1 78775 466 9

Printed and bound by CPI Group (UK) Ltd, Croydon, CR0 4YY

Jessica Kingsley Publishers' policy is to use papers that are natural, renewable and recyclable
products and made from wood grown in sustainable forests. The logging and manufacturing
processes are expected to conform to the environmental regulations of the country of origin.

Jessica Kingsley Publishers
Carmelite House
50 Victoria Embankment
London EC4Y 0DZ

www.singingdragon.com

Contents

Foreword

Jess Glenny has shown up strong for the yoga community by writing this much-needed text for a population who will benefit from it for years to come. Modern postural yoga has become synonymous with flexibility, an asset that many appear to possess while silently living in discomfort, confusion and a diminished sense of embodiment. Likewise, flexibility has become synonymous with hypermobility, a complex condition that is defined by a collection of symptoms far beyond just appearing to be good at yoga. Jess clearly articulates why these associations are incomplete at best and inaccurate at worst.

During my last decade of writing about tissue mechanics for the yoga population, I clearly recognised the lack of available research on hypermobility. There was just enough information to help me articulate that the condition was not a function of stretching and that stretching need not be vilified indiscriminately. Jess takes this basic premise and expands upon it tenfold, providing the reader with a comprehensive guide on how different styles of yoga can safely and effectively benefit hypermobile practitioners.

Only in recent years is hypermobility becoming more recognised by the medical community, resulting in a wide range of possible diagnoses under the hypermobile umbrella, as well as an awareness of how hypermobility expresses differently across individuals. Jess patiently outlines all the potential challenges someone with hypermobility might face and how they might choose to approach their yoga practice in response. Her book is full of personal anecdotes and includes insightful quotes from not only researchers and yoga educators, but also the students themselves. She truly grasps how important it is to hear directly from those whom the book is intended to benefit.

Because yoga tends to select for individuals on the hypermobility spectrum, Jess Glenny's work is especially important. She brings awareness to a crucial topic while maintaining her position as a yoga teacher rather than a medical professional or scientific researcher. For this reason alone, her book will serve many who might otherwise not have to access to this information. *Hypermobility on the Yoga Mat* will help yoga teachers and students navigate the practice we love while empowering us to make informed decisions about when to seek further care.

Jules Mitchell MS, LMT, RYT
Yoga Educator, Research and Adjunct Faculty, Arizona State University
Author: Yoga Biomechanics: Stretching Redefined
www.julesmitchell.com

Acknowledgements

Thanks go first and foremost to the many hypermobile yoga practitioners I have worked with over the years – one to one, in Mysore rooms, in restorative yin yoga classes and in yoga and hypermobility workshops – in collaboration with whom I have gradually evolved a body of knowledge about teaching hypermobile students. Your input has been invaluable.

Thank you to all those readers who have responded to my blogposts and articles about yoga and hypermobility and whose questions and comments have informed this book.

Thank you to members of the Hypermobility on the Yoga Mat, Yoga Teachers Support and Mentoring, Yoga Teachers UK and EDS Dancers Facebook groups for generously responding to my research questions and sharing your experiences.

Thank you to those yoga teachers and students who generously gave their permission to be quoted in this book.

Thank you to children's yoga teachers Iris Waller and Melissa Palmer for sharing your experiences of working with hypermobile children.

Thank you to Darren Higgins, practice principal of Vanbrugh Physiotherapy Clinic in London, for reading and checking the biomechanical information in this book. Any errors that remain are mine. Darren is also my main man when it comes to keeping my own body in motion. Working with him over the years has contributed to a huge uplift in my own proprioception and embodied understanding of biomechanics, for which I am very grateful.

Thank you to Stephen James, consultant in cardiothoracic anaesthesia and exercise capacity at King's College Hospital London and director of The Breathlessness Clinic, for responding to my questions about POTS and breathing.

Thanks to Jules Mitchell, yoga educator and author of *Yoga Biomechanics: Stretching Redefined*, for contributing the foreword to this book.

Thanks once again to the team at Singing Dragon for being a friendly and supportive bunch of people to work with and for always upholding excellent production values.

Thank you to Professor Rodney Grahame CBE, former consultant in rheumatology at University College London Hospitals, who diagnosed me with what's now called hEDS, and has been instrumental in creating awareness and recognition of the joint hypermobility syndromes among medical professionals, in particular in the UK. When I was assessed by Rodney, he asked me if yoga was a good thing for a hypermobile person to be doing. I hope this book provides a slightly more extended answer than the one I was able to give at the time!

Finally, thanks to my body, the crazy wisdom teacher that always has a new trick up its sleeve. I wouldn't have it any other way.

Notes on the Text

Terminology

At present, there is no word in English to denote those who are not genetically hypermobile. For this purpose, I have coined the term CT-typical. CT stands for 'connective tissue'.

Disclaimer

Many of the first-person quotations that head up chapters and sections are from actual yoga teachers and hypermobile yoga students who have kindly agreed to have their words included in this book. Others are fictionalised amalgamations of the experiences of different teachers and practitioners, and any resemblance here to real teachers and real students is only that.

Introduction

When I set out my stall, in 2003, I had no intention of specialising in hypermobility teaching. Hypermobile students came anyway. At that point, there was little awareness of the joint hypermobility syndromes in the yoga world, and most of us with genetic hypermobility were very poorly served by the existing attitudes and approaches to working with what, at the time, was rarely identified as a physiological condition. Historically – and continuing on today – yoga teaching has been geared towards CT-typical practitioners, for whom increasing flexibility may be a genuine need in creating biomechanical balance. The cues that serve this population are obviously very different from those that are helpful and appropriate for a hypermobile person, whose main needs are for structure and stability. I had no formal training (none existed) or particular experience in teaching hypermobile people, but I did have some knowledge about hypermobility – more than most other yoga teachers – and a familiarity with the territory in my own body, gained through practising yoga with hypermobile Ehlers-Danlos for over 20 years. And so it began.

I wasn't then, and I'm not now, a medical professional, a scientific researcher or any kind of expert on hypermobility. The suggestions in this book grow out of my own practical experience of making yoga friendly, accessible and helpful to hypermobile people ranging from elite professional dancers to those who are very incapacitated. Together we have generated a body of knowledge. Good movement strategies are key here, but they're not everything. An authentic practice resonates, repatterns, informs and pleasures. It leads us into the centre of our experience and reveals increasingly subtle sensations, emotions, and mental and nervous-system activities, so that over a period of time, the practising body becomes an ever-more intelligent system, a place where we can feel at peace and be at home. This is a process that encompasses but is much bigger than biomechanical recalibration.

Words have the tendency to nail thoughts down. Nevertheless, it's not the intention of this book to circumscribe what or how a hypermobility-aware practice should be. Ultimately, this is something that can only be discerned by the individual. As Body-Mind Centering® founder, Bonnie Bainbridge Cohen, says:

> The real key is to perceive what you're doing. I really can't teach you, but I can help you focus on your awareness so that you can discover what you are doing. Then you have choice.[1]

Practice is an intimate process. The role of the teacher is to offer relationship based on witness and informed suggestion, appropriate to the knowledge and experience of the student. That said, there is a great hunger for information and guidance among hypermobile yoga practitioners. I receive many requests, from all over the world, for advice about how to practise in ways that tend towards kinetic integrity rather than pain and dysfunction. If you are a hypermobile student of yoga, I hope that the signposts in this book will point you down generative pathways.

Yoga teacher training and hypermobility

While consciousness of genetic joint hypermobility has increased greatly in the yoga world during my time on the mat, the need for education among yoga teachers about what hypermobility is and how to work with it is still great. Once you have a hypermobility-aware eye, a quick glance around pretty much any general yoga class will reveal a considerable over-representation of hypermobile people relative to the population at large. However, yoga teacher training may include little or no content on working with hypermobile students. To get some idea of the current situation in this respect, I conducted a straw poll among teachers in two large online yoga teacher groups.

The earliest yoga teacher training reported was in 1972 ('we hadn't heard of hypermobility then'). The most recent was ongoing (in 2019). One trail-blazing, and CT-typical, British Wheel of Yoga teacher trainer, Andrea Newman, was including fairly extensive information about working with hypermobility in the early nineties. However, the majority of teachers graduating in 2016 or earlier had not received any hypermobility education. It was heartening to see that graduates in 2017 and onwards were much more likely to have received some input on working with hypermobility. However, in terms of what was taught and how knowledgeable and experienced the trainers were in the area of hypermobility themselves, things were still pretty patchy. Very few of even the recent graduates had been given any information about co-existing conditions and the multi-systemic nature of hypermobility. Training generally focused quite narrowly on biomechanics – mainly on limiting end range of motion, 'fixing' hyperextensions and building strength rather than working for flexibility – a lens that gave some graduates a rather skewed idea of what hypermobility actually is and what kinds of experiences hypermobile students might be having in their classes. Some teachers had sought to address this knowledge gap through continuing professional development (CPD) and discovered that – although the situation is improving slightly – there is a dearth of good-quality post-graduation training in hypermobility available for yoga teachers.

Difference versus pathology

One of the challenges for me in writing this book has been walking the teeter-totter line between acknowledging the very serious, sometimes life-threatening and definitely life-affecting experiences that the joint hypermobility syndromes can entail…and honouring those aspects of hypermobility that also bring gifts. These may be not only (paradoxically) capacities in the physical arena, but also differences in how we perceive the world that offer access to expanded cognition, deepened awareness and altered states. I was introduced to disability culture by the autism self-advocacy movement, which widely espouses the social model of disability, in which limitation resides not within the disabled person, but within the constraints imposed by a society unwilling to accommodate their disability. I tend to see hypermobility in this light, and wherever possible prefer to choose the language of natural human diversity over that of pathology.

How to use this book

This book is written with the needs of both yoga teachers and hypermobile yoga practitioners in mind. While some sections are addressed to teachers and others to hypermobile students, actually the whole book is for all of you. You don't need to be a teacher to implement the suggestions in Chapter 3 in your own practice, for example. And if you are a CT-typical teacher, Chapter 7 will inform you about some of the issues your hypermobile students may be facing when they attend yoga classes. If you are a beginning yoga practitioner, some of the information may be a little technical. Don't worry. Work with what you can currently understand. The rest will start to make more sense over time. If you can find a hypermobility-aware teacher to help you decode and apply the more difficult material, that's ideal. Chapter 7 is written more with beginning hypermobile yogis in mind.

Repetition

You will notice that there is some repetition in this book, as we look at things from different perspectives and through different lenses. When I trained to teach yin yoga with Paul Grilley, he always emphasised that repetition is important for assimilation, pointing to the oral traditions of the ancient Indian teachers. I hope that receiving information several times in different contexts, will likewise enable you better to understand and integrate it.

1

What Is Hypermobility?

Being hypermobile makes me struggle constantly to retain overall strength and core musculature. Not to mention, I can't always find where I am in Downdog (adhomukhasvanasana), for example. My range of motion is sometimes beyond my proprioceptive control. I really struggle in endurance exercises and am prone to feeling bouts of anxiety.

Elaine (yoga practitioner with HSD)

In this chapter, we will be defining terms, looking at the genetic and biological origins of hypermobility in so far as we currently understand them and considering some of the physical consequences of being hypermobile. The joint hypermobility syndromes are complicated and have many ramifications – not all of which there is space to go into in this chapter. The intention here is to present a general overview and to simplify some of the complexities in order to make them easily comprehensible to yoga practitioners and teachers. Please be aware that I am not a doctor. I have researched widely and have done my best to ensure that the information in this chapter is accurate and up to date, and I hope that it may join up some dots for you if you are, or believe you may be, hypermobile. However, if you have symptoms you think may be serious, seek the help of an appropriate medical professional, ideally one who is hypermobility informed.

Defining terms

When we talk about 'hypermobility' in the musculoskeletal system, we are referring to a greater than normal range of motion in any given joint. This expanded range of movement can be available for various reasons:

Injury

Significant physical trauma can cause individual joints to become lax due to damage to the structures designed to keep them intact. For example, if you tear a cruciate ligament – designed to tether the femur (thigh bone) and tibia (shin bone) together – the stability of your knee will be compromised. Your knee may become hypermobile because the cruciate ligaments are no longer able to do their job effectively.

Skeletal shapes

Each of us is born with our own uniquely shaped skeleton, and there is a surprising amount of variation in sizes, angles and proportions of individual bones. If the socket of a particular joint is broad and shallow, and the bone end that inserts into it is small, there will be lots of room for the bone end to move within the socket – and possibly even to move out of the socket partially (a subluxation) or totally (a dislocation). Where a person with shallow joint sockets has also inherited connective tissue (CT) laxity (see 'Differences in the connective tissue' below), they are more likely to experience repeated dislocations and subluxations – because the ligaments intended to stabilise the joints are overly elastic and don't hold the bones in place properly.

Differences in the connective tissue

Genetic differences in the coding of components of the connective tissue can cause that tissue to be lax, resulting in a general over-extensibility in the musculoskeletal (and other) body systems – too much 'give' that allows more movement in the joints than is healthy for their integrity. This type of hypermobility is generalised; in other words, it affects *all* the connective tissue (rather than only specific joints). However, this doesn't necessarily mean that a person with genetic hypermobility will be experiencing pain, dislocation or other problems equally in all the joints in their body, because many factors intersect to determine how hypermobile people are affected by connective tissue gene differences. We'll be talking more about this later in the chapter (see 'Hypermobility compared with hypermobility syndrome').

Genetic hypermobility is something the person was born with and (barring gene therapies that do not currently exist) will die with. They didn't get it by doing yoga – although what and how they have practised may have had an influence (for good or for ill) on how hypermobility affects them.

While some of the information in this book may be helpful for people with other kinds of hypermobility, it's really aimed at people with genetic tissue differences. In this book, when I refer to 'hypermobility' and to 'hypermobile people', I'm talking about those with a genetic tissue difference.

Genetic tissue differences

To date, more than 200 genetic (or heritable) disorders of the connective tissue have been identified: disorders affecting the joints, skin, bones, blood vessels, heart, lungs, ears and eyes.[1] Many of these disorders are rare, but the ones we are mainly focusing on in this book, hypermobile Ehlers-Danlos Syndrome (hEDS) and Hypermobility Spectrum Disorder (HSD) are relatively common. Marfan Syndrome (MFS), which we will also be discussing, is somewhat less prevalent. Some of the suggestions offered here may also be helpful in working with other genetic connective tissue disorders, but always check with medical professionals that your approach is likely to be beneficial, and if you're a yoga teacher, also work collaboratively with your student – be in ongoing dialogue with them about how your suggestions are working.

The specific gene mutations that cause some forms of hypermobility have been identified. For example, we know that:

- the vascular type of Ehlers-Danlos (vEDS) is caused by a mutation in the collagen-forming COL3A1 (or rarely COL1A1) gene;[2] we'll be talking more about the different types of Ehlers-Danlos (EDS) later in this chapter (see 'Other types of Ehlers-Danlos Syndrome')

- Marfan Syndrome is caused by a mutation in the FBN1 gene, which provides instructions for making a protein called fibrillin-1.[3] Fibrillin-1 is a component of thread-like filaments called microfibrils, which provide strength and flexibility to connective tissue.[4]

However, the genetic mutations causing the most frequently occurring forms of hypermobility, hypermobile Ehlers-Danlos and Hypermobility Spectrum Disorder, are as yet unmapped. While we do know that the mutated genes affect the protein collagen, a component of connective tissue, we don't yet know which specific genes are involved. As the symptoms, effects and presentation of hEDS/HSD are so diverse, it's very possible that a range of different genetic mutations, or groups of mutations, are responsible. At the time of writing, recruitment is ongoing for the Hypermobile Ehlers-Danlos Syndrome Genetic Evaluation study (HEDGE), the objective of which is to identify the underlying genetic markers of hEDS.[5] I'm enrolled in the study, so if there are significant findings, I'll be the first to tell you. Prior to the COVID-19 pandemic, results were expected in 2022, but I imagine they may now be delayed.

Types and more terminology

Historically, the classification of the hypermobility syndromes has been complicated, to say the least. In part, this is because the characteristics of hypermobility have been recognised by experts in the different and distinct medical specialisms of rheumatology and genetics, each of which evolved separate terminology and diagnostic criteria. In order to try to resolve this situation, in May 2016 a group of around 250 hypermobility experts from around the world came together in New York with the aim of redefining the classification and diagnosis of the Ehlers-Danlos group of conditions. The new names and criteria were published in March 2017 and are now in standard use. The Ehlers-Danlos Society explains:

> To recognise the continuum of joint hypermobility (JH), the hypermobility spectrum disorders (HSD) were created, ranging between, at one end, asymptomatic JH – someone who has no symptoms apart from their joints' capacity to move beyond normal limits – through to hypermobile EDS (hEDS), at the other end. The spectrum acknowledges that there can be severe effects on lives, whether they're the direct result of JH, or because they are known to be associated with having JH.[6]

Hypermobile Ehlers-Danlos Syndrome (hEDS)

HEDS was previously known as Ehlers Danlos Hypermobility Type (the diagnosis I was given in 2007, by Professor Rodney Grahame), and also as Ehlers-Danlos Syndrome Type III. It has also been referred to as 'benign' hypermobility, on the grounds that you're unlikely to die of it (some other forms of hypermobility may be life-limiting, as we will see). However, the effects of hEDS often feel far from benign to those experiencing them, and so the 'benign' word has now been dropped. Key diagnostic criteria for hEDS – the ones you may fairly easily observe in yourself – include:

- generalised joint hypermobility

- unusually soft and velvety skin, and/or mild skin hyperextensibility

- stretch marks without a history of weight loss or pregnancy

- piezogenic papules (bumps due to the protrusion of fat through herniated fascia) on both heels

- recurrent or multiple hernias

- dental crowding and high or narrow palate

- musculoskeletal pain in two or more limbs, recurring daily for at least three months

- recurrent subluxations or dislocations, in the absence of trauma

- exclusion of alternative diagnoses.

This list is not comprehensive. For full diagnostic criteria, see The Ehlers-Danlos Society's, 'Hypermobile Ehlers-Danlos Syndrome (hEDS) vs. Hypermobility Spectrum Disorders (HSD): What's the Difference?' at https://ehlers-danlos.com/wp-content/uploads/hEDSvHSD.pdf.

Other types of Ehlers-Danlos Syndrome

Prior to 2017, the various types of Ehlers-Danlos were categorised by number (in Roman numerals). They are now known by name, with 13 types having been identified, five of them being classified as rare conditions. This is confusing, because many medical professionals believe (wrongly in my view) that hEDS and HSD are themselves rare. These five rare forms of EDS are even rarer. While each type of Ehlers-Danlos has distinctive traits, there are a lot of commonalities. From the point of view of practising or teaching yoga, many of the suggestions offered for working with hEDS will also be applicable to the other forms of EDS, but always double-check with your student or, ideally, their medical team – there may be additional recommendations and contraindications. We'll be looking at special considerations for working with vascular Ehlers-Danlos Syndrome (vEDS) in the next section.

The 13 formally recognised types of Ehlers-Danlos Syndrome (EDS)

Current name	Abbreviation
Hypermobile Ehlers-Danlos Syndrome	hEDS
Classical Ehlers-Danlos Syndrome	cEDS
Classical-like Ehlers-Danlos Syndrome	clEDS
Cardiac-valvular Ehlers-Danlos Syndrome	cvEDS
Vascular Ehlers-Danlos Syndrome	vEDS

Current name	Abbreviation
Arthrochalasia Ehlers-Danlos Syndrome	aEDS
Dermatosparaxis Ehlers-Danlos Syndrome	dEDS
Kyphoscoliotic Ehlers-Danlos Syndrome	kEDS
Brittle cornea Ehlers-Danlos Syndrome	BCS
Spondylodysplastic Ehlers-Danlos Syndrome	spEDS
Musculocontractural Ehlers-Danlos Syndrome	mcEDS
Myopathic Ehlers-Danlos Syndrome	mEDS
Periodontal Ehlers-Danlos Syndrome	pEDS

The genetic basis for all the rare types of Ehlers-Danlos has been identified. This means that, unlike hEDS and HSD, they can be diagnosed by a blood test. You can find the genetic variations and current criteria for all the different types of EDS at: www.ehlers-danlos.com/eds-types.

VEDS

In addition to musculoskeletal connective tissue, vEDS affects medium and large arteries, potential complications including aneurysm (enlargement of the artery) and dissection (tear to the artery). In vEDS, arteries can rupture spontaneously, without previous enlargement, and this can be life-threatening. The gut walls and uterus are also fragile and at risk of rupture. While bruising is a factor with all types of EDS, in vEDS it is particularly pronounced. People with vEDS may bruise without any apparent trauma, and where a trauma has occurred, bruises may be larger than would normally be expected.[7] In 2017, the life expectancy of a person with vEDS ranged from ten to 80, with the median being 53 for women and 49 for men.[8] This may sound alarming, and vEDS does need to be taken very seriously. However, many people with vEDS experience few problems and live long and full lives. Annabelle's Challenge is a helpful website for support and information about living with vEDS: www.annabelleschallenge.org.

People with vEDS are encouraged to take mild to moderate exercise, for example swimming, stationary cycling, light weights and running on a well-cushioned treadmill. They are advised to avoid contact sports, as well as activities involving rapid acceleration and deceleration – because of the increased risk of blood vessel rupture these pose. Strong isometric exercise is also contraindicated, because during isometric contraction, blood pressure rises, challenging the integrity of fragile blood vessels.[9] Conventional yoga *asana* practice consists mostly of isometric holds, so if you have vEDS and are thinking about practising yoga, or you are considering teaching someone with vEDS, it's important to get medical advice first. The risk to the person is somewhat individual, and whereas some people may be advised against any isometric exercise at all, mild isometrics may be considered safe for others. On the whole, low-to-medium-intensity yoga classes are going to be most appropriate, while long holds and strenuous postures should be avoided. Restorative and gentle somatic practices will be helpful for regulating the nervous system and facilitating rest and integration. Vulnerable areas may need padding to prevent bruising, and if you're a teacher, be extra careful if you offer any physical assists.

Whereas people coming to a yoga class with hEDS and HSD are often unaware of their hypermobility, students with vEDS are fairly likely to have experienced major complications at a relatively early age, and/or to know about family members who have experienced these, so may well be diagnosed (by genetic testing), regularly monitored by a medical team and aware of what they need to do and not do to decrease the risk of complications. However, this is not a given.

Hypermobility Spectrum Disorder (HSD)

HSD is a new term, created to cover those who fall outside the hEDS criteria and yet are significantly affected by joint hypermobility. Previously, people in this category might have been diagnosed with Joint Hypermobility Syndrome (JHS). It's important to be aware that the effects of HSD may be equally severe and debilitating as those of hEDS, or even more so. The Ehlers-Danlos Society says that both hEDS and HSD:

> ...sit on a vast spectrum and can cause the same symptoms. What is important is that the problems that arise, whatever the diagnosis, are managed appropriately and that each person is treated as an individual. Both can be equal in severity, but more importantly, both need similar management, validation and care.[10]

Hypermobility compared with hypermobility syndrome

Joint hypermobility may be completely asymptomatic – indeed, it may be an asset, enabling the person to perform at an elite level as a dancer, gymnast, acrobat, footballer, musician and so on. For some people, joint hypermobility never becomes an issue; for others, age and lifestyle changes can bring complications; for others still, hypermobility is problematic and life-affecting from early years onwards. Where hypermobility is present but is not problematic, it is referred to in medical terms simply as 'hypermobility'. When hypermobility causes pain or other symptoms, it is referred to as a joint hypermobility *syndrome* (the specific type – Hypermobility Spectrum Disorder, hEDS, etc. – depending on individual characteristics). It is not definitively known why joint hypermobility can be an asset for some people and a serious disability for others. However, the following are some possible reasons.

Many hypermobilities

As we have already seen (in 'Genetic tissue differences' above), it's likely that a wide variety of different genetic mutations are responsible for creating connective tissue hypermobility. If this is the case, it might be more accurate to think about hypermobilities in the plural, and it could be that the specific genetic variation a person has plays a role in determining how problematic their hypermobility will be for them.

The Threshold Model

According to the Threshold Model, there is a critical mass of factors additional to the gene mutation, which, once reached, tips the person over into a hypermobility syndrome. These might include:

- age and the ageing process

- privilege related to socio-economic group, race, gender, sexuality, etc.

- mental health and psychological characteristics – which may increase or decrease resilience

- neurotype – an autistic person, for example, will be dealing with additional sociocultural and environmental stressors

- lifestyle factors, such as diet and exercise

- periods of temporary immobility (for example, due to illness or surgeries)

- a history of developmental trauma.

Marfan Syndrome

Whereas the Ehlers-Danlos Syndromes involve mutations in the collagen component of connective tissue, Marfan Syndrome, as we have seen, involves a mutation in the fibrillin component (see 'Genetic tissue differences' above). From the point of view of joint laxity, the issues for practising and teaching yoga are the same as those for hEDS and HSD. However, MFS also affects the vascular system, and so has some similarities with vEDS. Possible vascular complications of MFS include an enlarged or bulging aorta (the main blood vessel that carries blood from the heart to the rest of the body), separation of the layers of the aorta and prolapse of the mitral valve (a valve in the heart that lies between the left atrium and the left ventricle). These are all potentially life-threatening, and as with vEDS, people with MFS may have family members who have experienced serious vascular issues at an early age. I used to tell yoga teachers that because of prevalence in the family, people with MFS will usually have been diagnosed (by genetic testing). However, it turns out this isn't the case. The Marfan Foundation says, 'Our community of experts estimates that nearly half the people who have Marfan syndrome don't know it.'[11]

In terms of exercise, the recommendations for Marfan Syndrome are similar to those for vEDS: avoid activities that increase the heart rate and blood pressure, including any that involve bearing down, as these can place added stress on the aorta. It's advisable to stay within aerobic range (about 50 per cent of capacity).[12] If the person is medically cleared to practise yoga, they should stick to a low-to-moderate-intensity practice and avoid strenuous, fast-paced classes. People with MFS are at increased risk of retinal detachment, so inversions (if practised) should be approached with additional caution and held for only short periods of time. The Marfan Foundation has a booklet on exercise for MFS at: http://info.marfan.org/physical-activities-guidelines.

Marfan Syndrome versus Marfan habitus

As we have seen, Marfan Syndrome is a form of genetic hypermobility in which the fibrillin component of connective tissue is different. While everyone with MFS has a unique individual appearance, there are some specific genetic characteristics that many people with MFS have in common:

- Long, narrow long-bones with big knobbly ends, giving rise to long arms, legs, fingers and toes, and a tall, thin body (the classic ectomorph).

- Small skull and long neck.

- Indented or bulging sternum.

- Small jaw and big crowded teeth.

- High arch to the palate.

- Big hands and feet – with feet often flat and pronated.

- Spinal curvature and scoliosis.

Picture the small head and long limbs of the typical ballerina. That's a Marfan habitus.

Now, here's the kicker: some people with Ehlers-Danlos (me included) also have a Marfan habitus. We don't have Marfan Syndrome (our genetic connective tissue difference is in our collagen, not our fibrillin), but we do look Marfanoid. A fair few people with hEDS and HSD have told me that clinicians initially refused to refer them for diagnosis because they didn't have the typical Marfanoid appearance. This is because not *all* hEDS/HSD people have a Marfan habitus. But some of us do.

'Hyperflexibility'

The term 'hyperflexibility' occurs in some writing and teaching about yoga, and participants in my workshops are often confused about what it means. So am I. 'Hyperflexibility' isn't part of the standard medical terminology of joint hypermobility. If you are a teacher, and a student mentions having 'hyperflexibility' or being 'hyperflexible', you need to clarify with them whether they are referring to genetic joint hypermobility, and if so whether it is suspected or diagnosed.

Demographics: who has hypermobility?

It's difficult to gain an accurate impression of the general prevalence of hypermobility because studies have produced very wide-ranging statistics – from 4 to 30 per cent of the general population in my quick and unscientific online review. According to The Marfan Foundation, the prevalence of Marfan Syndrome is estimated to be 1 in 5000.[13] In November 2019, the *British Medical Journal* published a controversial paper by Demmler *et al.*, finding that EDS/HSD appears in the medical notes of one in 500 people in Wales and concluding that EDS and HSD should no longer be seen as rare conditions.[14] While many clinicians protested that hypermobility could not possibly be so prevalent, in my view this is still a massive underestimate of the number of people actually affected.

To some extent, too, it depends which general population we're talking about. Joint hypermobility is more common among people of African and Asian ethnicity,[15] so studies based on a cohort of predominantly white European people are likely to produce an unrealistically low prevalence. Joint hypermobility syndromes are under-diagnosed in general, and I suspect that among ethnic minorities diagnostic rates may be even lower. In an article for The Ehlers-Danlos Society, Nia Hamm, an African American with EDS, cites research showing that doctors are less likely to take reports of pain seriously when they come from African-American patients. She notes too that:

> Many members of the black community are distrustful of medical professionals. This may have to do with the long and painful history of medical professionals exploiting black bodies. It dates back centuries to when slavery didn't just mean free labour, but also a license for medical experimentation.[16]

Biological sex

It's possible to have hEDS as a result of a *de novo* gene mutation – a new alteration appearing for the first time in the family. In the majority of instances, though, hEDS is passed on *autosomally*. This means that the gene is carried by one or the other parent (or by both), and that it can affect both male and female offspring. This presents us with an anomaly, because hEDS, along with HSD, is more commonly diagnosed in women. Why might this be?

- Men are protected from some of the effects of hypermobility by greater muscle mass and higher muscle tone, as well as greater innate tendon and ligament tensility.[17]

- Hypermobility may be exacerbated by hormonal factors. In *Understanding Hypermobile Ehlers-Danlos Syndrome and Hypermobility Spectrum Disorder*, Claire Smith says:

  > Women tend to be more supple than men of the same age and are therefore more likely than men to have hypermobile joints. Hormonal fluctuations at key points in females' lives, such as puberty, hormonal contraception usage, or the perimenopause can trigger symptomatic

hypermobility. It is now widely recognised that, for many women, symptoms also significantly increase at certain points during their monthly menstruation cycle.[18]

- Cis males may be unwilling to identify with a what is viewed as a predominantly 'female' condition and may not present for diagnosis.

- Diagnosis and diagnostic criteria are not wholly objective but are subject to gendering prevalent throughout the society that produces them. As K. Malterud notes, 'the diagnostic process [is] a matter of social construction, where diagnosis results from human interpretation within a sociopolitical context'.[19]

While hypermobility is less frequently identified in biological males, men certainly can be hypermobile – I've worked with a number of men with hEDS/HSD – and may be very severely affected. According to The Ehlers-Danlos Society:

> The research is clear. Men can and do endure [sic] EDS, HSD, and myriad related disorders. And, even though EDS/HSD are under-diagnosed, they can be just as severe and debilitating in men as they are in women.[20]

Marfan Syndrome is equally prevalent and equally diagnosed among men and women.[21] Perhaps the predominance of vascular components explains the absence of diagnostic gender discrepancy here.

Occupation

It's probably no news to anyone that a high percentage of competitive gymnasts, acrobats, contortionists, skaters and professional dancers are hypermobile. I couldn't find any figures for the prevalence of hypermobility among circus performers or gymnasts, but according to one study of elite Australian ballet dancers, 72 per cent were found to meet the criteria for generalised joint hypermobility.[22] A 2004 study of The Royal Ballet company found that a whopping 95 per cent of female dancers and 82 per cent of male dancers met the criteria for joint hypermobility.[23] Moira McCormack, who was for many years lead physiotherapist at The Royal Ballet School and is a specialist in hypermobility, says, 'All the dancers in a vocational school are chosen for their hypermobility', and among this hypermobile population, 'Every school will have a scattering of more extreme hypermobiles.'[24]

The role of hypermobility in dance and gymnastics is pretty self-evident, but its prevalence in some other occupations may be more surprising. In 1831, the pronounced hypermobility of the virtuoso violinist Paganini was remarked upon in a medical note as an important contributor to his outstanding ability as a musician.[25] I haven't been able to find specific statistics relating to hypermobility among musicians, but greater than average rates are seen and remarked upon repeatedly in the dialogue surrounding hypermobility, including by medical specialists and researchers in the field, and by music teachers educated about hypermobility. Singers I have worked with have told me that they observe a higher than average rate of hypermobility in their profession and that extra flexibility of the vocal chords and palate offer the ability to produce a wider than usual range of sounds.

The situation is similar in some sports. Dr Jane Simmonds, who leads the physiotherapy team at the specialist hypermobility unit of University College London Hospitals (UCLH) and has a specialism in sports rehabilitation, says that 40 per cent of footballers are hypermobile.[26] A Hypermobility on the Yoga Mat workshop participant with a rugby-playing nephew told the group she had learnt that a high percentage of rugby players are hypermobile (scrums: scary thought!). An article in *Current Sports Medicine Reports* notes that joint hypermobility may be an advantage for cricket spin bowlers, divers, hurdlers (who need a wide range of hip mobility) and swimmers (particularly in butterfly stroke, which requires a lot of shoulder mobility).[27]

There are no statistics relating to hypermobility and yoga as far as I know, but there is a lot of anecdotal evidence that hypermobility is more common in the yoga-doing population than in the general one and that among yoga teachers the incidence rises higher. This is my observation too. We will be looking at why hypermobile people might be particularly attracted to yoga in Chapter 2 (see 'Why do hypermobile people love yoga?').

Professional asset or professional risk?

It's well recognised that in some occupations hypermobility can be an asset, and perhaps even a prerequisite for a professional career or a place in elite competition. In The Royal Ballet study cited above, 74 per cent of girls and 82 per cent of boys tested positive for hypermobility in The Royal Ballet lower school (11–16 years). Higher up the school, the prevalence of hypermobility increased significantly for the female dancers, with 94 per cent of girls and 83 per cent of boys in the upper school (age 16–18) being hypermobile (consistent with the percentages in the actual company), suggesting that hypermobility was selected for and contributed to professional success.

Recognising that 'GJH [Generalised Joint Hypermobility] is highly prevalent among athletes, dancers, martial artists and gymnasts, as also among other professionals in performing arts, such as musicians', Scheper *et al.* have coined the term 'copers' for those hypermobile people who, although 'at more risk of developing musculoskeletal pain…are still able to demonstrate high levels of physical performance and motor control'. They emphasise that while for copers hypermobility is, 'not seen as a clinical sign that is associated with disease', they are not necessarily symptom-free and are more susceptible to musculoskeletal injury, fatigue and deconditioning than their CT-typical counterparts. Scheper *et al.* note that, 'Although these individuals spent a lot of effort on physical training, GJH was still associated with decreased muscle strength and endurance, as well as lower functional capacities.'[28] One eminent and highly successful coper is Sylvie Guillem. Considered to be one of the greatest ballerinas of her time and known to be diagnosed with hEDS, Sylvie danced at world-class level until the age of 50 (a decade or so later than most classical dancers). In an interview with the *Evening Standard*, she said:

> The pain was always there. It's just that now I'm fed up with it. When I was 25 it was painful. I was getting out of bed in the morning and couldn't walk. But when you are young you don't care, it will pass. But one year after another, it's like, come on, give me a break![29]

For some, the difficulties with creating and maintaining strength, the fatigue and the higher frequency of injuries are not cope-able with. Kate Schultz, a former dancer with hEDS, says:

> My dance teacher loved me because of my flexibility. I could slide down into the splits without realising anyone else struggled. I could stretch and contort my legs in more complex pretzels than anyone else in my classes. As I've gotten older, the flexibility has turned into instability. Joints that did me favours by being loose when I was younger are now unable to stay where they belong and are a detriment to my well-being.[30]

Roxani Eleni Garefalaki, a performance artist with hEDS, was once an aerial acrobat, appearing at the opening ceremony of the 2004 Athens Olympics. She says:

> I was very successful, but shows would be followed by a complete collapse. I'd be in great pain and have to rest. In the end, I was spending everything I earned on osteopaths and physiotherapists to help the pain in my joints.

Roxani has now exchanged gymnastics for Alexander Technique. She explains that:

> I know how careful I must be with myself. I still get symptoms, but I know not to go to extremes in terms of exercise.[31]

The asset/risk trade-off operates across occupations. Professional guitarist, Tomlin Leckie, says:

> I have hypermobile joints, or Hypermobility Syndrome if you will. On paper this is rather cool. It means I'm pretty stretchy and can hit those big extended chords without too much trouble. However, in reality it means that I have a higher likelihood of getting issues such as tendinitis.[32]

Felicity Vincent, a professional cellist and Pilates teacher with a specialism in exercise for cellists, confirms that, 'Some degree of hypermobility can be an advantage in playing but is a double-edged sword, because stretchy tissue is particularly vulnerable to injury when over-worked.'[33]

Whether it's yoga, dance or gymnastics, hypermobility-informed teachers and coaches are singing from the same song sheet in terms of the need to create strong and stable biomechanics that tend towards longevity as a mover and decreased risk of injury. Physiotherapist and former competitive gymnast, Dave Tilley, says:

> Many gymnasts are born naturally hypermobile but then continue to gain more range through gymnastics that can lead quickly to elevated injury risk, instability, or pain. I think instead these gymnasts are better served training dynamic stability and learning how to control the excessive motion they already have.[34]

Autism and neurodifference

In 1996, while I was experiencing a period of crushing Chronic Fatigue Syndrome (CFS) – known in the UK as myalgic encephalitis (ME) at that time – I began to have a sense that the fragile elasticity of my body (hypermobility), and the eccentric way I processed information and related to the world around me (autism),[35] and the overwhelming fatigue I was experiencing... were All The Same Thing. It felt true. It made sense of my experience. But it also felt outrageous. At that time, I sort of knew I was hypermobile but didn't have a diagnosis; I had no idea that the eccentric way I processed information and related to the world was autism; and there was no information out there about the exhausting nature of both these aspects of personhood and how they could crescendo in annihilating fatigue. My GP had told me the fatigue would get better in a few weeks. I was too dizzy, foggy and bone-weary to go back and explain that it hadn't. It was like being lost in an enormous forest without a map or a compass but with a dim and intermittent intuition of a path. During that year, I journaled repeatedly about my sense of how all these experiences were connected...they must be...and yet they couldn't be...and yet they had to be. I was way ahead of the curve.

Cut to 2020. Autistic people and those who work with us at grass-roots level have for some time been aware of an intersection between autism and hypermobility, and the medical profession is slowly beginning to catch on. Baeza-Velasco *et al.* explain that this time lag is in part due to compartmentalisation in medicine:

> These conditions are seen by different medical fields, such as psychiatry in the case of ASD, and musculoskeletal disciplines and genetics in the case of hypermobility-related disorders. Thus, a link between them is rarely established in clinical setting, despite a scarce but growing body of research suggesting that both conditions co-occur more often than expected by chance.[36]

The authors of a 2014 study note 'anecdotal case reports and clinical suspicion of a link' between 'hypermobility and neuropsychiatric disorders of developmental origin'. Their research found joint hypermobility and autonomic dysfunction – an aspect of hypermobility we'll be looking at in more detail below (see 'Dysautonomia and POTS') – to be more common in a group of 37 individuals with autism, attention deficit hyperactivity disorder (ADHD) and/or Tourette's Syndrome than in a control group. The authors conclude:

> ...rates of hypermobility and symptoms of autonomic dysfunction are particularly high in adults with neurodevelopmental diagnoses. It is likely that the importance of hypermobility and autonomic dysfunction to the generation and maintenance of psychopathology in neurodevelopmental disorders is poorly appreciated.[37]

And, I would add, vice versa.

While there is all sorts of speculation out there, the bottom line is that we still don't know why neurodifference and hypermobility frequently co-exist. The authors of the 2014 study suggest, plausibly, that:

...autonomic reactivity and interoceptive sensitivity predispose to the expression of psychiatric symptoms, particularly anxiety... Inefficient neural co-ordination of efferent autonomic drive [nervous-system impulses going outwards] with imprecise interoceptive representations [awareness of internal body experiences] may be amplified in hypermobile individuals. In hypermobility, this mechanism might explain increased vulnerability to stress-sensitive and developmental neuropsychiatric conditions.

Like hypermobility, autism is under-diagnosed and often poorly understood even by those who profess to be experts in the field. If you are hypermobile, I suggest finding out a bit about autism – not from psychiatrists or medical textbooks, which often present views of autism that those of us who in fact are autistic find alien and baffling, but by engaging with the experiences of actual autistic people. There is a huge and very active online autistic community, with many excellent blogs, forums and advocacy networks. You'll find some suggestions for places to start in the Resources section. If you're a yoga teacher, the important takeaway is that your new student disclosing hypermobility may also be autistic and/or neurodifferent in other ways...and your autistic/neurodifferent student may also be hypermobile... whether or not they have a diagnosis in both areas.

Some basic biology

In this section, we're going to be looking at the role collagen and fibrillin play in the connective tissue (where both these proteins have their greatest concentration); considering the intersections and distinctions between connective tissue and fascia; and looking at why hypermobility is not just about joints but encompasses muscle too.

Collagen

As we have seen (in 'Genetic tissue differences' above), hEDS and HSD are physiologies in which collagen is genetically different from the norm. Collagen is a structural protein, the most abundant in the human body, making up about 25–35 per cent of total body protein – a significant proportion in terms of the effects of any genetic collagen abnormalities. There are about 30 different types of collagen – present, for example, in the cornea, cartilage, bones, teeth, blood vessels, gut and intervertebral disks. From the point of view of musculoskeletal integrity, the most significant form of collagen is Type I, which occurs in skin, bones, ligaments and tendons. Which types of collagen are affected in hEDS/HSD and which are not is likely determined by the precise genetic mutation (or mutations) the individual person has.

The role of collagen is to provide strength and support. Yin yoga teacher, Bernie Clark, explains:

> Tendons and ligaments do not normally stretch more than 4–10 per cent because they are made up predominantly of collagen. Collagen is a ubiquitous and amazing substance found throughout our bodies. What makes this protein so useful are its strength and resistance to stretching.[38]

Clearly, then, collagen with a genetic mutation that makes it more stretchy than usual is going to compromise the stability of physical structures in a significant way.

Fibrillin

As we have seen (in 'Marfan Syndrome' above), in MFS hypermobility is caused by a difference in the gene that tells the body how to make fibrillin-1. Like collagen, fibrillin is a protein and occurs in fibrous tissues. It is an important component in the sheath that surrounds elastin – the elastic component of connective tissue structures.

Connective tissue

When we talk about hypermobility, we are referring to a set of genetic conditions with a major effect on the connective tissue (CT) – a group of tissues that maintain the form of the body and the internal organs, providing support and cohesion to the whole. CT is composed of:

- stationary and migrating cells.
- ground substance (gel-like matter surrounding the cells)
- extracellular fibres – the most abundant of which is collagen.

Some types of CT are richer in ground substance, and others (for example, bone, tendon and ligament) are richer in collagenous extracellular fibres.

In a biomechanically well-functioning body, connective tissue has some elasticity (provided by its elastin component) but also plenty of strength and resistance (provided by collagen and reticular fibres) – enough that joints are stable, muscles maintain sufficient resting tone, veins can return blood to the heart efficiently, the intestines can move food through the digestive process at an appropriate rate and so on. When CT is too lax, stretchy or floppy, as in hEDS/HSD/MFS, there is a general lack of tensility in the body, and these processes cannot happen in an optimal way.

Fascia

The relationship between connective tissue and fascia is complex and overlapping, and to some extent is a product of how, as individuals, we view the connective tissue. All fascia is connective tissue – but not all connective tissue is fascia. Fascia is the system of bands or sheets of CT beneath the skin that bind together, separate, connect and define the spaces of muscles, organs and other body tissues. It is connective-tissue-as-fascia that keeps our bones, nerves, organs and cells in place. It used to be believed that fascia was an inert substance, but, increasingly, fascial research is showing us that this is a sophisticated and multi-faceted network of tissues, about whose full range of functions we still have much to discover. As the Fascia Research Society says:

> Fascia is the most pervasive, but perhaps least understood network of the human body. No longer considered the 'scraps' of cadaver dissections, fascia has now attracted the attention of scientists and clinicians alike.[39]

Use of the word 'fascia' tends to denote an interest in the CT as a complex organ in its own right, and an engagement with the cutting edge of research in this area.

Fascia wraps around our bones, muscles and organs a bit like a fibrous form of cling film (Saran Wrap in the US), but whereas cling film remains lifeless and separate, fascia is organically integrated, or meshed into, the structures it embraces. There's no precise or identifiable dividing line between one tissue and the next, rather a process of morphing and melding. Fascia is continuous, with all the muscles, organs and tissues folded within and emerging out of it. Yin yoga teacher Norman Blair says:

> Fascia becomes denser, forming tendons that become bones. Instead of all those apparently individual muscles, the body could be perceived as a large sheet of fascia with different muscular pockets... We are much more cavities and continuities than stuff that is solid and split separately... Fascia is the most dominant tissue in the body... Fascia is everywhere... We are cocoons of this fabric of fascia... Fascia covers, wraps and swathes the entire body,

from top of head to soles of feet. Fascia transmits information around the body. In the womb, fascia is formed before the nervous system.[40]

Myofascia, muscles and why hypermobility is in our muscles as well as our joints

It's sometimes said that the difference between ordinary flexibility and hypermobility is that flexibility is about muscles whereas hypermobility is about joints. This is not really accurate. The only meaningful distinction we can make in this area is in terms of how tissues are genetically constituted in the individual person.

In order to understand this a bit more, we need to consider that fascia (collagen- and fibrillin-rich connective tissue) makes up about 30 per cent of muscle mass.[41] For this reason, muscle can more correctly be termed myofascia. In other words, a lot of muscle is actually fascia, particularly where muscles are strong and tendinous. If we look at a muscle in cross section, we can see that it is made up of bundles of fibres nested within larger bundles of fibres, like a babushka doll. Each bundle is enclosed in a connective tissue tube, as is the entire muscle. Connective tissue is crucial to the structure of the muscle from the deepest, finest fibre bundle (the CT tubing of which is called the endomysium) through to the fibrous CT capsule of the whole muscle (called the epimysium), which merges seamlessly into the tendon.

The takeaways here are that:

- we can't separate muscle out from the fascial network it is woven into

- collagen is intrinsic to the formation of muscle – as it is to most structures in the body – and therefore genetic differences to collagen also significantly affect muscles.

Hypermobility in different body systems

As we have seen in the section above, collagen is an important structural component in all body systems, and any differences in its genetic composition affect far more than just joints. As Isobel Knight says, in *A Guide to Living with Ehlers-Danlos Syndrome (Hypermobility Type)*, genetic hypermobility, 'is a multisystemic disorder and its symptoms are holistic and far-reaching.'[42] In this section, we'll be looking at how hEDS/HSD/MFS manifest in different body systems. The ramifications of being hypermobile are extensive and widespread, and some are anecdotally well known but have not been studied scientifically. The following is not an exhaustive list.

Skeletal system
Dislocation

It's pretty obvious how increased risk of dislocation – the displacement of a bone from a joint – might be a consequence of laxity in connective tissue structures designed to maintain joint stability and support. Other factors that predispose towards dislocation (and subluxation – see 'Subluxation' below) in hypermobility include:

- changes in muscle tone, which cause imbalance in joint biomechanics, with tight muscles pulling the joint out of true (we'll be discussing muscle tightness and why hypermobile people are prone to this in the 'Muscular system' section below)

- deficits in proprioception leading to poor joint co-ordination (more on this in the 'Proprioceptive difficulties and dyspraxia' section below)

- lots of stretching without adequate strengthening.

Some hypermobile people never experience dislocation; for others, it's a regular feature of being hypermobile, and may or may not be experienced as problematic. Dislocations can be excruciatingly painful and may even require hospital treatment. However, some regular dislocators know how to put themselves back in joint quickly, simply and painlessly. Linda, a yoga practitioner with hEDS, says:

> My hip goes out all the time. It looks quite scary to other people, as my leg kind of collapses, but actually it's really easy to deal with. I just need to get on the floor and do this little manoeuvre and it's all fine again.

In contortionism, many acts are based on the ability to dislocate and 'relocate' joints at will. Daniel Browning Smith, a.k.a. Rubberboy, holds the world speed record for passing through an unstrung tennis racquet three times. Rubberboy has a diagnosis of Ehlers-Danlos and says that, 'I can dislocate both arms, both legs, turn my torso 180 degrees and all kinds of crazy stuff.'[43]

A number of my hypermobile students, clients and workshop attendees have reported experiencing spontaneous dislocations (dislocation without impact trauma or other accident) that medical professionals dismissed as impossible or implausible – but which x-ray later showed had indeed happened. Claire Smith, in *Understanding Hypermobile Ehlers-Danlos Syndrome and Hypermobility Spectrum Disorder*, also notes that, 'Areas which many clinicians would think were "very unlikely" or "impossible" to dislocate, are frequently mentioned by those with hEDS/HSD'.[44]

Jason Parry, specialist hypermobility physiotherapist, offers good advice for dealing with dislocation (and subluxation) in his article, 'Managing Dislocations and Subluxations in Hypermobile Ehlers-Danlos Syndrome and Hypermobility Spectrum Disorders'. You can find it on the Ehlers-Danlos Support UK's website at: www.ehlers-danlos.org/information/managing-dislocations-and-subluxations-in-hypermobile-ehlers-danlos-syndrome-and-hypermobility-spectrum-disorders. The key, according to Jason, is to stay calm and relaxed – simples, eh? What prevents joints from spontaneously slipping back in is the high-alert nervous-system response that causes muscles to go into spasm, unhelpfully locking the joint in the out-of-place position. Contortionists can 'relocate' their joints at will because they have trained their nervous system not to ramp up when they take a joint 'out'.

For more on dislocation, see 'Students who dislocate' in Chapter 2.

Subluxation

A subluxation is a partial dislocation, in which the bone does not move entirely out of the joint. A subluxation may last only a second, with the bone shifting out of its optimal placement in the joint and immediately back, or the bone may get stuck in an uncomfortable, not-quite-in-and-not-quite-out situation. As a big-time subluxater myself, I can often 'relocate' a wandering bone by getting warm and playing around with different small movements of the joint; occasionally I need the help of a physio or osteopath to encourage the bone back into place. Bones will also often spontaneously find their way home, usually when I'm warmed up and engaged in physical activity, such as adjusting in the Mysore room.

As with dislocation, hypermobile people sometimes report subluxations that are not generally considered to be possible. Claire Smith notes that, 'Rib subluxations are…often described (including those that move out of position from front to back as well as inwards and outwards).'[45] I experience rib subluxation myself. It feels as if one of my lower thoracic ribs partially shunts underneath its neighbour at the costal cartilage – which should be a tough fibrous tissue not allowing for shunt, but in some hypermobile people appears not to be as tough and fibrous as all that.

Not strictly a subluxation, another excessive-rib-movement event

I experience myself, and have come across in other hypermobile yoga practitioners, is when the end of one of the floating ribs gets wedged underneath the costal cartilage during strong spinal flexion, for example *dwipada sirsasana* (Two Feet Behind the Head Pose) or *halasana* (Plough Pose). Even *paschimottanasana* (Straight-Legged Forward Bend) can be a culprit for some hypermobile yogis if it's practised with little hip flexion and lots of spinal flexion. Pregnancy, and the consequent shifting of ribs, has been a predisposing factor for me.

It was many years before I realised that the little clicks, the joint pain that suddenly appeared and just as suddenly disappeared, the sense of something being just not quite right in a joint…were subluxations. For a hypermobile person, subluxation can be the path of least resistance when carrying out ordinary physical tasks; I have myself, in the past, routinely subluxated some joints – for example shifting the humerus slightly forward out of the socket – in order to perform certain movements, without realising that I was doing anything unusual or biomechanically less than optimal. I try not to now! As I've worked with hypermobile people over the years, I've found that this is a common experience for many of us, and may not be perceived by the individual as in any way different from the norm – because for us it is the norm.

Osteoarthritis

In hypermobility, joints habitually move beyond normal range of motion, creating potential for excessive wear and tear that may progress to osteoarthritis. There is plenty of anecdotal evidence for increased rates and degrees of arthritis among those with hypermobility, and many of my hypermobile students and clients have been informed about a hypermobility–osteoarthritis connection by clinicians. Annie, a member of a support group for women with hEDS, says:

> *I'm 50 and was diagnosed with early-onset arthritis nine years ago. The consultant said it was due to my hips repeatedly dislocating and that arthritis is a common complication of hypermobility.*

According to Alan Hakim, consultant in rheumatology and a hypermobility specialist, early onset osteoarthritis is typically related to overworking of the joints at an early age and over a protracted period of time[46] – for example in physically challenging yoga practice, dance, gymnastics, manual labour and so on.

Not all specialists agree that hypermobility predisposes to osteoarthritis, however. Indeed, one 2018 study of multiple joint osteoarthritis (MJOA) in older hypermobile adults suggests that being hypermobile may have a protective effect. The authors conclude that, 'in this large community-based cohort of adults, joint hypermobility was inversely associated with at least one definition of MJOA and was not positively associated with either radiographic or symptomatic MJOA by any definition.'[47]

It may be helpful to note here that (in the general population) there is little relationship between degree of osteoarthritic degeneration and amount of pain experienced. Rheumatologist, Don Goldenberg, says:

> In osteoarthritis, the pain intensity often correlates poorly with the severity of peripheral joint damage. For example, 30–50 per cent of individuals with moderate-to-severe radiographic changes of osteoarthritis are asymptomatic, and 10–20 per cent of individuals with moderate-to-severe knee pain have normal findings on radiography.[48]

In other words, you can have very serious joint degeneration with no pain or loss of function, and you can have little or no joint degeneration with a lot of pain and loss of function. Just because osteoarthritis is present, it doesn't mean that it's the cause of your pain.

Osteopenia and osteoporosis

Osteopenia is the medical name for low bone density. When osteopenia progresses to the point where the reduction in bone density is severe enough to create an increased risk of fracture, it is termed osteoporosis. There is some evidence to suggest a relationship between osteopenia/osteoporosis and hypermobility, but the jury is currently out pending further research. One reason for a bone loss/hypermobility correlation might be that pain and debilitation give rise to a decrease in the kind of bone-loading exercise that maintains bone density.

Clicking and cracking

Joint clicks can have a variety of causes, some of them benign and others less so. One commonly cited reason is decavitation. This occurs when carbon dioxide builds up in a naturally occurring cavity in the joint and escapes with a pop when the joint is forcibly stretched or compressed. Cracking of the knuckles, neck, toes and so on is decavitation, as are some osteopathic manoeuvres. While some medical professionals consider decavitation harmless (and to date there appears to be no scientific research to indicate any risk),[49] others argue that, when habitual, this kind of clicking and cracking tends to further loosen ligaments and exacerbate joint laxity, and may contribute to arthritic degeneration. PhysioWorks, for example, argues that, 'Repeat manipulation or cracking destroys the supportive ligaments and eventually the joints fall out of position much easier [sic]' and advises that, 'You can achieve the same result with less long-term harm by gentle joint stretching and mobility techniques to gradually loosen stiff joints.'[50]

Yin yoga teacher, Paul Grilley, has a slightly different take on decavitation. He explains, 'If a joint is immobile long enough, then some of the [synovial] fluid between the bones squeezes out and a temporary vacuum, or fixation, occurs.' Paul compares this to 'when the bottom of a glass of water sticks to the surface it is resting on'. The pop occurs when the vacuum breaks, releasing the joint. Paul believes that defixation is 'beneficial, because it allows the free functioning of the joints'.[51]

Paul Grilley also describes a less helpful form of clicking that he describes as 'friction popping' and which happens due to bones catching and vibrating.[52] This kind of grinding and grating may be due to arthritic joint degeneration or simply to unhelpful biomechanics. In either case, good hypermobility-informed bodywork can help, and is advisable to protect against deterioration. PhysioWorks says:

> Joints are held under tight compression that results in the two bone surfaces grating back and forth… This can usually be easily fixed through some simple physiotherapy treatment and sticking to an exercise programme that improves your joint alignment, muscle strength and flexibility.[53]

A form of clicking I experience a lot is tendon catching on the bone. Sometimes this is benign and due simply to a naturally occurring bump on the bone. Sometimes, however, tendon clicking can be caused by less than optimal joint positioning. In this case, alignment and stabilisation work by a physio or other biomechanical specialist can help.

Scoliosis

Scoliosis – a sideways curvature of the spine – is more likely to occur where there is a connective tissue abnormality.[54] The curvature can be S-shaped or C-shaped, and as a result, one shoulder or hip may be higher than the other, and the back may have a humped look. Congenital scoliosis (one present from birth) is caused by a malformation of the vertebrae occurring in the first six weeks of the embryo's life,[55] but scoliosis can also appear in childhood or adolescence. The cause is not known;[56] however, it seems plausible to me that in hypermobile people, the fascial structures are too lax and the muscles too low in tone to support the spine in an upright position as it grows. In my experience (in working both with my own body and with clients), what has been identified as scoliosis in hypermobile people is sometimes actually a kind of collapse in the ribcage due to lack of muscular and fascial support. This can be corrected by appropriate strengthening, mobilisation and proprioceptive work. I have found the Thoracic Ring Approach™, a physiotherapy modality, very helpful here. It's gentle, and more like somatic work than the kind of thing you might expect to do with a physio. You can find a physiotherapist certified in the Thoracic Ring Approach™ here: https://ljlee.ca/connecttheraphy-certified-practitioners.

Spondylolisthesis

There is research evidence dating back at least as far as 1980[57] that spondylolisthesis – the forward slippage of one vertebra in relation to its neighbour below – is more common in those with hypermobility. Spondylolisthesis can occur due to a congenital difference in the shape of the vertebrae, or it can be acquired – for example as a result of multiple micro-fractures caused by repeated hyperextension (backbending).[58] It generally manifests as back pain and spasms due to nerve compression. Treatment is by rest from aggravating activities and physiotherapy to help with strength, support and good biomechanics.

For more information about spondylolisthesis, see the 'Spondylolisthesis' sections in Chapters 3 and 4.

Labral tears in the hip

The labrum is a ring of tough cartilage that lines the hip socket (you also have a labrum in each shoulder joint), helping to maintain joint integrity. Labral tears are associated with lots of mobility in the hip, sometimes as a result of the shape of the hip socket, and sometimes as a result of genetic hypermobility (usually together with a joint shape that increases vulnerability to labral wear and tear). The most common symptoms are a pinching sensation in the hip and pain deep within the joint. Walking and other movements may produce a clicking sound. If you think you may have a labral tear, it's important to have it properly evaluated by a physiotherapist.

Labral tears are a hot topic among yoga teachers and practitioners these days, and some believe that they have become more common because of the way we are practising yoga. Yoga anatomist and ashtanga vinyasa teacher, David Keil, says:

I'm hearing more conversations about labral tears in the yoga world recently.

Are the instances of labral tears increasing? Are we just getting more informed about accurately identifying pain and injury within the yoga community? Is it the yoga that is tearing the labrum? These are valid questions, however, the answers to questions like these are difficult to fully uncover.[59]

It's important to bear in mind that it's only in recent years, since the advent of magnetic resonance imaging (MRI), that labral tears have become diagnosable, and this in itself may account for the 'rise' in numbers of yoga practitioners presenting with this injury. That said, if you are genetically hypermobile and prone to hip dislocations, you are in a vulnerable population and may want to practise hip work conservatively. Hypermobile yoga practitioners in general will benefit from practising towards strength and stability in the pelvis and away from excessive 'opening' of the hips, which may damage the integrity of the pelvis.

For information on how to work with labral tears in a yoga class, see 'Labral tears of the hip' in Chapter 4.

Dental issues

As we saw earlier (in 'Marfan Syndrome versus Marfan habitus'), a high palate with big, overcrowded teeth is a feature of the hypermobility syndromes. Gum disease and mouth ulcers are more prevalent in hypermobility, due to fragility of the oral mucosa, and (like pretty much everything else in our bodies) teeth may move more than is normal for CT-typical people.[60] This has implications for dental braces, with teeth tending to lapse back to their original position once braces are removed, perhaps because of excessive stretching, tearing and slow repair of collagen fibres in the jaw.[61]

Dislocations, subluxations and pain in the temporo-mandibular joints (TMJ) – the joints of the jaw – are common in those with hypermobility, and where dental procedures are carried out there may be issues with anaesthetics. We'll be discussing anaesthesia in more detail below (see 'Anaesthetics').

Other skeletal system issues

- Increased risk of fracture (due to repeated trauma).

- Increased risk of disk problems (due to excessive mobility in the spine).

- Pubic symphysis dysfunction (instability of the pubic symphysis – the cartilaginous joint that unites left and right pubic bones at the front of the body). This may present a particular issue during and after childbirth.

- Over-pronating feet (dropped insteps). For more on over-pronation, see 'Knock-knees' in Chapter 3.

- Bursitis (inflammation of a bursa, a fluid-filled sac that provides cushioning within the joints).

Muscular system
Tears, sprains and strains

As you would expect, hypermobility gives rise to a greater risk of tears, sprains, strains and inflammation in fragile muscles, tendons and ligaments.[62] In many hypermobile people, the ligaments and fascia are not sufficiently tensile to support the skeletal structure efficiently, for example in the hip and shoulder girdles and in the neck. Dr Alan Pocinki says:

> Chronic neck strain affects nearly every patient with JHS for two main reasons. First, the ligaments that are supposed to support the head are too loose and therefore cannot do their job well. The muscles of the neck are forced to do more of the work of supporting the head than they are meant to do, so they become strained. Second, most JHS patients have shoulders that are too loose, that is the 'ball' of the upper arm is not held tightly in the 'socket' of the shoulder. Because of the weakness of the shoulders, almost any activity that uses the arm, including reaching, pushing, pulling, and carrying, pulls not only on the shoulder but also on the neck. For these two reasons, neck muscles are constantly being strained.[63]

Muscle strengthening can help but may not completely eliminate pain and muscle spasm.

Micro-tears can also be a source of chronic inflammatory pain in the muscular system. Dr Clair Francomano, a geneticist with a special interest in Ehlers-Danlos, says:

> High-resolution MRIs reveal microtrauma, microscopic tears that start up the inflammation... Because each joint can subluxate over and over in just a single day, these microtraumas happen over and over in the same tissue without healing successfully.

Dr Francomano notes that these tears are not visible on ordinary MRI.[64]

Low muscle tone/hypotonia

The National Health Service (NHS) website explains that in a healthy person:

> …muscles are never fully relaxed. They retain a certain amount of tension and stiffness (muscle tone) that can be felt as resistance to movement. For example, a person relies on the tone in their back and neck muscles to maintain their position when standing or sitting up.[65]

In hypermobility, muscle tone is generally reduced. There is a lack of tensility which makes activities like standing or unsupported sitting challenging. Low muscle tone is not the same thing as muscle weakness. Some hypermobile people have very strong muscles, and to some extent this can compensate for hypotonia (or low background muscle tone) and for general joint laxity – but it can only compensate. It isn't a remedy.

Fatigue

Being hypermobile is fatiguing for all sorts of reasons, which we'll be going into later (see 'Fatigue' below). In terms of the muscular system specifically, muscles may be overworking to compensate for hypotonia and laxity in the ligaments and fascial system. Just holding yourself up requires a lot more muscle recruitment for a hypermobile person than it does for the average CT-typical Joe. Ian, a yoga practitioner with hEDS, says:

> *One of the most challenging yoga postures for me is tadasana (Mountain Pose). Just standing up – so tiring! I feel as if my muscles don't have the fibre to do it.*

Despite strength building over many years, sitting or standing static continues to be a challenge for me. Where too much demand is placed on hypermobile muscles, for example in lengthy unsupported sitting for meditation practice, they may go into spasm. Like many hypermobile people, I find motion far kinder on my muscular system, and lean towards practices based on movement.

Spasms

For some of us (me included) muscle spasm is a chronic problem, and a major source of pain and restricted mobility. Yes, you read that right: hypermobile people experience restricted mobility, and this can be a significant issue. Because the musculoskeletal system is generally lax in hypermobility, muscles may spasm in order to create compensatory support. Perhaps spasming of this kind ought really to be placed under the 'Nervous system' heading below, as it appears to be driven by a nervous-system requirement for greater biomechanical stability. While some muscles are designed primarily to support postural stability, others are mainly movers. In a hypermobile body, movers may be inappropriately recruited as stabilisers, so creating distortions in biomechanics…which generate further muscle spasm…and a chain of musculoskeletal dysfunction ensues.

Other contributors to muscle spasm are nerve irritation and muscular guarding of injured areas – which may continue long after the injury is healed.[66]

Other muscular system issues

- Cramps.

- Tics.

- Tendinitis.

- Plantar fasciitis (inflammation of the plantar fascia, a fascial band connecting the heel bone to the toes and supporting the arch of the foot).

Nervous system
Proprioceptive difficulties and dyspraxia

Proprioception is the ability to know where we are in space and where our body parts are in relation to each other; to judge speed and distance (within our own body and in relation to objects outside ourselves); and to assess extension (how much a body part has stretched). Proprioception enables you to know without looking whether your arm is above your head or by your side.

It used to be believed that proprioception was a muscle function, but it is increasingly being understood that proprioception actually occurs primarily in the fascia. Warren Hammer, a chiropractor and soft tissue/fascia expert, explains that, 'One of the most relevant discoveries in the world of anatomy over these many years is that muscle spindles, the chief proprioceptive cell affecting our muscles, are not in the muscle, but in the fascia surrounding the muscle and its muscle bundles.'[67] It's not surprising, then, that genetic differences in the connective tissue create disturbances in proprioception.

Tom Myers, fascial expert and author of *Anatomy Trains*,[68] explains the biomechanics of proprioception:

The muscles have spindles that measure length change (and over time, rate of length change) in the muscles. Even these spindles can be seen as fascial receptors, but let's be kind and give them to the muscles... For each spindle, there are about 10 receptors in the surrounding fascia – in the surface epimysium, the tendon and attachment fascia.[69]

The receptors are:

- Golgi tendon organs, which measure load (by measuring the stretch in the fibres)

- Paciniform endings, which measure pressure

- Ruffini endings, which communicate sheer forces (those going in two different directions) in the soft tissue to the central nervous system

- interstitial nerve endings, which communicate all of the above, as well as, possibly, pain.

Proprioception can be cultivated, and mine has enormously improved, especially as a result of strength training. But still, for me as a hypermobile person, proprioceptive signals often feel distant and dim, like radar through deep waters. I imagine that for CT-typical people the signal is constant and reliable, relaying a seamless and reassuring stream of information about where, how much, how fast and so on, but for me it's constantly dropping out, leaving me uncertain about the boundaries of my body, the cohesion of its parts and its position in space.

There is a knock-on effect here for our sense of embodiment, which may be vague and intermittent. When I was a child, I loved cut-out dolls because they had thick black edges. I wanted a body boundary like that – an interface with the world that was clear and palpable. Instead, I felt amorphous, not consistently 'here' and unsure that others could see me. For most of my life, I had no idea why I felt so insubstantial and uncontained, and imagined it to be due to some kind of existential lacuna. With knowledge and growing awareness, however, I have become more able to feel into the experience of dysproprioception and to identify it as a cause of difficulties and anxieties. We'll be talking more about the relationship of hypermobility with anxiety later (see 'Anxiety' below).

Profoundly autistic people, who often experience extreme versions of dysproprioception, have articulated well the sense of disintegration this kind of dissolved embodiment can involve. In *The Mind Tree*, a book written when he was between eight and 11 years old, Tito Mukhopadhyay writes (of himself in the third person):

He felt that his body was scattered and it was difficult to collect it together. He saw himself as a hand or as a leg and would turn around to assemble his parts to the whole.

He spun round and round to be faster than the fan. He felt so that way!

He got the idea of spinning from the fan as he saw that its blades that were otherwise separate joined together to a complete circle, when they turned in speed.

The boy went to an ecstasy as he rotated himself faster and faster.

If anybody tried to stop him he felt scattered again.[70]

I think many of us who are hypermobile will identify with using movement as a way to gather up scattered parts and feel joined up as a body. I certainly do.

At the more severe end of the proprioception deficit spectrum, proprioceptive difficulties can warrant a diagnosis of dyspraxia, which – in addition to movement co-ordination challenges – also involves difficulties with sequencing and planning, and sometimes with organising thinking and language. Kaiya Stone, a University of Oxford student with dyspraxia, remembers:

When I was aged 16 and an office assistant, I put the company I worked with in a near-criminal position. My job involved 'simple' admin tasks, which I processed with the success of a malfunctioning computer, spitting out wrong answers no matter what combinations I tried. Once, I was seconds away from shredding some crucial documents before a colleague stopped me.[71]

Dyspraxia often occurs together with other neurodifferences, such as dyslexia, dyscalculia (difficulty with numbers), autism and ADHD. Kaiya was eventually also diagnosed with dyslexia and ADHD, and describes herself (like me) as 'thinking in pictures' (hyperphantasic).[72]

Neuropathic pain

Claire Smith describes neuropathic pain as, 'the result of a malfunction, or injury, in the peripheral or central nervous system'.[73] As distinct from other types of pain, neuropathic pain sensations are often described as shooting, stabbing, burning, lacerating and tingling, and may be associated with numbness or weakness. In hEDS/HSD/MFS, one cause of neuropathic pain may be the impingement (or squeezing) of a nerve, perhaps because of subluxation, inflammation or osteoarthritis. I've certainly experienced short-term, localised nerve pain as a result of impingement. Whether impingement can account for chronic, generalised neuropathic pain is less clear.

Pain is a major issue for many with hypermobility and the causes are usually complex and various. We'll be talking more about pain in 'Restorative yoga for pain management' in Chapter 5.

Restless Legs Syndrome (RLS)

Restless Legs Syndrome is described by the Restless Legs Syndrome Foundation as, 'a strong urge to move your legs (sometimes arms and trunk), usually accompanied or caused by uncomfortable and unpleasant sensations in the legs'.[74] This most often occurs at night and can interfere with sleep. (For more on sleep disturbances, see 'Sleep' below.)

Chiari malformation Type 1 (CMI)

Chiari malformation Type 1 is a condition affecting the tissue around the brainstem. Non-profit organisation, Conquer Chiari explains that, 'The bottom part of the brain, the cerebellum, descends out of the skull and crowds the spinal cord, putting pressure on both the brain and spine and causing many symptoms'.[75] Henderson et al. add that, 'Obstruction of fluid circulation may flatten the pituitary gland, leading to hormone changes'.[76] An association between CMI and connective tissue disorders was first noted in 2007 by Milhorat et al.,[77] but more research is needed to ascertain prevalence here. Where hypermobility is involved, excessive mobility of the head and neck make CMI more difficult to manage, with increased risk of fluid leaks.[78]

People with CMI may not be aware of any symptoms or they may experience headaches and neck pain. Other symptoms can include dizziness, muscle weakness/numbness/tingling, problems with vision including involuntary movement of the eyes, tinnitus, problems with swallowing, and nausea.[79] Where neurological issues are worsening, urgent surgery is recommended, but where CMI is relatively mild, surgical intervention may not be necessary, and the condition can sometimes get better spontaneously.[80] The condition can often be managed with physiotherapy to improve muscle tone (and release tight muscles), create greater stability, and train posture and proprioception.[81] For information on how to work with CMI in a yoga practice, see 'Chiari malformation Type I (CMI)' in Chapter 4.

Other neurological system issues

- Headaches.

- Impaired sensation and hypersensitivity.

Cardiovascular system
Dysautonomia and POTS

Dysautonomia is an umbrella term encompassing any abnormality in the functioning of the autonomic nervous system – the branch of the nervous system that regulates unconscious body functions such as heart rate and respiration. There are many forms of dysautonomia, but the one that figures most prominently in hypermobility is Postural Orthostatic Tachycardia Syndrome (POTS). Most if not all people with hEDS/HSD/MFS experience POTS to some degree. When I was diagnosed with POTS myself, I asked the cardiologist if he had personally ever seen a patient with Ehlers-Danlos who didn't also turn out to warrant a POTS diagnosis. He said, no.

The most commonly experienced symptoms of POTS are:

- fatigue (again – we'll be totalling up the fatigue-generating aspects of hypermobility later – see 'Fatigue' below)

- dizziness

- brain fog

- palpitations.[82]

Other symptoms include:

- headaches

- nausea

- shortness of breath

- insomnia

- body temperature and sweating abnormalities

- chest pain

- fainting (according to POTS UK, experienced by about 30 per cent of people diagnosed with POTS).[83]

POTS is a complex and only partially understood condition. One plausible mechanism for some of the symptoms is in the venous return to the heart, which is accomplished partly through the muscle pump (the squeeze and release of active muscles in the extremities) and partly through valves (made of connective tissue) inside the veins. In hypermobile people, both valves and veins may be slack, making the blood return sluggish. In order to maintain circulation, the body reduces blood volume and produces adrenaline, which causes the heart to beat faster.[84] Another driver is hyperventilation[85] (when we exhale more than we inhale, causing a reduction of carbon dioxide in the body). I was investigated for this in the course of my POTS diagnosis and was discovered to be routinely hyperventilating. It's important to note that in the case of POTS this imbalance is happening on an autonomic-nervous-system level rather than as a result of something the person is 'doing' and can change by doing differently.

There are plenty of people with atypical POTS presentations, but the most usual POTS profile is normal-to-lowish blood pressure together with a high resting heart rate (even when the person is very fit and a low resting heart rate would be expected). It's important to be aware that POTS is *not* caused by low blood pressure, and is different from the kind of dizziness and fainting that occurs when blood pressure is unhealthily low.

People can be affected by POTS in quite individual ways, but I'm probably fairly typical in experiencing being upright and static as very challenging. Queuing or standing on the street to talk to a neighbour, for example, make me feel dizzy and faint. (Where possible, I sit on the floor, or if I have to stand, I look for something to lean on.) Likewise, if I stand up too fast or reach my arms above my head too quickly, I feel faint and may have to get my head down immediately. Despite being very fit, I experience periodic shortness of breath, accompanied by mental cloudiness and the desire just to lie down. While some people with POTS sweat to excess, I barely sweat at all (no, I *really* don't need a towel, hot yoga teacher), and am usually wearing at least one more layer of clothing than everybody else.

In yoga practice, the effects of POTS are typically seen in fast head-up exits from head-down postures, for example standing up out of *parsvottanasana* (Intense Side Stretch) or *prasarita padottanasana* (Wide-Legged Forward Bend). Standing up out of a dropback to *urdhva dhanurasana* (Upward-Facing Bow Pose) is another dizziness inducer. *Pranayama* can also be difficult and contraindicated for people with POTS. We'll be talking more about how to work with all of this in a yoga practice in 'Postural Orthostatic Tachycardia Syndrome (POTS)' in Chapter 4.

Despite this impressive array of symptoms, it's common for people with POTS not to know they have it – even when they are experiencing a fairly severe version. Until I was somewhere in my forties, for example, I thought it was normal to feel faint when standing. I just assumed that everyone in the supermarket queue was struggling not to pass out. One reason may be the invisibility of POTS: the typical POTS person doesn't appear from the outside to be different from the norm in any way, and so may find it hard to recognise their own difference. When I was in the cardiology unit for one of the diagnostic tests, a nurse mistakenly directed me to the staff toilets, because, 'You look much too healthy to be a cardiac patient.' And I am very healthy. I'm a very healthy person with POTS. Another reason may be the overlapping nature of POTS, hEDS/HSD/MFS, Chronic Fatigue Syndrome, and autism/neurodifference, with some of the same symptoms being allocated to all the conditions in the cluster. It can be difficult to separate things out, to work out what belongs where and to pinpoint which of the conditions your own particular group of symptoms may be indicative of.

POTS is poorly recognised by the medical profession, and it can be even harder to get a referral to an appropriate diagnostician if you suspect you have POTS than if you suspect you have a form of joint hypermobility. Research by myheart.net found that, 'Postural Orthostatic Tachycardia Syndrome is often misdiagnosed by doctors as anxiety, panic attacks, depression, or some other psychological disorder.' Seventy-eight per cent of those surveyed had been told during the diagnostic process that the source of their symptoms was not physical.[86]

The diagnostic route for POTS is referral to a cardiologist, via your GP. I was diagnosed at King's College Hospital London, where the consultant cardiologist, Nicholas Gall, has a particular interest in POTS and the investigations are more thorough than in many other cardiology departments. POTS UK has compiled a list of cardiologists with a POTS specialism. You can find it at: www.potsuk.org/doctors.

General recommendations for managing POTS include:

- increasing salt in the diet, or by supplementation, to between 3,000 and 10,000 mg (assuming that blood pressure is on the lowish side)

- drinking 2–2.5 litres of water a day

- eating small, frequent meals

- using compressions stockings.

Raynaud's Syndrome and chilblains

Raynaud's Syndrome is the result of decreased blood flow to the extremities in low temperatures. Most often it affects just the hands, occasionally also the feet, causing them to be chronically cold. The fingers (and/or toes) may turn white, blue or red, and there may be numbness, pins and needles or general discomfort.[87] Raynaud's is most common in – but not exclusive to – women under the age of 30. (I'm 57 and I've still got it.) It's thought that Raynaud's is caused by disruption to nervous-system control of blood vessels in the fingers and toes, although exactly how and why this occurs is not clear.[88] As you might imagine, Raynaud's can be a symptom of POTS, where it may occur during inactivity of the hands/feet without low temperatures.[89]

Raynaud's can also predispose to chilblains, small, itchy, reddish-blue bumps which develop on fingers and toes, sometimes with blisters, when the skin is exposed to cold and humidity.

Other cardiovascular system issues

- Varicose veins.

Cardiological issues specific to Marfan Syndrome and vEDS

As mentioned above, there are specific cardiovascular implications for people with Marfan Syndrome and vEDS (see 'Marfan Syndrome' and 'VEDS' for more information). People with Ehlers-Danlos (even the hypermobile type) *can* also experience these problems, but they are far more common in MFS and vEDS.

Respiratory system
Asthma

Some specialists believe that asthma (or asthma-like symptoms) can be caused (or exacerbated) by connective tissue laxity. Paediatricians, E. Soyucen and F. Esen, for example, hypothesise that:

> Asthma may also be caused by a connective tissue defect. Changes in the mechanical properties of the bronchial airways and lung parenchyma may underlie the increased tendency of the airways to collapse in asthmatic children… We postulate that BJHS [Benign Joint Hypermobility Syndrome] may lead to persistent childhood wheezing by causing airway collapse through a connective tissue defect that affects the structure of the airways.[90]

Difficulties with voicing

Speech and language therapist, Angela Hunter, explains that, 'posture, breathing and the voice box need to co-ordinate to achieve a voice' and that, 'Any general body hypermobility or fragility of tissues could, therefore, upset the smooth working of the voice by making these movements more difficult or by the tissues of the voice box becoming more easily inflamed.'[91] Some hypermobile children do not achieve reliable voice production until into their second decade, and adults may have difficulty with maintaining voice, the vocal cords and related structures fatiguing quickly.[92]

Obstructive sleep apnoea

When the hypermobile person relaxes during sleep, fragile cartilage may cause collapse in the upper airway (at the base of the tongue and the soft palate), creating interruption to normal breathing and sleep disturbances – or obstructive sleep apnoea. Verywell Health reports that:

> A 2017 study of 100 suggests that 32 per cent of those with Ehlers-Danlos syndrome have obstructive sleep apnoea (compared to just 6 per cent of controls). These individuals were identified as having hypermobile (46 per cent), classical (35 per cent), or other (19 per cent) subtypes [of Ehlers-Danlos].[93]

Guilleminault *et al.* explain that, 'In ED patients, abnormal breathing [obstructive sleep apnoea] during sleep is commonly unrecognised and is responsible for daytime fatigue and poor sleep.'[94]

Respiratory issues specific to Marfan Syndrome

- Sudden lung collapse (pneumothorax), is a condition in which the lung detaches from the chest wall. It can be recurrent for some with MFS. Symptoms include shortness of breath, a dry cough, chest pain that worsens when the person takes a deep breath and chest pain that worsens with coughing.[95]

- According to The Marfan Foundation, about 70 per cent of people with MFS have restrictive lung disease, in which the chest is not able to expand fully and oxygen intake is limited. Symptoms include shortness of breath, coughing, wheezing and chest pain.[96]

- Emphysema.[97]

Reproductive system
Pelvic floor dysfunction

Pelvic floor dysfunction is a difficulty with contracting and relaxing the pelvic floor muscles in a biomechanically helpful and effective way, and often involves hypotonicity (weakness and lengthening) in some muscles and hypertonicity (tightness and spasming) in others. While the scientific research paints a confusing picture, anecdotal evidence suggests that pelvic floor dysfunction is more prevalent among the hypermobile population. Given our general tendency to primary hypo- and secondary hypertonicity, along with proprioceptive difficulties, this is not surprising. We'll be looking later at how yoga can potentially help here – as well as how it can actually cause or exacerbate pelvic floor dysfunction when practised inappropriately (see 'Pelvic floor dysfunction' in Chapter 4).

HYPOTONICITY (TOO LOOSE)
Signs of pelvic floor hypotonicity include:

- stress incontinence – urine leaking during coughing, sneezing, jumping, running

- urgency in urinating/defecating

- organ prolapse (see also 'Uterine prolapse' below)

- 'fanny farts' – air enters the vagina…and on exit makes a noise similar to passing wind

- reduced vaginal sensation

- difficulty with keeping tampons in

- 'bulging, aching, heaviness, dragging, pulling, discomfort or dropping' in the vagina/pelvic region, which may feel worse towards the end of the day[98]

- pelvic instability, presenting as feelings of looseness or stiffness, or as 'clicking, grinding or crunching sensations'[99]

- lower back/hip pain.

Risk factors for hypotonicity include hypermobility, being overweight and having had multiple pregnancies.

HYPERTONICITY (TOO TIGHT)
In hypermobile people, the pelvic floor may, paradoxically, be too tight because it's too loose (muscles contract to compensate for connective tissue laxity). Signs of pelvic floor hypertonicity include:

- urge incontinence

- urinary frequency

- slow or delayed flow of urine

- painful urination/cystitis

- constipation, straining and incomplete emptying of the bowels

- pelvic pain

- lower back pain

- coccyx pain

- vulva pain (vulvodynia)

- pain on penetration or insertion of a tampon (vaginismus)

- pain while sitting.

Risk factors for hypertonicity include history of sexual abuse and history of practising strong core strength exercises without appropriate attention to softening and release.

Dr Uchenna Ossai of the O.School has a great user-friendly introduction to the pelvic floor and sexual function (which doesn't focus solely on straight, white, able-bodied people). You can find it here: www.o.school/originals/pelvic-floor-health.

Uterine prolapse

In uterine prolapse, the cervix or uterus slips down into the vagina. It's not hard to see how connective tissue weakness can predispose to uterine prolapse (and prolapses of all kinds). Joint hypermobility is well recognised as a risk factor for pelvic organ prolapse.[100]

A 2012 study of 120 women – not everyone with a womb and vagina is a cis woman, but it's difficult (impossible) to find research that takes this into account – found that:

A large number of women with BJHS [Benign Joint Hypermobility Syndrome] have prolapse symptoms which significantly affect their quality of life. POP [Pelvic Organ Prolapse] is more severe in women with BJHS.[101]

In my family, we have uterine prolapse in two generations of the hypermobile line, and I'm working to avoid it myself if I possibly can. We'll be looking at how yoga can help here in 'Pelvic floor dysfunction' in Chapter 4.

Painful periods

Dysmenorrhoea (painful menstrual cramping) is common among those with hypermobility. A 2012 Italian study by Castori *et al.* found that 82 per cent of participants with hEDS/HSD experienced dysmenorrhoea.[102] In 2016, a study by Hugon-Rodin *et al.* reported that 72 per cent of 386 participants with hEDS experienced dysmenorrhoea.[103] According to Claire Smith, one possible reason for this prevalence is that, 'Defects in the collagen structure may result in the muscles of the womb having to contract much harder…in order to shed the unused womb lining.'[104] I recall, many years ago, reading an article by an ayurvedic doctor who attributed dysmenorrhoea to laxity in the ligaments designed to hold the womb in place – a revolutionary suggestion at a time when those of us with hypermobility generally received little validation for our sense that many of our body parts (not just our joints) were too loose. In this hypothesis, the womb is suspended akilter, with the result that blood pools and the womb contracts spasmodically in the attempt to clear it.[105]

Hormones, more periods and menopause

I've noticed in my yoga practice that there seems to be a relationship between where I am in my menstrual cycle and how likely I am to feel pain, dislocate or get injured. I have to be very careful when I'm premenstrual.

Victoria (yoga practitioner with hEDS)

Oestrogen tends to stabilise collagen, while progesterone tends to increase collagen laxity. Androgens, the main sex hormone in cis males, have little impact on collagen either way, but do tend to increase muscle bulk around joints and so can have an indirect stabilising effect.[106] Among hypermobile people who menstruate, spiking of hypermobility-related issues around the (progesterone dominant) time of bleeding is often noted. Professor of rheumatology, Howard Bird, notes:

Many hypermobile patients, though not all, noticed [sic] a worsening in symptoms, more pain in the joints, clumsiness or a greater tendency to dislocate in the five days leading up to menstruation and in the few days after menstruation. This is exactly the time when the progesterone compounds far exceed the stabilising oestrogen compounds.[107]

This was also my experience during my menstruating years – whereas from end of bleeding to ovulation, my body generally felt less painful, and more stable and able to take on physically challenging activities.

Given the destabilising effect of progesterone, it will be no surprise that progesterone-based forms of contraception can be problematic for those with hypermobility, causing a general exacerbation of laxity, joint pain and so on.[108] Isobel Knight says:

> The fact I felt more hypermobile leading up to menstruation, and the fact my back pain and fatigue increased and my injury risk also seemed to increase around my menstrual period, are entirely related to higher progesterone rates which impacted substantially on my HMS [hypermobility syndrome] symptoms. The implications for the way in which progesterone can affect HMS women is therefore critical to take into account when doctors consider contraceptive and other hormonal treatments.[109]

At menopause, when oestrogen levels fall, joint laxity can also increase.[110] We'll be looking more at hypermobility and menopause in Chapter 7 (see 'Menopause and beyond').

Other reproductive system issues

- Endometriosis.

Digestive system

For some hypermobile people, digestive difficulties eclipse musculoskeletal problems in severity, and the relationship between hypermobility and gastrointestinal disorders has been recognised by researchers since at least 1969.[111] According to Dr Heidi Collins (whose pdf presentation on gut health and hypermobility is accessible and well worth a look):

> Gastrointestinal complications of EDS are:
>
> - **Common**.
> - Potentially **disabling**.
> - **Well-documented** in existing literature.
> - **Under-appreciated** by clinicians.[112]

Well recognised by experts in the field, the association between hypermobility and gut disorders is slowly beginning to disseminate out into the wider medical profession.

Irritable Bowel Syndrome (IBS)

Connective tissue is a major component of the gastrointestinal tract (the long twisting tube of hollow organs extending from the mouth to the anus), so it should perhaps come as no surprise that connective tissue differences can give rise to problems with digestion, causing sluggishness in the passage of food through the body. Qasim Aziz, professor of neurogastroenterology, says:

> This sluggishness is likely to be due to the increased elasticity of the gut due to abnormal connective tissue… The increased elasticity of the gut would make it more compliant (floppy) and hence the peristalsis (sequential movements that push the food through the gut) would be less effective.[113]

According to the NHS, the major symptoms of IBS are:

- stomach pain/cramps
- bloating
- diarrhoea
- constipation.

And secondary symptoms may include:

- flatulence
- passing mucus
- tiredness/lack of energy
- nausea
- back ache
- urinary problems
- incontinence.[114]

Even where a diagnosis of IBS is not warranted, hypermobile people may experience mild forms of some of these symptoms.

Hernia

Overly extensible connective tissue increases the risk of hernia. According to the Hypermobility Syndromes Association (HMSA):

> Hernias (bowel pushing through the abdominal wall) are common [among those with hypermobility]. Perhaps most familiar to the public is the hiatus

hernia – part of the stomach squeezes into the chest through an opening in the diaphragm. This can cause symptoms of pain, heartburn, fullness and nausea and vomiting. A hernia might also be found, for example, in the midline of the abdominal wall, around the belly button, or at the groin. Most often they present as a tender lump that might also expand on straining or coughing.[115]

Research by Z. Al-Rawi *et al.* found a positive correlation between the presence of hiatus hernia and joint hypermobility.[116]

Acid reflux (heartburn)

Given the hiatus hernia–hypermobility correlation, it isn't surprising that acid reflux is often an issue for hypermobile people. Laura Brockway, specialist registered neurogastroenterology nurse, explains that:

> Some preliminary research suggests that people with hEDS are more likely to have a small hiatus hernia at the lower end of the oesophagus. This means that the upper end of the stomach slips into the chest cavity through a small hole (hiatus) in the diaphragm (the large muscle that separates the chest cavity from the abdominal cavity. This is quite a common finding and is not usually dangerous, but it can mean that the muscle that closes to stop food or liquid contents of the stomach from escaping back up into the oesophagus is somewhat inefficient, resulting in the acid reflux and/or heartburn symptoms.[117]

Poor absorption of nutrients

Many hypermobile people have difficulties with absorption of nutrients. Marco Castori *et al.* state that:

> Nutrient deficiencies may participate in the onset or worsening of selected clinical manifestations of JHS [Joint Hypermobility Syndrome]/EDS-HT [Ehlers-Danlos Syndrome, Hypermobility Type] (e.g., pain, fatigue, osteoarthritis, reduced bone mass, and skin and mucosal features), and… tailored nutritional supplementations may improve patients' quality of life.[118]

More research into the relationship between diet/nutrition and hypermobility is needed – and, at time of writing, Ehlers-Danlos Support UK (together with Professor Qasim Aziz and Lisa Jamieson of Queen Mary University of London) is seeking funding to run a study on the effect of dietary changes on EDS.[119] In the meantime, many of the hypermobile people I work with have benefited from high-dose, highly absorbable vitamin and mineral supplements. Interestingly, even though I can eat anything and don't have any digestive symptoms, I have experienced clear improvements to immunity and general resilience as a result of supplementation. A significant number of my students, clients and workshop attendees report having improved their gut and general health by following a gluten- and dairy-free diet. Jeannie Di Bon, a movement therapist specialising in hypermobility, Ehlers-Danlos and chronic pain says:

> One piece of advice every person with a chronic illness must be tired of hearing is that they 'just need a healthier diet'. We all know that eating more fruit and veg is not going to suddenly cure hypermobility and EDS, however much kale we eat! But, paying attention to food and nutrition is an essential 'small step' in properly managing the symptoms of hypermobility and EDS. It's one thing I found really helped my symptoms and energy levels. There's no one-size-fits-all approach, but nutrition and diet do have a part to play in managing or even alleviating certain symptoms.[120]

Difficulties with chewing and swallowing

Laxity in the temporo-mandibular joints can give rise to difficulties with chewing and cause delays in triggering the swallow reflex, leading to food being left behind in the throat and delayed movement through the oesophagus.[121]

Other digestive system issues

- Rectal prolapse (rare).

- Incontinence (rare).

Urinary system

Frequency and urgency

The need to urinate frequently and/or urgently may be due to inadequate support from lax collagen in the bladder wall and pelvic floor. Neurological factors, affecting the autonomic control of the bladder, may also play a role.[122]

Nocturia

Nocturia is the need to urinate during the night. Again, insufficient CT support and neurological factors may be a cause. Anxiety can also exacerbate the situation. It's often recommended that people with nocturia reduce fluids before going to bed, but for those with POTS this may not be advisable (see 'Dysautonomia and POTS' above).

Stress incontinence

Stress incontinence is involuntary urination that happens when pressure within the abdomen increases suddenly, for example when jumping or sneezing. It's common after childbirth, when it may be a more serious issue for hypermobile birth-givers. Whereas stress incontinence is generally somewhat rare among those who have never given birth, it can affect nulliparous (having never given birth) hypermobile people.[123] For more information on urinary incontinence, see the 'Pelvic floor dysfunction' sections in this chapter and Chapter 4.

Bladder diverticulum

A bladder diverticulum is a kind of hernia, in which part of the bladder lining protrudes through the bladder wall. It may be completely unproblematic, but can cause urinary tract infections, bladder stones, urine reflux (flowing backwards), bladder tumours and difficulty urinating.[124] Bladder diverticulum is more common in male urology.

Immune system

Lowered immunity

One of the biggest challenges of the hEDS/autism/POTS cluster for me has been with immune system function. At one stage in my life, it was normal for me to have flu throughout the winter – not the kind of flu where you feel a bit rough, but the kind where you lie in bed sweating and shivering, and it takes a couple of hours to summon the energy to crawl (literally) to the toilet. It took me a number of years and multiple strategies (less work, more rest, supplementation, herbal antivirals and an annual flu vaccination among them) to arrive at the point now where I have a strong and resilient immune system and am rarely ill. Jo Rawston, who blogs about her experience with EDS, and in particular with immunity, explains that:

> People with EDS often have a lowered immune system. Part of this is probably related to being generally unwell for a long time, but there also seems to be a specific deficiency in IgG-3, which is one of the antibodies that fights infection. This can result in a vulnerability to infection, especially those mentioned above [ear, sinus, chest, bladder, kidney, skin and wound], and especially [those] caused by viruses and certain (gram negative) bacteria.[125]

According to Castori *et al.*, digestive issues and malabsorption may play into immune problems in hypermobile people. They conclude that:

> If supported by more robust data in adequately selected samples, the link between gut mucosal integrity and immune dysregulation, and JHS/EDS-HT may open a new era of investigative studies aimed at understanding the pathologic bases of many JHS/EDS-HT associated complaints.[126]

Autoimmune conditions

Autoimmune conditions, in which the immune system attacks the body, include Type I diabetes, rheumatoid arthritis, psoriasis, multiple sclerosis and Hashimoto's thyroiditis. There has long been a suspicion in the hypermobile community that autoimmune conditions are more prevalent among those with hypermobility. Recent research bears this out. A 2017 study by Rodgers *et al.* found that:

> Autoimmune/inflammatory diseases (psoriasis, PsA [psoriatic arthritis], AS [ankylosing spondylitis], RA [rheumatoid arthritis], inflammatory eye disease, autoimmune thyroiditis, SLE [systemic lupus erythematosus], Crohn's disease, pernicious anemia, and TRAPS [tumor necrosis factor receptor associated periodic syndrome]) were significantly more prevalent in the CWU [comprehensive workup: detailed dermatological markers, radiographic studies, etc.] hEDS population than in the general population of the US.[127]

Ocular system

Ocular discomfort

According to Dr Diana Driscoll, collagen makes up 80 per cent of the structures of the eye,[128] so it's easy to see why many of those with EDS and HSD experience ocular discomfort – dry eyes, irritation and general eye pain that doesn't indicate any serious pathology. For me, ocular discomfort manifests as frequent stabbing sensations in the eyeball and something that feels like deeply embedded grit.

High myopia

High myopia (nearsightedness) is more common among hypermobile people due to a flattening of the cornea and an elongation of the eye.[129]

Retinal detachment

Retinal detachment is more common in hypermobile people, especially those who also have myopia. Diana Driscoll explains that in Ehlers-Danlos:

> The retina (neural tissue) doesn't stretch with the sclera [the white of the eye] but rather gets 'pulled along for the ride' and can become thin resulting in retinal holes, tears, staphylomas, retinal degenerations, and detachments. Dilation of the eyes is recommended annually, or any time the patient notices a sudden increase in floaters, flashes of light (usually out to the side of the vision), or immediately if it seems as if a curtain is coming up over one eye. These can be symptoms of a retinal detachment and may need to be treated on an urgent basis.[130]

According to The Marfan Foundation:

> Head trauma can cause retinal detachment in anyone, and those who are highly myopic (near-sighted) are always at risk for retinal detachment. For people with Marfan syndrome, however, retinal detachment can happen spontaneously.[131]

Spontaneous retinal detachment is also a possibility for those with hEDS/ HSD.

Keratoconus

In keratoconus, the cornea bulges outwards in a cone shape, which is gradually pulled downwards by gravity, blurring the vision. Keratoconus may require specialised contact lenses, and occasionally, a corneal transplant may eventually become necessary.[132]

Blue sclera

Sclerae (or eye whites) are the protective outer layer of the eye and are composed of collagen and elastic fibres. It's normal for children under the age of two to have blueish eye whites, because their sclerae are thinner and so the blood vessels are more visible, giving a more blue than white appearance.[133] Blue sclera is also frequently mentioned in the literature of hypermobility conditions. MedicineNet explains that:

> The blue colour is caused by thinness and transparency of the collagen fibres of the sclera, allowing the veins in the underlying tissue to show through. Blue sclerae are characteristic of a number of conditions, particularly connective tissue disorders. These include osteogenesis imperfecta, Marfan

Syndrome, Ehlers-Danlos syndrome, pseudoxanthoma elasticum, and Willems De Vries syndrome, among others.[134]

The blue tone is easiest to see in a dim room with a light shining onto the eye and the person looking down towards their nose.

Dislocation/subluxation of the lens

This is most common among people with Marfan Syndrome or Marfan habitus[135] and is rare in the general population. Symptoms include nearsightedness (which may be mild or severe, blurred vision, double vision and fluctuating vision. Lens dislocations/subluxations usually happen before the age of 20.[136]

Epicanthic folds

An epicanthic fold is a fold of skin across the inner corner of the eye, as in Down Syndrome. While some authorities describe epicanthic folds as a feature of Ehlers-Danlos Syndrome, others argue that the typical Ehlers-Danlos eyelid shape observed in some – but not all – people with Ehlers-Danlos is not truly epicanthic. Diana Driscoll describes this type of eyelid as having, 'redundant skin on the upper lids' and 'downward slanting eyes' (towards the temples)'.[137] In Caucasian people, this eyelid type looks slightly East Asian.

Fibromyalgia (FM)

Fibromyalgia is a portmanteau diagnosis for chronic pain with no perceivable organic cause (there are no abnormal blood tests, scans, biopsies or other investigations to indicate a pathology). Like hEDS/HSD/MFS, it often involves headaches, fatigue, abnormal sleeping patterns, digestive issues and disturbances to the autonomic nervous system (heart rate, breathing, temperature, etc.). In my experience as a yoga teacher/therapist, it's very common for the hypermobility syndromes to be misdiagnosed as – or lumped into – fibromyalgia by doctors who are not familiar with the particular presentation of hypermobility. If you are a yoga teacher, this is something to be aware of if a student with FM comes to one of your classes. My student, Judith, says:

I had chronic pain and difficulty sleeping for years and was eventually diagnosed with fibromyalgia. I had no idea I was also hypermobile until I started doing yoga with Jess. She noticed that the way I moved looked loose-jointed, and suggested that my digestive issues, immune problems, dyslexia, joint pain and so on might all be linked. I eventually managed to get referred to a rheumatologist, who confirmed that I had HSD. Now that I know there's a problem with my collagen, everything makes a lot more sense, and I don't feel like a hypochondriac any more with all my different health challenges.

Dr Alan Hakim and Professor Rodney Grahame concur:

Fibromyalgia (FM) is probably the most common diagnosis given to people with CWP [chronic widespread pain]. However Ehlers-Danlos Syndrome (particularly hypermobile Ehlers-Danlos Syndrome) and the related Hypermobility Spectrum Disorders can also present with a similar picture.

They add that:

...it is important that your doctor does not ignore hEDS/HSD just because FM is present. Aside from the fact that hEDS/HSD has other problems not seen in FM that could be missed, the physical therapies used to help FM might cause harm if not adapted for the hypermobile individual.[138]

Mast Cell Activation Syndrome

Mast Cell Activation Syndrome (MCAS) was only defined as a condition in 2010 (although it has been proposed in medical literature for decades),[139] and is now something of a hot topic in the communities of hypermobile people and professionals in the field.

Mast cells were discovered by Paul Ehrlich in 1879[140] and are a component of the immune system. Their function is to defend against allergens and pathogens (bacteria, viruses, parasites and the like) by releasing a variety of chemical mediators, such as histamine. They also play a role in wound healing. Mast cells are found within connective tissue wherever the body interfaces with the external environment. Mast-cell-rich sites include the skin, the respiratory system (mouth, nose and lungs), the digestive system (stomach and intestines), the urinary system, blood vessels, lymphatic vessels, nerves and the brain[141] – a lot of places!

Over-activation of the mast cells can be triggered by a range of external factors, for example heat or cold, exercise, fatigue, stress, environmental toxins, drugs, cuts and wounds, and insect bites. The results are described by Mast Cell Action as, 'a wide range of unpleasant, sometimes debilitating, symptoms in any of the different systems of the body, frequently affecting several systems at the same time.'[142] These symptoms may include:

- flushing

- chronic fatigue

- painful, gritty, red or watering eyes

- rashes and hives

- swelling

- IBS-type digestive pain

- allergies and sensitivities

- muscle pain

- wheezing, runny nose and respiratory system difficulties

- headaches

- anxiety and panic attacks (due to an adrenaline response to over-production of histamine)

- brain fog.

Some people are relatively mildly affected by MCAS and may experience just one or two of these symptoms, while others may experience many.

Awareness is growing that people with Ehlers-Danlos – and perhaps especially those with Ehlers-Danlos together with POTS – are somewhat likely also to have MCAS. In a 2014 pilot study of 15 women with EDS and/or POTS, 66 per cent of those with both EDS and POTS (nine participants) also met the criteria for a mast cell disorder.[143] Making a diagnosis of a mast cell disorder is not easy. As Mast Cell Action notes:

> [MCAS may mimic] many other conditions and [present] a wide range of different symptoms that can be baffling for both the patient and their physician. Often there are no obvious clinical signs since MCAS confounds the anatomy-based structure underpinning the traditional diagnostic approach.[144]

EDS and POTS are equally complex, with overlapping symptoms that are also common to MCAS. As Claire Smith comments, 'It would seem that this is a complicated intersection of two [or three] poorly understood illnesses for which further investigation is crucial, not only to validate patients' symptoms, but also to improve the treatment approach for those affected.'[145]

Pain

For some people – particularly in the earlier phases of life – hypermobility is completely pain-free, but for those who progress to a form of hypermobility syndrome, some sort of pain, to some degree, is going to be a factor. Often the causes and types of pain are various and interwoven.

Musculoskeletal pain

Probably the most routinely experienced type of hypermobile pain is musculoskeletal. According to Castori *et al.*, 'Musculoskeletal pain is extremely common in JHS/EDS-HT…and is strongly related to functional impairment.'[146] There is often a general pattern of creeping pain that begins in one individual joint and gradually extends around the body, settling into the shoulders, hips, knees, usually on one side rather than both or affecting one side in a different way from the other. Castori *et al.* describe this dissemination of pain:

> Initially recurrent myalgias [muscle pain] and arthralgias [joint pain] are limited to a few joints and muscles and may have a migratory pattern. Thereafter they become persistent and assume a more generalised distribution, although asymmetry between the two sides of the body are frequently reported for both intensity of pain and number of painful foci.[147]

In healthy people without hypermobility, an injury typically leads to initial acute pain – pain that subsides as the injury heals – and eventual resolution. In hypermobile people, injury may not heal within the expected time frame and may result in chronic pain – pain that persists beyond the point where full recovery would be expected. Sometimes this is because hypermobile tissues are fragile and tend to repeated re-injury, perhaps on a micro level. Sometimes, the cause appears to be a dysfunction of the central nervous system (CNN), in which – rather than producing pain in a time-limited way, as an alert that something is wrong – the CNN perpetuates, or even amplifies, pain. Claire Smith describes this as like, 'a fire alarm relentlessly ringing.'[148]

A further probable reason for the generalisation of pain in hypermobility lies in the nature of the myofascia, which, as we have seen (in 'Fascia' above) is continuous and interpenetrating. Therefore a force in one part of the body, for example a repeated dislocation or a chronic muscle spasm, may have a ripple effect throughout the whole myofascial system, producing tension in diverse areas of the body. This can happen in a non-hypermobile body too, but in the hypermobile person, the myofascia may have reduced capacity to resist this kind of disruption and may be much more seriously affected.

Chronic musculoskeletal pain can lead to feelings of physical vulnerability and anxiety with regard to movement. Castori *et al.* note that, 'Pain catastrophising, fear of pain, and kinesiophobia [fear of moving] are among the most known maladaptive cognitions', as well as 'fear of falling'.[149] Can you be surprised when moving in what you might expect to be a very ordinary and innocuous way can lead to injury and pain flare-ups potentially lasting months, or even never being fully resolved? I have become much more conservative with regard to movement as I've got older and chronic pain has become more of a factor for me. I'm concerned about creating new pain complexes, and scared of falling and of being bumped into, and I'm not convinced that this cognition is as maladaptive as all that! The dilemma is that radically reducing amount and types of movement is probably the most harmful of all approaches to hypermobility – and so I do keep pressing into the edges of what feels feasible and helpful in terms of movement practice. Some of my most debilitated hypermobile clients have gradually decreased their activities until they are very disabled – and need help to expand their range of physical possibility in ways that not only *are* safe and manageable but also *feel* that way to the person. For more information, see 'Deconditioning…and reconditioning' in Chapter 7.

Neuropathic pain

Neuropathic pain is generally caused by damage to nerves. According to the Brain and Spine Foundation:

> The pain is usually described as a burning sensation and affected areas are often sensitive to the touch. Symptoms of neuropathic pain may also include excruciating pain, pins and needles, difficulty [with] correctly sensing temperatures, and numbness. Some people may find it hard to wear thick clothes as even slight pressure can aggravate the pain.[150]

A 2011 study of 44 people with Ehlers-Danlos by Camerota *et al.* found that neuropathic pain is a common feature of EDS.[151] In the hypermobile population, however, nerve pain may be present without any diagnosable evidence of injury to the nerves.[152] It seems plausible that small subluxations, and even fascial constrictions, could cause impingement (trapping) of nerves.

Autism and pain

It is well recognised that autistic people tend to experience pain differently from allistic (non-autistic) people. In an article for the website Spectrum,

'Unseen Agony: Dismantling Autism's House of Pain', Sarah DeWeerdt explains that, 'Although some people with autism are insensitive to pain, others are unusually vulnerable to it.'[153] Paradoxically, an apparent lack of pain response may be the result of a learnt numbness as a result of hypersensitivity. Noah, a counsellor and psychology teacher with Asperger's Syndrome (part of the autism spectrum), explains that as a child he experienced physical pain when his mother vacuumed the house: 'She would put the vacuum on the wood floor, not the carpet, and that's really loud, so it would really freak me out.' Initially, Noah says, he, 'would scream and yell for her to stop', but after failing repeatedly to have any effect on the noise, he eventually came to understand that he had no control over the sound of the vacuum cleaner – nor over many of the other sensory experiences he found painful. His response was to shut down sensory channels. He says: 'I was very numbed off. I could handle really intense cold or even pain.'[154]

Baeza-Velasco *et al.* comment that painful conditions are generally under-researched and under-diagnosed in the autistic population. Indeed, for many years, it was a common view among medical professionals that autistic people did not experience pain. Nevertheless, there is evidence that chronic pain is common among those with autism.[155] A 2017 University of Dallas study led by neuroscientist, Dr Xiaosi Gu, has established a link between Autism Spectrum Disorder (ASD) and enhanced sensitivity to pain, demonstrating that when autistic people experience a painful stimulus, our brains generate a greater response in the anterior cingulate cortex.[156] While autistic people may be experiencing considerable pain, however, we may not be experiencing it in the same way as allistic people – Noah feels pain as, 'an all-encompassing, irritating process that envelops your whole brain'[157] – or expressing it in the way that allistic doctors expect.

Sleep

Jeannie Di Bon comments:

> Whilst much of the discussion around hypermobility and EDS focuses on movement, a common source of anxiety, frustration and stress for those living with such conditions comes from the other half of our lives – sleep. Many people living with EDS have huge difficulties when it comes to getting enough quality sleep.[158]

According to EDHS.info, 'When studied in the sleep lab, [hypermobile people] often have a relative and sometimes complete lack of deep sleep, and/

or an increased number of sleep-disrupting "arousals".[159] There are a number of reasons why hypermobile people may have difficulty getting plentiful and refreshing sleep.

Getting comfortable

If you're hypermobile, it can be very difficult to find a comfortable sleeping position, and lying still for a period of time can sometimes become acutely painful as muscles start to tighten up. Jo Southall, an occupational therapist with hEDS, says:

> If I sleep on my side I can't relax or my hips cause problems. So, I have a maternity pillow with extra lumbar support, I've got a pillow to go under and between my knees and another one to prop up my wonkier shoulder. I've made it into bed, surrounded by pillows. Trouble is I still can't get comfy. After a while I roll over stealthily, so as not to lose track of my pillows or wake my slumbering boyfriend. This new position is better for my back but worse for my shoulder, so I change the pillow arrangement and try to think of something besides the pain. I count sheep, make up stories in my head, run through relaxation protocols and generally try to avoid thinking about the time. After another three position changes... I'm finally starting to feel genuinely sleepy.[160]

Injury

I sometimes tell people that for me sleeping is a dangerous activity. This is not entirely a joke. Jeannie Di Bon comments that, 'Just getting into bed and moving around while in bed can cause dislocation, subluxation or trapped nerves.'[161] It's not unusual for hypermobile people to get out of bed with a new injury that they didn't have when they got in the night before.

Obstructive sleep apnoea

For more information, see the 'Obstructive sleep apnoea' section above.

Restless Legs Syndrome

We have already noted that a significant number of hypermobile people experience Restless Legs Syndrome and other night-time cramps (in 'Restless Legs Syndrome (RLS)' above). Jo Southall says:

Nocturnal cramps (mostly in my legs) have been an issue since I was about five. I'm told I'll grow out of them, but at 26 years old I'm starting to doubt that.[162]

Nocturia

As we have seen (in 'Nocturia' above), nocturia – waking up needing to pee – is more common among hypermobile people – and, obviously, disruptive of sleep patterns.

Adrenaline

Raised adrenaline levels may make it hard to fall asleep and stay in deep sleep. For more on adrenaline see 'Adrenaline levels, hypermobility and PTSD' below.

Brain fog

As you might imagine from the name, brain fog denotes confusion, clouded thinking, difficulty concentrating, forgetfulness and inability to process information. Neurogenetics nurse, Jenny Morrison, explains that:

> In hEDS/HSD, it is thought that brain fog may be related to lack of blood flow to the brain due to blood pooling in the legs because of stretchy veins… Brain fog also appears to be more common in those with POTS secondary to their hEDS/HSD, suggesting that there may be a link there.[163]

As someone with both hEDS and POTS, this hypothesis feels right to me. I associate episodes of brain fog with periods of POTS-related breathlessness.

The Mighty invited Facebook followers with chronic illness to describe what brain fog feels like to them. These were a few of the responses:

> My mind feels as slow and achy as my body, struggling to take each step. (Barb)

> It's like looking all over the house for your cell phone, purse and keys when all of them are in your hands. Or looking at a banana and only being able to call it 'that yellow thing'. (Sue Elizabeth)

> I used to be able to spell very well. Now I change sentences because I can't remember how to spell. I can't say words that are in my brain. I know what I want to say but the bridge from my brain to my mouth is broken. (Roni)

It feels like my head is stuck in a daydream and I'm constantly fighting to get back to reality. Sometimes I'll ask a person a question and think I'm listening, and then suddenly realise I haven't heard a single word they've said. (Out of Loop)[164]

Anxiety

According to EDHS.info, 'Individuals with hypermobility are (up to 16 times) over-represented among those with panic or anxiety disorders'.[165] The link between hypermobility and anxiety-related mental health difficulties is well substantiated by research. In an evidence-based review for *Current Psychiatry*, doctors, Andrea Bulbena-Cabré and Antonio Bulbena, state:

> Psychiatric symptoms are being increasingly recognised as a key feature of JHS/hEDS. Our group published the first case control study on the association between JHS/hEDS and anxiety in 1988. Additional studies have consistently replicated and confirmed these findings in clinical and nonclinical populations, and in adult and geriatric patients. Specifically, JHS/hEDS has been associated with a higher frequency and greater intensity of fears, greater anxiety severity and somatic concerns, and higher frequency of the so-called endogenous anxiety disorders [anxiety due to internal stressors].[166]

Practical anxiety triggers

Given the background of pain, fatigue and other debilitating symptoms, for many of us hypermobility brings a plethora of anxiety-generating pragmatic life concerns. For example, a hypermobile person might understandably worry about:

- working enough to make a basic living

- applying for (appealing rejection…and regularly reapplying for…) state benefits – a process which feels to many disabled people like institutional gaslighting

- taking care of children, elderly parents and other dependants

- maintaining a household – cleaning, paying bills, organising repairs and so on

- managing health – making medical appointments, communicating with sceptical doctors, exercising, eating well

- dealing with periodic flare-ups and age-related progression of symptoms

- processing and adapting to the loss of things they may once have loved but now are no longer able to do (martial arts, gymnastics, running, hiking).

Proprioceptive anxiety triggers

It's easy to see why being unsure where you are in space, where your body parts are in relation to each other and whether an ordinary activity is going to cause dislocation or injury might lead to a state of constant low-level anxiety. As Isobel Knight says:

> In many ways it is no wonder that people with HMS suffer from anxiety. It is constantly difficult being in a body that feels chaotic and out of control.[167]

Mary, a hypermobile Pilates teacher, describes this general and ongoing bodily insecurity: 'This sense of not knowing where you are in space is basically eroding a sense of identity... [It's] not knowing who and where you are literally, which makes the condition so debilitating.'[168]

Interoceptive anxiety triggers

While proprioception is compromised in hypermobility, interoception (awareness of internal body states) is generally heightened. There is a scientifically well-recognised association between interoceptive capacity and anxiety. In a 2014 neuroimaging study of 36 hypermobile people, Mallorquí-Bagué *et al.* found a clear link between joint hypermobility and, 'the presence of anxiety symptoms through the expression of enhanced interoceptive sensitivity'. They also found that the degree to which participants felt able to regulate their attention to interoceptive experience, and their capacity to trust that what they noticed was not malign or dangerous, had an impact on their anxiety, suggesting that, 'enhancing awareness of bodily processes, e.g., through mindfulness approaches, may be used therapeutically for managing anxiety'.[169] Somatically based yoga – which invites a curious, even-gazed witnessing of our embodied experience and all our responses to it – could also be very helpful here.

Brain differences

There is evidence that brain structure is different in hypermobile people and more productive of anxiety. In a 2012 neuroimaging study, Eccles *et al.* found structural neurological differences between hypermobile and non-hypermobile participants: 'Strikingly, bilateral amygdala volume distinguished those with from those without hypermobility.' They noted, 'observed differences in the structural integrity of specific emotional brain regions' in hypermobile people and concluded that:

> Our findings specifically link hypermobility to the structural integrity of a brain centre implicated in normal and abnormal emotions and physiological responses. Our observations endorse hypermobility as a multisystem phenotype [the product of genetic and environmental influences] and suggest potential mechanisms mediating clinical vulnerability to neuropsychiatric symptoms.[170]

Anxiety and certain kinds of heightened emotional responsivity are also a feature of autism. Eccles *et al.* note that some of the differences they observed in the brains of hypermobile people (in the superior temporal cortex) also characterise autistic brains. Differences seen in the inferior parietal cortex may be linked to dyspraxia (no surprises there). All in all, the research reinforces the intersecting cluster view of hypermobility, autism and the other neurodiversities: 'Our findings suggest that processes compromising function in neuro-developmental conditions may occur in individuals with hypermobility, putatively enhancing vulnerability to stress and anxiety.'[171]

Perfectionism

In a study of adolescent dancers, those with hypermobility were found to score more highly for perfection than those without.[172] Reports of perfectionism by hypermobile people are common. It's easy to understand that if your body feels chaotic, creating a sense of control in other arenas may be a priority. Perfectionism is a frequently found trait among autistic people too, suggesting once again that both hypermobility and autism inhabit intersecting territories and involve overlapping ways of being in the world.

Eating disorders and self-harm

When I work with hypermobile people, experience leads me to expect that they may also have a history of eating disorders and/or self-harm. Isobel Knight recalls being told by the medical liaison officer at the Hypermobility Syndromes Association that self-harm was – anecdotally – common among hypermobile people,[173] and social media groups for hypermobile people document many experiences of cutting, picking, starving, purging and bingeing. Given the awareness of these correlations by those of us who are hypermobile or who work with hypermobile people at grass-roots level, the lack of research (that I could discover) into the relationship between hypermobility, eating disorders and self-harm is striking.

For people with hypermobility, eating disorders and/or self-harm may be a way of creating a sense of connection and coherence in a body experienced as falling apart, uncontained, permeable or distant. In *A Guide to Living with Ehlers-Danlos Syndrome (Hypermobility Type),* Isobel discusses her own history of self-harm through skin-picking:

> I have some very serious scars which can now only reflect my despair. I started to harm myself from the very young age of five... I frequently remember having this sensation of feeling at odds with my body, feeling disconnected with it, that it felt 'unreal' not knowing where I was and feeling out of control, which I think might just link to having a very poor sense of proprioception. I would have self-harmed to 'get back into' and connect with my body. Seeing blood and mess and then sensing pain helped me to regain control. I self-harmed for 27 years before finally obtaining the right psychological support for me.[174]

Undiagnosed autism may also be a factor here – it was for me. There is a growing awareness of the relationship between autism and anorexia nervosa – Heather Westwood and Kate Tchanturia have reviewed the recent research on this subject[175] – and there is abundant anecdotal evidence that (due to the gendering of diagnosis) cis women and girls are more likely to be diagnosed with an eating disorder than with autism when they meet the criteria for both, even though in this situation eating disorders are generally a response to the experience of being autistic in a neurotypical (NT) world. My first episodes of disordered eating were triggered by the all-enveloping stress of starting school (the noise, the smells, the baffling social rules). They continued in various forms for 46 years, impervious to insight, therapy, mindfulness, moving, drawing, writing, process work...only finally ebbing away shortly after I had been diagnosed as autistic. Understanding the nature of, and reasons for, my hypersensitivity, social confusion and overwhelm enabled me to take a step back, place fewer demands on myself and respect my real limits.

The majority of my hypermobile clients with mental health issues (which are not due to developmental trauma or Post-Traumatic Stress Disorder (PTSD)) are autistic and diagnosed, or clearly (to me) autistic but not diagnosed, or somewhere close to the edge of the autistic spectrum, missing some of the criteria required for full autisticy,[176] but presenting as highly sensitive and easily overwhelmed.

Adrenaline levels, hypermobility and PTSD

A link between hypermobility and raised adrenaline levels is well recognised by researchers and hypermobility-informed medics. Pain, stress and fatigue all stimulate production of adrenaline. The Move Daily website suggests, plausibly, that, 'there are also arguments to be made for direct musculoskeletal sources of stress and anxiety based on how and where a hypermobile person seeks structural stability.'[177] With hypermobility it's easy to find yourself in a negative feedback loop in which adrenaline generates further stress, anxiety and fatigue…which generates further adrenaline…which generates further stress, anxiety and fatigue… In this situation, gentle somatic practices, such as restorative yoga and yoga nidra, which shift the nervous system out of sympathetic (adrenalised) and into parasympathetic (rest, relax and integrate) mode, can be very helpful. More on this in Chapter 5.

Dr Alan Pocinki observes:

> The body's tendency to overreact to stresses by making too much adrenaline can lead others to think that hypermobile people are 'too sensitive', 'irritable', or 'anxious'. Patients themselves may notice this, saying, 'I've always overreacted to little things. I can't help it.' It is very important to recognise two things about this phenomenon. First, it is a physical reaction, so that counselling usually will not be effective in treating this type of anxiety. Similarly, adrenaline highs and lows may be mistaken for the mood fluctuations of bipolar disorder… Second, while a feeling of anxiety can be produced by emotional stress, it is just as likely that such symptoms have a physical cause, most often fatigue, pain, or dehydration, and less commonly by a drop in blood sugar or blood pressure.[178]

In my experience of client work, dysregulation of adrenaline production may predispose hypermobile people to PTSD, a condition in which the body becomes stuck in the adrenalised fight/flight/freeze response following an experience (or experiences) of trauma. There is a growing realisation that PTSD can sometimes arise out of cumulative experience of micro-trauma – a kind of slow attrition. Some hypermobile people appear to be experiencing ongoing low-level PTSD due to the stress inherent in living in an unstable body which may feel adrift in space, and perhaps also in time if the person has significant dyspraxia. This is another area in which anecdotal evidence is plentiful but scientific research is lacking.

Fatigue

Researchers Castori *et al.* comment that for hypermobile people, 'The impact of fatigue on daily life is often equal [to] or more dramatic than the impact of pain.'[179] Hypermobility is indeed very, very tiring and has an enormous impact on the capacity for work and social life. @illnesscantstealjoy, a college student with EDS and POTS, comments:

> I used to never take naps. Never stop. Never slow down. Never turn down an opportunity to hang out with a friend or add another organisation to my load. I used to always take more than 16 credits a semester. But now I take naps. Instead of meeting up with people between every class, I go back to my room and allow myself to rest. I turn on soft music and let my brain slow down. Sometimes I cry and sometimes I'm just perfectly content in simply being. I turn down positions and delegate tasks that don't have to be done by me. I dropped from 18 credits at the beginning of the semester to now only 13.[180]

We have seen that multiple factors make hypermobility fatiguing. As promised, here is the tally-up:

- Defective collagen structures (in ligaments, tendons, fascia, etc.) and...

- Hypotonic resting muscle tone, which together necessitate extra musculoskeletal work to keep the body upright. Castori *et al.* state that, 'Muscle weakness due to postural control muscle overactivation is probably the earliest pathological process contributing to chronic fatigue.'[181]

- Pain and anxiety.

- Poor digestion leading to suboptimal nutrition.

- Poor sleep.

- Immune system difficulties leading to repeated illness.

- Co-existing POTS/orthostatic issues – heart beating too fast, too little CO_2 in the system, brain fog.

- Co-existing autism, in which the brain has to work much harder to process social information, sensory sensitivities, language, etc.

- Co-existing MCAS, in which the body is dealing with inflammatory autoimmune responses.

In the face of so much potential exhaustion, resting sufficiently and setting sensible limits on how much we take on (as @illnesscantstealjoy describes above) are essential. Equally so, though, is maintaining a level of fitness. Strengthening muscles, tuning proprioception and building stamina in appropriate ways are crucial to creating optimal health and quality of life with hypermobility.

Chronic Fatigue Syndrome

Whereas fatigue is manageable and its impact on daily life *relatively* low-level, Chronic Fatigue Syndrome – the condition previously known in the UK as myalgic encephalitis (or ME) – is a more pathological development and is severely life-affecting. People with CFS are generally unable to work, socialise or carry out routine daily tasks like preparing a meal or making a bed. Angie Ebba, an artist with CFS, describes it like this:

> CFS is so much more than 'just tired'. It's a disease that impacts multiple parts of your body and causes exhaustion so debilitating that many with CFS are completely bedbound for varying lengths of time. CFS also causes muscle and joint pain, cognitive issues, and makes you sensitive to external stimulation, like light, sound, and touch. The hallmark of the condition is post-exertional malaise, which is when someone physically crashes for hours, days, or even months after overexerting their body.[182]

Nijs *et al.* have found that generalised joint hypermobility is more common among those with CFS,[183] and it is believed that hypermobility is an undiagnosed driver of CFS in some instances.[184] We'll be looking in more detail at CFS in Chapter 4 (see 'Chronic Fatigue Syndrome/ME').

Anaesthetics

Consultant rheumatologist, Alan Hakim, reports for the Hypermobility Syndromes Association that:

A large proportion of people with Joint Hypermobility Syndrome (JHS) and Ehlers Danlos – Hypermobility Type appear to be resistant to local anaesthetics either as topical creams or injections. In one large survey JHS patients were three times more likely to report the poor effectiveness of local anaesthetic compared to people without JHS.[185]

Research carried out by Jane Schubart *et al.* in 2019 found that among a sample of 980 respondents with EDS who had undergone a dental procedure under local anaesthetic, 88 per cent had experienced inadequate pain prevention (as compared to 33 per cent in a control group of 249 people without EDS). According to the study, 'The agent [local anaesthetic] with the highest EDS-respondent reported success rate was articaine (30 per cent), followed by bupivacaine (25 per cent), and mepivacaine (22 per cent).'[186]

A BBC article entitled 'The People Who Can't Go Numb at the Dentist's' quotes Jenny Harrison, who has Ehlers-Danlos and works as an EDS nurse:

[Local anaesthetic] works for a few minutes and wears off very quickly... In some people it doesn't work at all, but for me it probably lasts about 10 minutes.

According to the article, 'Some of her patients have told her that their doctor or dentist simply won't believe them when they say, "Local anaesthetic doesn't work on me."'[187] Research in this area is needed, but one hypothesis is that the anaesthetic solution diffuses away from the injection site more slowly in lax tissues.[188]

Ehlers-Danlos also has implications for general anaesthesia. These are complex and are summarised in a review by Wiesmann *et al.*, 'Recommendations for Anesthesia and Perioperative Management in Patients with Ehlers-Danlos Syndrome(s)'. If you have EDS, are about to undergo surgery and would like to show this article to your anaesthetist, you can find it here: www.ncbi.nlm.nih.gov/pmc/articles/PMC4223622/?fbclid=IwAR0L Trz7TF4EOciIDsU-Yjd_wbg8uT5u0SOVo0ALfpINKurW8kgQO2Yfgn4.[189]

Diagnosis

Last week I got my diagnosis. I am thrilled. It was absolutely brilliant to get a medical professional to believe all my symptoms and connect the dots. The years of subluxations; sprains; anorexia; POTS; back, knee and shoulder issues; the exhaustion; the fibromyalgia; the food intolerances; the inflammatory bowel disease... The list goes on, all of it just because of my faulty collagen.

Hannah (yoga practitioner with HSD)

If you are experiencing:

- pain (local and generalised)
- fatigue
- regular soft tissue trauma (sprains, strains and bruises)
- dislocations and subluxations
- injuries of overuse
- gastric problems...

...you may be genetically hypermobile. Strongly suspect hypermobility if you also have diagnoses of:

- fibromyalgia
- autism/dyslexia/dyspraxia
- Chronic Fatigue Syndrome.

As Professor Rodney Grahame has said, 'Joint Hypermobility Syndrome is a common clinical entity which is much misunderstood, overlooked, misdiagnosed and mistreated.'[190] Awareness of the joint hypermobility syndromes is growing among medical professionals, but it is still often not easy to get a diagnosis. At the time of writing, The Ehlers-Danlos Society is running a social media campaign to raise awareness of the length of time diagnosis can take. I was lucky. I approached my GP, who referred me to the hypermobility service at University College Hospital London – no longer possible these days – where I was diagnosed by Rodney Grahame. For many people, though, the route to diagnosis can take decades to traverse and involve weathering disbelief and disaffirmation. @callumjarvisgroves says:

From the first time I googled 'why is my skin so stretchy' as a 12-year-old, I knew I had Ehlers-Danlos syndrome. It was just the constant dismissal, being told to man up or that I have Munchausen's that stopped me from believing and searching for answers… Now that I am diagnosed and an adult, I feel sorry for the child that got dismissed at every opportunity, because years of pain could have been avoided because the care I needed was never given. My issues just got chalked up to 'behavioural problems'.[191]

For @claircoult, diagnosis was a similarly frustrating and protracted process:

I was misdiagnosed with ME aged 15. I was finally diagnosed with EDS aged 38. For 23 years my symptoms were completely ignored, my health deteriorated and I became disabled. When I raised the subject of EDS, my NHS doctors said, no, that's rare, you don't have that. I had to pay to see a private doctor to get my diagnosis.[192]

The current diagnostic path in the UK is referral to a rheumatologist by your GP. Go to your GP armed with a comprehensive checklist of your symptoms and don't necessarily expect them to be familiar with the different hypermobility conditions. It may be helpful to point them in the direction of the Ehlers-Danlos Syndromes Toolkit, a diagnostic tool devised by the Royal College of General Practitioners. You can find it at www.rcgp.org.uk/clinical-and-research/resources/toolkits/ehlers-danlos-syndromes-toolkit.aspx.

Having jumped the GP hurdle, you're still not home and away. Not all rheumatologists are familiar with the hypermobility conditions either. My suggestion is that you do some research locally. Ask in online hypermobility forums (there are many groups on Facebook). Find out which rheumatologists in your area have diagnosed hypermobility and been knowledgeable about it, and ask to be referred to them.

Once they have diagnosed you, theoretically a rheumatologist can further refer you to the UCLH hypermobility service for more specialised help. At the time of writing, however, the hypermobility service has closed its waiting lists. It is hoping to redesign services to increase capacity. The place to get updates is: www.uclh.nhs.uk/ourservices/servicea-z/medspec/rheum/hmc/pages/home.aspx. If it is suspected that you have one of the rarer forms of Ehlers-Danlos, you might alternatively be referred to the EDS National Diagnostic Service, which has centres at Sheffield Northern General Hospital, and Northwick Park and St Mark's Hospital in London.

Beighton Criteria

The Beighton Criteria is a simple scoring system that measures joint hypermobility on a nine-point scale. You can find the Criteria at: www.ehlers-danlos.com/assessing-joint-hypermobility. The Criteria are much discussed on social media and sometimes touted as a way to self-diagnose. While they *may* give you an idea about whether you are hypermobile, it's important to be aware that medical professionals do not assess based on the Beighton Criteria alone, and if they did, many instances of hypermobility would be missed. Older and more debilitated hypermobile people may not be able to touch their wrist with their thumb or bend forwards and put their hands flat on the floor. As Rosemary Keer (senior physiotherapist and hypermobility specialist) and Katherine Butler (hand therapist and hypermobility specialist) say:

> Hypermobility may be masked when range of movement is decreased due to fear, pain or stiffness following injury or inactivity or in the case of an older person who may have lost their normal degree of flexibility with age.[193]

Indeed, some of the stiffest students I've taught have had a hypermobility diagnosis, and would probably not have scored a single point on the Beighton Criteria.

Blood tests

While the genetic markers for Marfan Syndrome and the rarer types of Ehlers-Danlos are known, at present those for hEDS and HSD have not been discovered. Most joint hypermobility cannot therefore be diagnosed by genetic analysis of a blood sample. In the UK, you will only be asked to take a blood test if it is suspected that you have MFS or one of the rare EDS subtypes.

Is it worth it?

Given the difficulty of accessing diagnostic services, I'm often asked whether there's any point in getting diagnosed. I think it all depends. I was initially self-diagnosed. I sought 'official' confirmation because I found it hard to really believe myself and to set appropriate boundaries around what was and was not appropriate for my body. It's very common for hypermobile people to be told by doctors that there isn't any point in seeking diagnosis because 'there isn't any treatment' – an attitude that demonstrates the limited perspective of many in the medical profession. While it's true that there isn't a magic chemical bullet that will eliminate hypermobility, diagnosis offers an explanation, understanding and awareness, as well as, with luck, access to specialist services and benefits. With hypermobility, management is all – and good management can make an enormous difference. Rosine, who was diagnosed with Ehlers-Danlos at the age of 59, says:

> The hEDS diagnosis changed my life in many respects. It gave me some emotional relief and the unparalleled understanding of the causes of a life plagued with health issues. Additionally, whereas until then doctors had never seemed to find the cause of my ailments, suddenly the word EDS seemed to add meaning to my medical chart.[194]

Knowing can put us in touch with important aspects of our embodiment, as well as with communities of people who are 'like us'. For me, a hypermobility diagnosis was also the entry point into exploring my neurological differences and finding belonging in my neurotribe. Rosine was also able to make links with neurodivergence, in her case dyscalculia and synaesthesia. She says, 'Until I read about it, I thought that everybody was like me, never realising that I was the only one computing using a colour spectrum and feeling emotions instead of conceptualising numbers.'[195]

What does hypermobility feel like?

It may come as a surprise to the non-hypermobile population, but it's unusual for a hypermobile person to feel flexible, even when they are an elite dancer or acrobat able to get into pretzel positions. 'Floppy' tends to be more relatable than 'flexible' to many hypermobile people, and most of us can identify with feeling collapsed, hanging from our bones, or ramshackle – struggling to hold ourselves upright and keep the structure together. People who clearly (to observers) are very, very bendy are also sometimes unable to identify themselves as such. One reason for this lack of perceived flexibility is that the typical felt experience of a hypermobile person is one of stiffness and restriction: as we have already seen, in a hypermobile body, muscles are often overworking to the point of spasm to provide compensatory stability and keep the structure upright. Another is that hypermobility is genetic, so we tend to grow up in families where other people are also hypermobile and so the particular traits, capacities and deficits of hypermobility are normalised. And then there is the familiarity of our own particular embodiment – it just feels natural. Rosine (who we heard from above) says, 'Throughout my life I always thought that everybody had the hypermobility that I had.'[196] I have many vivid memories of instances in my life when I realised that a hypermobile movement capacity I had taken for granted was not available to the majority of people. At the age of 18, for example, in my first ever yoga class, we were invited into *virasana* (Hero Pose). I duly plonked down in what was my most comfortable sitting position, wondering when the yoga was going to start, and was stunned to observe that the majority of the class were unable simply to sit down 'normally'.

When hypermobility progresses to a hypermobility syndrome, key experiences are of pain, difficulty, anxiety and fatigue. Members of the Hypermobility on the Yoga Mat Facebook group described having a hypermobility syndrome like this:

Imagine you don't feel a great sense of where you are in space, so you wobble a lot, trip, bump into things, and clip yourself on corners. And if you've ever had that feeling of leaning your neck too far back and it gets really sore and tight...that's how my joints feel most of the time unless I do an astonishing amount of movement. Imagine that almost every time you stand up, you almost black out a little. And sometimes you do. Imagine that if you don't open the door the right way, you might dislocate your shoulder. Imagine that to sleep, you need a minimum of five pillows so you don't wake up having seriously messed up your body. Imagine some days you just wake up with weird, random symptoms, and you've learned to shrug most of them off because doctors don't believe you a lot of the time. 'Oh, I guess I'm gonna be a little blind in one eye today, shrug city.'

Clare (yoga teacher with hEDS)

Hypermobility is thinking I know my body and its limitations and then finding I've still managed to accidentally do something to trigger an issue, and a new part has joined the party. It's people assuming that I'm absolutely fit and completely well because I teach and practise yoga, when I'm actually often struggling to stand up in one place (if not moving, doing yoga or dancing) for any length of time, and not able to sit still for any length of time either.

Ali (yoga teacher with HSD)

Being hypermobile means having pain and not being believed. I often worry that I'm making it up or catastrophising, even though deep down

I know I'm not. Then there are the injuries that should have healed but haven't…and the movements that shouldn't have injured me in the first place.

Zenobia (yoga practitioner with hEDS)

For most people in the group, struggles to be heard, believed and accurately diagnosed were a key part of the hypermobility experience. Rosemary, a yoga practitioner with vEDS, recalls that, 'my prolapsed and collapsed bowel was misdiagnosed as an eating disorder, and autism was misdiagnosed as obsessive compulsive disorder'. Zenobia says:

After a while, I gave up looking to conventional doctors for help. They clearly had nothing to offer. I started consulting alternative practitioners and learnt about herbal medicine. I use natural methods to look after myself as much as possible.

✳ ✳ ✳

This chapter has focused on the challenges of being hypermobile – deliberately. Hypermobile people ourselves are often not initially able to identify the full range of difficulties we are facing, because we're so used to dealing with them, because they are often minimised or attributed to psychological issues by others and because we lack the information to assemble all the pieces of the jigsaw puzzle. While knowledge about the hypermobility syndromes has grown hugely in my lifetime, Hypermobility on the Yoga Mat workshops are still characterised by the clink of pennies dropping. Validation through community is one of the most powerful aspects of these trainings.

It's not all bleak though. Despite the many ongoing challenges, I wouldn't swap my hypermobile body for one with more stable collagen. I often refer to my body as a crazy wisdom teacher. As I get older, the ways it finds to pull the rug out from under my feet get crazier. My response to the injuries, pain and fatigue that come with being hypermobile has been to get interested in it all. We may envy those blessed with a smooth practice trajectory, but too much facility can make it difficult to engage deeply and subtly with embodied practice. Hypermobility offers many opportunities to learn – on biomechanical, emotional, psychological and spiritual levels – and these learnings seep outwards into the rest of our life. This is the very heart of yoga.

Teaching Yoga to Hypermobile Students

It took 15 years of searching, but I have finally found a teacher who knows about hypermobility and can work with it – a teacher who is kind, empathetic and patient, and understands the challenges that come with being hypermobile. I'm so grateful for his support.

Jenna (yoga practitioner with HSD)

In this chapter, we will be considering what makes a hypermobility-aware yoga teacher. We'll be looking at how to identify hypermobile people in a yoga class, how to spot situations where hypermobile students may be at risk (and guide them towards greater safety) and how to create generative relationships with our hypermobile students – the real essence of yoga teaching. This chapter is less about techniques and practicalities (we'll be discussing these in Chapter 3) and more about outlining some general principles for teaching hypermobile students in an effective and appropriate way.

Why do hypermobile people love yoga?

Yoga teacher, Amber Wilds, writes:

During my teacher training I was told, you probably won't see hypermobility in your yoga classes very often, but it became apparent over the duration of our training that many of my fellow students were hypermobile (to varying degrees). While some had been diagnosed, others hadn't been aware of their hypermobility prior to our training. I therefore began to question whether, rather than being a rarity in a yoga class, hypermobility was actually far more common than initially thought.[1]

Indeed, as we have seen, hypermobile people are one population you are pretty much guaranteed to encounter in significant numbers in any yoga class you teach. Why is this? Why do people whose range of joint motion is so excessive as to be considered pathological flock to an activity with the potential to increase it further? There are a number of reasons.

Embodiment

What drew me to yoga and dance practices initially was a dimly felt but deep disconnect from my body, experienced not on an intellectual level but in some much more fundamental place in myself. Only many years later did I understand that this sense of being not securely contained within my body or consistently visible to others in it was the product of a lack of proprioceptive feedback – that it was biological and neurological in origin. Practising yoga required me to cultivate close and steady attention to my body, and being in movement seemed to turn up the proprioceptive dial, so that I felt a clearer and more frequent sense of physical cohesion. Many of the hypermobile people I teach report similar experiences on first coming into contact with yoga. Sura, a yoga practitioner with hEDS, says:

> *Even just lying on the floor in my first yoga classes was amazing for me. It was as if I felt connected into my body by all the points where I could feel the floor, whereas at other times it seemed as if I could easily float out of my body and get lost.*

Dimitri, a yoga teacher with hEDS, says:

> *I started to feel all this sensation, and it was as if I was actually 'in' my body for the first time. I was getting all this new feedback, and it was very satisfying.*

Being 'good' at yoga

As a teacher, you won't need to be told that yoga is a whole-person practice in which we move towards integrity, not a stretching competition. Nevertheless, for some hypermobile people first encountering yoga, flexibility is experienced as an asset, enabling them to access postures (albeit in a rather ramshackle way) that others struggle even to approach. Their flexibility may be admired by other students and they may be told they are 'good' at yoga –

all of which can be a great incentive to go on practising. Hypermobile yoga teacher, Bernadette Birney, says:

> People tend to enjoy things we're good at. Speaking from my own early yoga experience, I equated being limber with being 'good at yoga'. I enjoyed my practice more because I felt successful. That early 'success' encouraged me to stick with it.[2]

Perhaps on the face of it, this might seem a little shallow, but we need to bear in mind that for many hypermobile people, physical activity is a site of repeated failure. As a child, I dreaded PE (physical education) so intensely that I felt sick throughout the day preceding a lesson, and PE-anxiety dominated my week. Running even short distances made me dizzy and breathless (POTS) and hurt my joints (hEDS), and I was unable to kick or catch a ball (dyspraxia). I failed to pick up the rules of games that no one ever actually taught me (dyspraxia), and as an autistic person, I also struggled to understand the dynamics of teams. I didn't want to play and no one ever wanted me on their side. I kidded myself that I didn't care, but I still flinch every time I see a game of park rounders.

These are not unusual experiences for people with hypermobility, and many of us just stop moving much at all, believing that we're 'useless' at anything physical. Discovering an activity that you can not only do but are actually praised for can therefore be a momentous – even life-changing – experience, as Kara, a yoga practitioner with HSD, explains:

> *I'm rubbish at sports, and by the age of 30 I had become some sort of sloth. Then I discovered yoga. It was the first physical activity I was good at and got approval for. Of course, I know now what the point of yoga is, and I was probably hanging in my joints and all that, but being praised still made me feel good. I could actually participate, even excel.*

Feeling 'tight'

To people who know nothing about genetic hypermobility, the idea of excessive flexibility often suggests a sense of freedom and capacity; in fact, as we saw in Chapter 1, the experience of being hypermobile is often one of tightness and restriction (see 'What does hypermobility feel like?'). As specialist hypermobility physiotherapist, Rosemary Keer, and occupational therapist, Katherine Butler, explain, 'Hypermobile patients often complain of "stiffness"'; however:

What they feel has no relation to the common definition of stiffness that may be experienced by anyone with arthritis or a healthy person who over-exerts themselves. Upon examination, unlike a patient with arthritis, they will often appear to be mobile with a range of movement equal to or greater than average and therefore have no apparent functional deficit.[3]

As we have seen in Chapter 1, where there is structural hypermobility, the nervous system tends to seek to create tension – and it does this in ways that are often uncomfortable and unhelpful to functional biomechanics. Excessive mobility may also cause multiple micro-tears with accompanying inflammation, and there may be early-onset joint degeneration present too. All in all, it's not surprising that one hypermobile person I talked to described stretching as 'blissful'. Especially on initial contact, yoga may seem like an opportunity for endlessly stretching out all the endlessly tight places. Over time, of course, this becomes problematic. We'll be talking more about the role of stretching in yoga practice for hypermobile people later in this chapter (see 'Stretching').

Calming a hyperactive nervous system

The capacity of yoga to alter mind state and emotions, promoting a sense of calm and general well-being, often feels like a godsend to an over-adrenalised and chronically anxious hypermobile person. Vera, a yoga practitioner with MFS, says:

I initially went to yoga for fitness. The thing that kept me coming back, though, was the way it made me feel. Since going to yoga, my self-harming has reduced drastically and I generally feel more positive and less stressed.

The quiet and tranquillity of yoga practice (in most settings, anyway) also contributes to nervous-system regulation and is widely appreciated, providing a kind of sanctuary to many hypermobile people. Derek, a yoga practitioner with HSD, says:

Even though the class was in a community centre, and there was lots of activity going on in the building, in the yoga room it felt so calm and peaceful. All the noise from outside fell away. It was just me and myself in this safe space.

Finding structure

As practice progresses, yoga can be a place where hypermobile practitioners find strength, structure and stability – without pushing too hard or working to the point of exhaustion. As a controlled and mostly low-impact movement form, in which slower and steadier responses are valued over quick-fire reactions, it may be safer than other types of physical activity, presenting less risk of tripping, straining and moving in biomechanically unhelpful ways. Lucy, a yoga teacher with HSD, says:

> *I think at first the sensation of stretch in the joints gives us a way of actually feeling our bodies in a good way. Then we learn not to overdo it and strengthen instead of stretching, but all the time improving our embodiment and proprioception.*

Student intake

If you work in a gym or teach for a studio, you may not have the luxury of a student intake form. If, on the other hand, you run your own classes, I recommend that you ask about hypermobility, along with other health conditions, in your written intake material. If you need your form to be brief, you could simply include the hypermobility syndromes and their co-occurring conditions in a general alphabetical list of injuries and ailments, and ask any necessary follow-up questions verbally. If you have room to expand, the hypermobility section of your form might look like this:

1. Are you hypermobile or do you suspect you may be hypermobile?

   Are you:

   - diagnosed with Hypermobility Spectrum Disorder?

   - diagnosed with Ehlers-Danlos Syndrome? If yes, which type?

   - diagnosed with Marfan Syndrome?

   - diagnosed with a different hypermobility syndrome?

   - not formally diagnosed?

   Please tell me briefly about any ways in which hypermobility may affect your participation in the class and let me know about anything I can do to help.

2. Do you have Postural Orthostatic Tachycardia Syndrome (POTS)?

3. Are you autistic or do you have dyslexia, dyscalculia, dyspraxia, ADHD or any other form of neurodifference?

These are some things to bear in mind:

- Asking about hypermobility in general will catch those students who have been told informally (by a physiotherapist or another yoga teacher, for example) that they are hypermobile but don't know which type of hypermobility they have – and may never have heard of Ehlers-Danlos, Marfan Syndrome and so on.

- It can be very difficult to access diagnostic services for joint hypermobility syndromes, so do take suspected but undiagnosed hypermobility seriously.

- It's important to know if your student has Marfan Syndrome or the vascular type of EDS because this will have a significant impact on the type of practice that is safe – i.e. not life-endangering – for them, so if they don't specify which type of hypermobility on the form, do check this specifically. (For more information, see 'Marfan Syndrome' and 'VEDS' in Chapter 1.)

- Although neurodifference such as dyslexia and dyscalculia may not on the face of it seem all that relevant to participation in a yoga class, its presence is an indicator of a student who falls into the 'likely to be hypermobile' group, so I always ask about it.

- Other physical issues that often co-occur with hypermobility – for example IBS and general digestive issues – will probably be covered elsewhere in your form (if they aren't currently, it's a good idea to add them). Where you believe a student may be hypermobile, do look out for co-occurring conditions, as they will be suggestive that your assessment is correct.

The intake form does not replace talking to your students about their health and history – and this is something you may be able to do even if you work in a setting where it isn't possible to ask your students for written information. If at all possible, have a short, friendly conversation with any new student who is (or may be) hypermobile to check out what their past experiences have been and what their current needs are. Don't expect to learn everything at once. Disclosure is an aspect of relationship and as such it happens over time. More information will emerge as trust grows between you and the student. This is an ongoing conversation.

For more information about student intake forms in general, see my book *The Yoga Teacher Mentor*.[4]

Responding to a disclosure of hypermobility

The way you respond when a student tells you they are hypermobile can be crucial for your relationship and may make a big difference to whether the student feels able to trust you and is willing to come back to your class. Bear in mind that hypermobile students have sometimes had previous bad experiences in yoga classes. They may have been pushed, pathologised or disbelieved; their pain, fatigue and other difficulties may have been minimised; and they may have struggled to dispel the teacher's ignorance about what genetic hypermobility actually entails. So how can you welcome hypermobile students into your class in a way that reassures them that they have entered a safe space? These are a few suggestions:

- Thank the student for telling you about their hypermobility. Full disclosure from a hypermobile student may be long. If the student has trusted you sufficiently to be comprehensive, appreciate that too: 'It's really helpful to have all the details.' A hypermobile student may have been considered neurotic, hypochondriac or self-dramatising in the past, so show them that you understand the range of issues that may be involved in living with a multi-systemic condition.

- Reassure the student that they can be included in the class (assuming that they can). If you're not sure that they can be included safely, explain that the class may not be appropriate for them but that they are welcome to give it a try, and if it turns out not to be right for them, you can suggest other teachers or classes that might work better. Make it a point to know about appropriate classes and teachers in your local area to refer to. For more information, see 'Including and referring' below.

- Ask clarifying questions about any particular issues the student has raised, for example:

- Have you noticed any movements that tend to make the back pain worse?

- Have you had a diagnosis for the knee pain from an orthopaedist or physiotherapist?

- What tends to trigger the dizziness?

• Reassure the student that it's fine to come out of any posture at any point and to rest in *balasana* (Child's Pose) or *savasana* (Corpse Pose), or in some other appropriate way.

• Invite the student to ask if they need help at any point and to give you feedback on how any of your suggestions are working for them. Let the student know that this is a collaborative endeavour and that you value their input.

• Ask the student if there is anything else they need in order to be comfortable and fully present in the class.

'You must find yoga really easy'

If I had a pound for every time I've heard this response to a disclosure of hypermobility... It often comes from other yoga students (or would-be yoga students), but teachers sometimes also share the belief that genetic hypermobility is a golden key to yogic attainment – assuming yoga to be a sub-category of acrobatics. If you've read this far, it should be crystal clear to you by now that while some hypermobile people do have an initial facility in yoga as stretching, once the honeymoon period is over and we have begun to encounter the bigger *asana* project, for most of us yoga is really not easy. In fact, hypermobility presents many additional challenges in *asana* work (including fascial and ligamentous instability, muscular hypotonia, proprioceptive deficits, dysautonomia, frequent dislocations and injuries, chronic pain and fatigue).

Unfortunately, the expectation of this kind of reaction sometimes mitigates against disclosure by hypermobile students. It's very difficult to frame a simple, in-the-moment response to such a complex agglomeration of misunderstandings, first off about what actually constitutes yoga and what it might mean to be 'good at it', and second about the actual nature of joint hypermobility. For many hypermobile students it feels easier just to keep shtum.

Spotting hypermobility in your students

While some hypermobile students will arrive at your class with a diagnosis, the majority will not. While a yoga teacher is not a diagnostician (and we need to be clear about this in our interactions with our students), nevertheless we are trained to work with bodies in movement and it is within our remit to identify particular movement styles and deficits, to notice where biomechanics are out of synch and to help our students to practise more effectively in this regard.

It's not always the case that hypermobile people can contort themselves into unfeasible-looking positions. You will encounter a range of hypermobile students in your classes, from those who appear to move well and are able to perform highly gymnastic postures, to those who are very deconditioned and lack the strength and control to carry out even very basic movements. So what are some common denominators? How can we identify hypermobility in our students? The following are some clues:

- Hypermobile people may appear floppy, wobbly, gangly or out of control of their own limbs. Think of a new-born foal making its first attempts to stand up.

- They may 'hang' in their joints. Their legs may appear banana-shaped (concave at the knee) in standing, for example, and their elbows may seem to swivel inside out.

- They may seek to prop themselves up (for example leaning on a wall or a chair) rather than standing or sitting under their own steam, and they may slump if they do have to sit or stand without support. Rosemary Keer and Katherine Butler note that:

  > Even if they are initially able to stand or sit in a good position, it is difficult [for hypermobile people] to sustain the position for long periods. It is easier for their bodies to take the path of least resistance and settle into a position which requires decreased muscle work, resting on tension in their soft tissues. Familiar postures are slumped sitting, standing with hyperextended knees and hips, and hanging on the hip.[5]

- They may show signs of dysautonomia, for example feeling dizzy in head-down to head-up transitions such as coming to standing from *parsvottanasana* (Intense Side Stretch).

- They may appear clumsy – all hands, elbows and feet. Where the person is proficient at yoga *asana*, this may be more evident when they are outside these well-rehearsed and controlled movement patterns and doing something common or garden, like getting props from a cupboard or making a cup of tea. Think of my alter ego, Olive Oyl, tripping over her feet and tangling herself up in her own arms.

- They may find it difficult to learn forms and sequences and to implement movement cues.

- They may flop into the most challenging variation you have set (or one you haven't) – but without structure or control.

- They be poorly co-ordinated.

- They may appear saggy in standing postures, and have difficulty engaging muscles to create more stability, even when guidance is offered.

- They may have the classic marfanoid appearance – think Olive Oyl again – but remember that you don't have to have a Marfan habitus to be hypermobile (see 'Marfan Syndrome versus Marfan habitus' in Chapter 1).

- They may be very sensitive to what they perceive as criticism and may quickly become overwhelmed and upset by input from the teacher, even when it's well meant.

- They may exhibit signs of neurodifference: extreme sensitivity to sounds, textures, incense or fluorescent lights, for example, and difficulty with divining class rules. They may be perceived as the 'difficult' student, the one who always does their own thing, and may even be labelled as disrespectful, a show-off, lazy or uninterested. (I've written in a lot more detail about working with 'difficult' students and the relationship between 'difficult' and hypermobile, neurodivergent and traumatised in *The Yoga Teacher Mentor*.[6])

Be aware that not all hypermobile people will obviously fit this profile. Good proprioceptive training and strength building may give the person an appearance of stability and control. Excessive muscle spasm and ongoing inactivity can also make a hypermobile person appear very stiff. On the whole, though, a cluster of these characteristics tends to suggest that the person may be hypermobile and may benefit from hypermobility-friendly teaching techniques. This approach is generally good practice and will be beneficial to most students, so there's no harm in adopting it with a possibly hypermobile student, even if your assessment turns out to be wrong.

The chief risks for a hypermobile person in a yoga class

We generally think of yoga as a pretty safe activity, and on the whole it is. However, there are some factors that can increase risk considerably for the hypermobile population in a yoga class. While it definitely is possible for a hypermobile person to tear a ligament or dislocate a joint doing yoga, the more usual issue is the long-term deleterious effects of practising too much yoga (without including other types of activity to add in strength, stamina and different movement patterns) and practising yoga in ways that do not tend towards stability and support. Some of the things that can pose a risk in a yoga class include:

- emphasis on working towards an ever-greater range of motion in the joints (a.k.a. too much stretching), which increases the risk of dislocation, chronic muscle spasm, micro-tears and general pain

- encouragement to work too hard or in too large increments for strength and stamina

- dogmatic teaching which seeks to impose inappropriate alignment 'rules', set sequences of postures and by-the-book practice structures

- teaching that overrides the hypermobile person's somatic intelligence and sense of what is appropriate for them, encouraging them to do more and go further

- strong physical adjustments aimed at manipulating the hypermobile person into position

- very hot practice

- very fast practice

- passive practice without appropriate support from props

- lack of individual feedback from the teacher

- lack of sensible, informed guidance towards stability

- lack of knowledgeable input regarding helpful and effective biomechanics

- inappropriate *pranayama* (breath practices) (for more information, see 'Pranayama' in Chapter 4).

Some of these risk factors can be mitigated by the way you approach teaching the hypermobile person, others cannot. If you teach a very stretch-oriented form of yin yoga without props, hot yoga or fast vinyasa in a large group with few opportunities for offering individual help and guidance to students, your class is unlikely to be suitable for a hypermobile student and you will serve them best by referring them to a teacher and setting where they can practise in a safe and beneficial way (see 'Including and referring' below).

Where to start...

When a student shows up in your class with hypermobility that has never been addressed, there are often so many areas where they are out of kilter that it can be hard to know where to begin. My suggestion is that you pick one or two key things which are foundational to basic postures, for example, placement of hips to feet in standing postures, positioning of shoulders relative to hands and feet in quadruped postures or creating central body engagement. What you choose will depend on the style of yoga you're teaching and the individual presentation of the student. If you try to 'fix' everything at once, you are likely to overwhelm the student with Too Much Information.

Remember that this student has proprioceptive deficits which mean it will take them longer to embody biomechanical changes than it would a CT-typical student. Proprioceptive challenges, together with interoceptive overload (which can act as a kind of interference), will generally make this student's threshold for integrating outside input fairly low, so go slowly and offer sparingly: drip, drip, drip, not a bucketful. Somatic processes are by nature gradual and go at an organic pace – which will be slightly different for each individual. There's no rush and there's no destination to get to.

No postures are contraindicated

When yoga teachers contact me for help in working with hypermobile students, they often want to know which postures are going to be helpful and which they should avoid. Whereas for some health conditions there is a menu of recommended postures and another menu of postures that are contraindicated, it doesn't work like that with hypermobility. Each hypermobile person is an individual with unique biomechanics and has to be evaluated as such. A posture that is an absolute no-no for one hypermobile person may be the one that ensures, for example, a well-functioning pelvis for another. And this may shift in line with changes in the person's age, fitness, strength, range of general activities, health, work and so on. Perhaps this complexity is one of the reasons that hypermobility is sometimes ignored in teacher training. Making this kind of evaluation, in collaboration with the hypermobile student, requires a good eye for movement patterns, experience and some biomechanical nous. Which brings us on to...

Including and referring

Ideally, students with joint hypermobility require a skilled and experienced teacher. At the same time, hypermobile people are highly likely to turn up to all sorts of yoga classes with all sorts of teachers without any diagnosis or any awareness that they may be in need of specialist teaching. Where hypermobility is not producing a lot of symptoms and difficulties for the person, a little general knowledge about how to include students with hEDS, HSD and MFS in a low-risk and helpful way may be adequate – in the right kind of setting (small class, slow-to-medium speed, plenty of time to address individual needs). Where the person is in pain, dislocating frequently, struggling with limited proprioception and on the whole experiencing a wide range of hypermobility-related issues, they need referral to a suitably skilled and experienced teacher. Continuing to try to integrate the person into a class when they are clearly working beyond their capacity for strength and stability (and you are not able to reel them in or offer them suitable modifications) will not serve them and, indeed, will put them at risk of injury and further general exacerbation of symptoms. Bear in mind that these students by definition have fragile tissues, and that where carrying out a movement in a suboptimal way might not have too much of an effect on a CT-typical person, for someone with a genetic collagen or fibrillin difference, it may be, or quickly become, harmful. If you don't know or feel out of your depth, it's not only OK, but also ethical and professional, to refer – no matter how much the student likes you and loves your class. Explain to the person clearly and kindly why you feel unable to teach them and why you feel that X would be a more appropriate teacher.

Referring to allied professionals

It's also important to recognise when the person needs referral to a different kind of professional. While there are many things that as yoga teachers we can uniquely offer our students, there are others we cannot, even when we are knowledgeable about and experienced at working with hypermobility. When your classes have a significant hypermobile population, it's particularly important to have a list of tried and trusted, hypermobility-aware professionals to refer out to. These might include a:

- physiotherapist
- massage therapist
- osteopath
- yoga therapist
- body-based psychotherapist.

It's also helpful to know the diagnostic pathway for the joint hypermobility syndromes so that you can point any students interested in receiving a formal diagnosis in the right direction. See 'Diagnosis' in Chapter 1 for information about this.

Framing yoga appropriately

Many beginning students share the popular view of yoga in our culture as a kind of esoteric contortionism, and even experienced students are often overly focused on flexibility. Framing *asana* practice as a movement towards balance and integrity will be helpful to any new hypermobile students who think they have just joined a stretching programme, as well as to those who have been around the block a few times and are looking for yoga situations where they can work in a sensible, rounded way. Set out the context for practice in a kind and neutral way, being careful not to pathologise innate flexibility or blame students for having it. You don't want to undermine the fragile confidence new hypermobile students may have established in their capacity to 'do' yoga. Explain to your students that for some people balance and integrity will mean working primarily for strength, stamina and stability; for others it will mean leaning into increasing mobility. This approach will serve not only the hypermobile people in your class, but also your stiffer students, who may feel that they are 'bad' at yoga because they are not flexible.

By asserting the real biomechanical aims and objectives of *asana* practice, you may be going against the grain of many students' beliefs about yoga, based on what they have seen in advertorial and on social media, and you will probably need to keep gently redirecting everyone towards the actual project. Think about this as gardening: cultivating the ground of practice you want to offer your students.

Yoga versus asana

Asana is a tool of yoga, but yoga itself is, of course, a much larger field of practice. Where hypermobile (and other) students are overly taken up with extreme flexibility and exotic postures, it's helpful to refer them, kindly and gently, to the internal – energetic, somatic, psychological – dimensions of yoga. Remind them that the intention of physical practice is to create a simulacrum for life, in which our habitual patterns (*samskharas*), so naturalised as to be transparent to us, can become opaque, and once visible may be worked with consciously. This doesn't mean that we shouldn't take pleasure in the physical sensations of *asana*, or that it's wrong to enjoy working towards challenging postures; it does mean that we need to understand the larger context of the endeavour. Physical practice is an opportunity in which yoga may occur; it is not itself yoga.

Working for strength and stability

According to hypermobility specialist physiotherapists, Rosemary Keer and Jane Simmonds, a main objective in the management of hypermobility is, 'improving the endurance and strength capacity of the postural support and joint-stabilising muscles'.[7] Likewise in yoga, a key remit of hypermobility teaching is guiding students to engage postural muscles, so that they are better able to support themselves structurally. As we saw in Chapter 1, this kind of engagement is difficult for hypermobile people because:

- hypermobile musculature is generally hypotonic (lacking in tone)

- hypermobility entails a deficit in proprioception.

Many hypermobile students will lack the proprioceptive capacity to engage particular named muscles, even when they know theoretically where those muscles are and what they do, and it can be helpful to use imagery and (appropriately negotiated) touch to indicate where and how the muscle activation needs to happen.[8]

Be aware that while developing strength is desirable for hypermobile people, EDS, HSD and MFS are genetic conditions of the connective tissue. While muscle strength can compensate to some degree for lack of tensility in the fascial tissues, it can never create the kind of stability that is inherently present for CT-typical people. This compensatory form of stability is not automatic and must be consciously turned on and maintained. For this reason, stabilising their body can be physically and mentally exhausting for hypermobile people. Over time, the situation can improve somewhat, with gains in resting muscle tone from practising consistently towards strength and improved neural mapping of movement pathways as a result of proprioceptive work, but the hypermobile person will still be genetically different from their CT-typical peers and will still have to work harder to achieve the same movement.

While strengthening is an intention, it's extremely important not to push hypermobile students or set overly demanding goals. Kathryn Bruni Young, the creator of Mindful Strength, explains that neurological adaptation to new movement patterns can happen very quickly, in as little as five days in the general population[9] (probably slightly longer in the proprioceptively challenged hypermobile one). This means that if you introduce a student to a different way of practising, say, *chaturanga dandasana* (Four-Legged Staff Pose), they will be able to embody the new pattern and see results relatively quickly. But it takes much longer for muscles and tendons to adapt, and between 12 and 24 months for the fascial system to remodel.[10] In this period of lag between neurological learning and tissue change, students – especially hypermobile ones – are vulnerable to injury if they try to ramp up the load, repetitions and intensity of their physical practice. The catch-up phase may feel like a plateau, but really it's an important time of soft tissue consolidation.

When working with hypermobile students, be particularly careful to break strength work down into easy, manageable pieces, and expect progress to happen in very small increments. Err on the side of conservative here. Flare-ups and reversals are part of the process and are to be expected. It can be helpful to frame them for your student as part of a larger arc of practice, in which slow positive change is visible – and yet is not the objective. We're really here to feel, notice and bear witness to our own experience.

Stabilising at end range of motion

While some hypermobility-aware physiotherapists see their work with hypermobile clients as centred on training to stay out of end range of motion, others take the view that in normal activities in real-life conditions a hypermobile person is highly unlikely to be able to stay out of end range consistently. They therefore consider it more beneficial in terms of general stability, pain reduction and acute trauma prevention to train for strength at end range. Rosemary Keer and Jane Simmonds, for example, feel that, 'It can be more useful, especially if the individual is experiencing significant pain, to start with static exercises in the hypermobile range.'[11]

This is sometimes surprising to yoga teachers, who have been told that they should keep their hypermobile students out of end range of motion at all times – and on the whole, I suggest that this is indeed what you do. Stabilising out of this range is for the most part specialist work. Just know that if your hypermobile student has been given an exercise that involves repetitions in hyperextension, it may not be because their physiotherapist lacks knowledge about hypermobility. Bear in mind, too, that much of the training for elite athletes and dancers consists of working for strength at very extreme ranges of movement.

Stretching

Most of our students probably imagine that when they stretch they are elongating muscles. In fact, however, a muscle is not extensible, like a piece of chewing gum, but has a fixed length.[12] Much remains to be discovered about what actually is happening here, and interpretation of what we do know definitively is frequently contested among sports, fitness and movement professionals. For a review of the current state of play in the science of stretching, have a look at the work of yoga teacher, Jules Mitchell, who specialises in redefining stretching for yoga in the light of current evidence-based research.[13]

While there are many different stretching techniques in use by personal trainers and physiotherapists, these tend to be outside the remit of regular yoga teachers offering general yoga classes. In this section, I'm going to keep it simple and non-technical. There is little if any hypermobility-specific research into the role of stretching, so the following information is mostly pragmatic – based on my own experience of working with hypermobile people and on what has generally been found helpful by other yoga and movement professionals working with this population, as well as, of course, by hypermobile yoga practitioners ourselves.

Passive stretching

The image that comes to the mind of most lay people if you mention yoga is one of passive stretching – a stretch assisted by gravity (or by some other external means, such as a weight or an adjustment by a teacher). In a passive stretch, the idea is to relax completely and allow the external force to do its thing. The obvious danger of passive stretching, especially for a hypermobile person, is that the external force will prove stronger than the tissues being stretched, with the result being a tear or strain.

We have probably all come across hypermobile students whose yoga practice looks like pulling taffy – hanging out at end range of motion, with no muscular support, tugging on their joints – and who are reluctant to rein in the stretch and re-orient towards structure. Passive stretching is the kind most usually beloved by hypermobile people, at least, those who are not yet well educated about how to work in more helpful ways with their body – and the kind most often considered to be contraindicated for hypermobility. You see the problem here?

Why do hypermobile people love passive stretching? One reason is that extreme stretch may be one of the few proprioceptive feedbacks we can feel clearly. As a result, it may give us a sense of containment and of being 'in' our body. Another is that passive stretching may feel good, especially to a hypermobile body that is often full of aches and pains and muscular contraction. Deirdra, a hypermobile yoga practitioner with HSD, says:

> Holding my joints together for 52 years has been such hard work. Stretching releases all that tension from my body, and it's fabulous just to let go. For a little while, nothing hurts.

Where a muscle is in chronic spasm, passively stretching it can be as hard to resist as scratching a mosquito bite. Unfortunately, as with the scratching, relief is usually short-lived, with the longer-term consequence likely to be that the muscle clamps down harder. This is because, on the whole, spasming muscles in a hypermobile body are *weak* and tight, and really require sensitive strengthening accompanied by gentle mobilisation rather than lots of stretching (for more on the difference, see 'Mobilisation versus stretching' in Chapter 7).

That said, passive stretching has its place when done sensibly and in tandem with strengthening work. As I have oriented myself more thoroughgoingly towards strength and stability in my repertoire of practices, I have felt more need for regular stretching, usually with some simultaneous muscle engagement (so you could say this isn't really passive), and into end range for short periods of time. And sometimes stretching has even been a long-term fix for niggling pains. But it's all about balance. Passive stretching should be the side, not the main dish. Strength work is the meat and potatoes.

Active stretching

Not all stretching is created equal. Many movement specialists, including the legendary Shirley Sahrmann (Professor of Physiotherapy at Washington University School of Medicine and expert in movement system impairment syndromes) advocate active stretching as a way to create greater gains in flexibility and maintain them for longer. Orthopaedic surgeon and founder of Bandha Yoga, Ray Long, explains that:

> In active stretching, one improves muscle flexibility by contracting the opposing muscle group while stretching the target muscle.[14]

An example might be lifting a leg and holding it extended – as in the final, hands-free part of *hasta padangushtasana* (Hand to Big Toe Pose) in the ashtanga vinyasa standing sequence. The front of the leg – hip flexors and quads – engage to lift the leg, so that the back portion of the leg – hamstrings and gluteals – can stretch.

Now you may be thinking that hypermobile students don't need to be making gains in flexibility, and that's kind of true, but it's also kind of not. Hypermobile biomechanics are often way out of kilter, in part because of excessive tightness in some parts of the movement system (and excessive weakness and flexibility in others). An active stretch enables a hypermobile person to:

- focus on a specific muscle that needs to be released

- strengthen the agonists (the muscles that oppose the ones being stretched) – because contracting the agonists is what holds the stretch.

Active stretching is generally considered a lot safer than passive stretching, particularly for those who are hypermobile, because the force of the stretch is limited by the person's strength. An active stretch is challenging to maintain for more than 10 seconds (just think about holding *hasta padangushtasana* hands-free), and the optimal hold time is rarely more than 15 seconds.

When we cue our students to engage muscles, or to feel resistance in a standing posture, we are moving them into active stretch. Hypermobile students will often struggle to create any kind of muscular support at first;

however, even a little engagement builds strength, and gains in strength improve proprioception, which improves the capacity to engage muscle...so with patience and repetition, it's possible to initiate a positive spiral. Bodies respond to other bodies, and this is a situation where using hands on can be very helpful (with consent). In the best case scenario, the nervous systems of student and teacher can synch through touch, enabling the student to 'read' proprioceptive information through the teacher's hands. (For more information, see 'Touch' below.)

Strength is flexibility

It can be helpful to articulate for any hypermobile students who are fixated on stretching that the key to creating useable, relatively pain-free and long-term flexibility is generally through strength. That is: by working for strength they are actually cultivating flexibility, rather than limiting it. The Australian Ballet leads the way in functional, research-based fitness for dancers – the majority of whom, as we saw in Chapter 1, will be hypermobile (see 'Occupation'). The conclusion of principle company physiotherapist Sue Mayes and team is that, 'For dancers, the message is clear: strengthening the muscles is the safest and most effective road to flexibility.'[15] Advice that is totally transferrable to the yoga world.

Where a hypermobile student is strong and stable and has good control over their movement, personally I take the view that it's fine for them to work, carefully, with their full range of motion – if this is their objective and if doing so isn't problematic for them. Some hypermobile people aren't interested in this level of physical challenge and can't be bothered with the amount of strength training it requires, and that's fine. There are plenty of practice styles that don't go there. If the person is experiencing a lot of pain and subluxation/dislocation, they are not strong and stable – even if they appear to be – and need to be working:

- more slowly

- in smaller increments

- for shorter periods

- in more basic shapes.

As well as:

- limiting the amount of yoga practices they do in a week (as a rule of thumb, more than three is too many)

- looking outside yoga for exercise forms that can improve strength and stability, such as weight training, Functional Range Conditioning® and Pilates. (For more on cross training, see 'Yoga addiction versus cross training and supportive practices' in Chapter 7.)

Proprioceptive problems

I'm just about at the end of my tether with one of my students. I go over the same alignment with her week after week, often several times in one class, and none of it sinks in. After six months, she still looks all over the place in every posture. She just doesn't seem to be able to get it.

Judy (CT-typical yoga teacher)

As we saw in Chapter 1 ('Proprioceptive difficulties and dyspraxia'), hypermobile people, by definition, have difficulties with proprioception, the ability to sense:

- the position of their own body in space

- the orientation of one body part to another

- the range of movement in a body part

- the degree of effort required to carry out a movement

- which muscles need to be switched on or off, and in which sequence, in order for a movement to be made in the most economical way.

At the further end of the continuum, proprioceptive difficulties may be severe enough to warrant a diagnosis of dyspraxia.

Unlike sight, hearing and so on, proprioception is a largely silent sense. When functioning normally, it runs in the background, outside our awareness, so freeing up our attention for other things. Because of this, it can be difficult for a teacher with normal proprioception, and without the relevant education, to recognise where a student is experiencing impaired or intermittent proprioceptive feedback and to understand their difficulty with carrying out simple movements. CT-typical teachers often end up exasperated with proprioceptively challenged students because they don't recognise what the student is experiencing as an intrinsic disability and therefore lack the will or imaginative capacity to empathise and teach appropriately. It's a bit like getting angry with a blind student because they repeatedly fail to see what you are demonstrating. Students with proprioceptive difficulties are often the subject of projection from the teacher – that they don't listen, can't be bothered with proper alignment and are stupid or disrespectful of the teacher's time, energy or instruction.

Clues that a student is experiencing proprioceptive issues include the following:

- It takes them a long time to learn postural shapes and sequences.

- They confuse left and right and generally have a problem with spatial directions.

- They find it difficult to know how much they are stretching or to feel an edge.

- They find it difficult to engage specific muscles to support themselves.

- They are clumsy, drop things and trip over a lot.

Even where a hypermobile student appears to be well co-ordinated, the likelihood is that they are using learned coping methods in an (apparently) seamless way. With practice, many hypermobile people can compensate well for proprioceptive deficits, particularly when carrying out familiar movements in a focused way; however, this does not mean that they are no longer experiencing problems with propriocepting. Jenifer Ringer, former principal dancer with New York City Ballet, notes that, 'We ballerinas can be very clumsy "on land" when trying to do such simple things as walking'.[16] I don't know whether Jenifer is hypermobile, but we do know that most ballerinas are (see 'Occupation' in Chapter 1).

When you are teaching someone with a proprioceptive deficit, the key thing to remember is: they are not doing it deliberately. These students may be trying really hard, 'failing' repeatedly and still coming back and trying again. Wowza! That's a lot of grit and determination! Take it as a given that a proprioceptively challenged student will need to see, hear and feel a cue (ideally all three) many more times than a 'regular' student in order to embody it. Engagement and control come very slowly to those with limited proprioception.

Patient, committed teaching is required, as well as the ability to notice, articulate and celebrate small gains. These are often students who have bailed out of other fitness and exercise settings, having been repeatedly chastised for their inability to run, stay on the beat or catch a ball, and they may be very appreciative of a teacher with the capacity to slow down and make a welcoming space for them, irrespective of how many times they need to be reminded to place their shoulders over their hands or check that their feet are parallel.

'Listen to your body'

'Listen to your body' has become something of a yoga platitude, frequently bandied about by teachers but rarely examined or explained. Yoga is an embodiment practice, so naturally we want to encourage our students to pay attention to somatic information and prioritise their own embodied experience. As a mentor of yoga teachers, however, I'm sometimes concerned that 'listening to your body' is being advocated as a preventative against all physiological ills (which it certainly isn't) and as a means of absolving teachers of the responsibility of engaging with their students' biomechanics and understanding how to work with them intelligently. The expectation that 'listening' will necessarily produce safe and intelligent movement strategies without external intervention is particularly misguided where hypermobility is concerned.

When hypermobile students 'listen', we tend to hear a wealth of interoceptive information but only rather sporadic proprioceptive feedback. For a certain type of somatic practice this is rich material, but if the intention of your work involves guiding your student towards producing postures in a more balanced and stable way, you will need to be proactive as a teacher in offering information and feedback. Hypermobile practitioners often have gappy and circuitous mapping of body movements – even very basic ones, and left to our own devices will tend to utilise the same unhelpful approaches again and again. Bear in mind that these are students who may not have passed through all the stages of infant movement acquisition in the normal way and may be lacking certain basic kinetic patterning. (For more on hypermobile infant development, see 'Early movement acquisition' in Chapter 6.)

Especially in the early stages of practice, hypermobile students require a clear template for each posture (which can evolve as the student's capacities change). A template isn't a series of rote-learned alignment rules. It's an intended shape, the production of which is informed by the teacher's skills and knowledge about movement, and by the student's in-the-moment experience in the posture, as well as by anything else they already know about their body. Even students with a lot of practice under their belt will often still need your feedback, as their internal experience of where they are in space, and what they are engaging in order to be there, may not always match with what is actually happening.

Students who dislocate

To most people, dislocation sounds painful and dramatic – and, indeed, it can be. For some hypermobile people, however, dislocating is an everyday occurrence and really may not be a big deal, as we saw in Chapter 1 ('Dislocation'). If you are working with a student who regularly dislocates (and may also easily be able to put themselves back in joint), keep teaching towards structural integrity and avoid communicating any sense of fear, horror or fascination. The capacity to put oneself back 'in' is contingent on being able to relax the muscles around the joint – so terrifying your student with the awful consequences of what has just happened is going to be counterproductive!

Most dislocators cannot help it. However, you may come across the occasional 'performance dislocator' – who will show off their capacity to rearrange their limbs on a whim. Sometimes these students have no idea that what they are doing is unhelpful for their general biomechanics and dangerous for their long-term joint health. Once you have talked to them about integrity in the joint capsule and maintaining bony surfaces, they will usually welcome help with stabilising. If they don't care or don't believe you, you may need to explain how yoga is different from a stretch or contortionism class, and set some boundaries around the intentions for practice in your teaching. If these are ultimately just not a fit with the practice intention of the student, they will probably vote with their feet.

In my experience, many hypermobile people do not identify dislocation (or subluxation) as being such. When a student says, 'My hip goes out of alignment and then goes back in by itself' or 'My shoulder clicks in and out', they are describing a dislocation or a subluxation (which it is depends on how severely 'out' the joint goes and for how long). If you ask about dislocation/subluxation (verbally or on your intake forms) it will be helpful for most hypermobile students to clarify what kind of biomechanical events you are referring to. For some students, recategorising routine slippage and travel of parts can be a game changer, enabling them to take their own hypermobility seriously and understand that it needs special care-taking and attention.

If they don't already have a relationship with an experienced and hypermobility-aware physiotherapist, this could be a good referral for a student who dislocates frequently. As we saw in Chapter 1, dislocation is often exacerbated by patterns of muscular looseness and tension around the joint that pull it out of true. These can be complex and subtle, and need to be diagnosed by an appropriate professional.

If a student experiences a traumatic dislocation in your class – one in which they are seriously out of joint and cannot get back in again, calling an ambulance may seem like the natural first line of response. However, according to hypermobility specialist physiotherapist Jason Parry, there are only two, fairly uncommon, situations in which a dislocation requires immediate hospital treatment:

- the limb starts to change colour due to lack of blood supply

- the limb goes completely numb.

Otherwise, Jason recommends that in a situation of dislocation hypermobile people avoid hospital at all costs. The reason for this is that the chief remedy for dislocation is relaxation, to enable muscles to release, so allowing bones to slip back into place – whereas in A&E, the person is likely to be immobilised on an uncomfortable plastic chair in a tense and anxious state for a long time! A further problem is that medical staff may forcibly 'relocate' the joint under anaesthetic…only for it to pop out again a short time later, because the myofascial situation that created the dislocation in the first place has not been addressed. Alternatively, medics may put the dislocated joint in a cast, making it impossible for the out-of-place limb to find its way home again. Instead, Jason suggests that the person:

- stays as calm as possible and breathes normally

- uses relaxation techniques

- takes appropriate analgesia

- supports the joint with pillows or a sling

- sits/lies in a comfortable resting position

- uses heat (warm wheat bags, hot water bottles, etc.) to relax muscles

- distracts themselves from the pain if possible (by meditating, chatting, reading, watching a movie, etc.)

- massages the area gently.[17]

I would add that, in my experience, staying in gentle movement within the range of comfort is also very helpful, in alternation with supported resting.

As well as encouraging muscles to find more optimal functioning, movement can also help to diffuse nervous-system overstimulation. Jason reassures dislocators that once the joint is out, it's out: the worst-case scenario has already happened, and the only way onwards is upwards. Although repeated dislocations can cause cumulative joint degeneration, traumatic damage is very unlikely from a one-off dislocation. It's a waiting game – it may take a few hours or a few days for the joint to go back in.[18]

That in mind, my suggestion is that if your student is not back in joint by the end of the class, rather than insisting they depart in an ambulance, help them to call a friend, relative or taxi to take them home. Check in with the person the next day to see how they're doing. It should go without saying, but I'll say it anyway: unless you have specific training (and insurance) do not ever attempt to manipulate a student's dislocated joint back into place – even if they ask you to. Follow the protocols above and trust the natural intelligence of the person's body and the passage of time to put things right.

Touch

As yoga teachers, most of us are used to negotiating touch with our students – both explicitly, in words, and in more intuitive and usually non-verbal ways. I've discussed the ethics of using touch in a lot more detail in *The Yoga Teacher Mentor*,[19] so here I'm just going to flag up that for hypermobile students, the process of negotiation is particularly important. These are students who, on the whole, are highly sensitive on multiple levels and who may have processing styles that are significantly different from the norm. Make sure that you check in with your student if you are intending to use touch. With some students, this may need to be a conversation; with others, the communication may happen on a kinaesthetic or energetic level and almost instantaneously. Your student needs to be sure that their preferences are paramount, that they have control over how they are touched and that a wish not to be touched will not get in the way of the work of the class or offend you. Be aware that verbal consent in particular may be fairly superficial and not reflective of what the person actually wants. Make sure you take the time to feel into the message the student is really communicating and check that it's congruent with what they're saying.

That understood, touch can be a particularly useful tool when working with hypermobile people because of the proprioceptive difficulties (sometimes coupled with verbal processing issues) of this student group. Here are some examples:

- Touching a muscle that needs to switch on can help the student to engage it.

- Touching a muscle that needs to release can help the student to relax it.

- Holding a hyperextending joint in a neutral position can help the student create neural maps for the new alignment.

- Adding in some of your own strength can help the student to feel the structure of a more challenging version of a posture and build towards creating it for themselves.

- Offering some gentle physical pressure can help the student to find the muscles they need to create resistance.

- Putting a hand on can generate more proprioceptive feedback, helping the student to sense better where a body part is in space and in relation to other body parts, and enabling them to feel more contained in their body.

- Putting a hand on can communicate emotional support, reassurance or safety.

Where the system of the teacher is very attuned to the system of the student, touch can also generate a kind of *shaktipat* (or energetic transmission), by which the student receives information from the teacher on a body-to-body level. I've experienced this with several teachers and – most markedly – with a physiotherapist. For me in the teacher role, too, my hands are a crucial giver and receiver of somatic information. To some people this may sound magical, but when we are engaged in cultivating embodied awareness, this kind of transmission can be a pretty normal occurrence.

Bodies vary immensely in their genetically determined density. If you use touch a lot in your teaching, you will probably be used to feeling into the texture, resistance and extensibility of your students' tissues and will have developed a high degree of sensitivity in this area. If this is not a capacity you have cultivated, take time to develop your 'hands' in low-risk situations – ones in which you are not moving, pushing or extending a joint and in which the intention is primarily to tune in. Never pull on a hypermobile joint, and bear in mind that hypermobile tissues are delicate and joints are often tender, so squeezing or pressing may hurt too. Be receptive, be mindful. What is a firm touch for most students may be painful for a hypermobile practitioner.

For information on the particular issues of touch and autism see 'Touch' in Chapter 4.

Adjustment

When I straw polled an online group of hypermobile yoga practitioners about what they look for in a yoga teacher, the number one requirement was that the teacher asks before adjusting. For most respondees this didn't mean that they didn't want to be adjusted at all, but they needed negotiation around each adjustment, and they needed to know that the teacher was skilful, hypermobility aware and able to tune in to their tissues.

If hypermobile practitioners are nervous of physical adjustments, this is often with good cause. Many of us have had bad – even injurious – experiences of adjustment in the past. Sometimes this was not because the adjustment was aggressive or the desire of the teacher to carry out the adjustment was overly forceful. Proprioceptive difficulties make it hard for hypermobile people to know when to say 'stop' because our stretch receptors don't signal that we have gone beyond safe limits until several beats after the event. For this reason adjustments aimed at 'going deeper' or increasing the amount of stretch in a posture are very high-risk for hypermobile students and almost always inappropriate.

We'll be talking more about the practicalities of adjustment in Chapter 3 (see 'Adjustment: speaking in hands').

Working with edge

Hypermobile students who persistently practise at end range of motion – even when they have been guided into more stable and sustainable versions of postures – are probably not:

- stupid

- not listening

- showing off.

As we have seen, hypermobile people have limited proprioceptive capacity, and this is physiologically determined, not an aspect of their personality or an area where they have agency. Stretch receptors in a hypermobile body generally do not fire until the person has already exceeded safe range. As a result, the harder edges on the spectrum may be the only ones the person can feel, and they will need to develop alternative strategies for creating a brake on excessive degrees of movement. As the teacher you can help by offering feedback repeatedly, with patience and without judgement, and by educating hypermobile students about edge as a range of possibilities. I'll be discussing working with the edge in detail in Chapter 7 (see 'Edge'). All of this information is for teachers too, and the experiential work presented there can be incorporated into a general yoga class – it will also benefit your CT-typical students.

Students who want to follow you

Proprioceptive deficits make the process of learning alignments and sequences slower and more arduous. Some hypermobile students may have no faith in their ability to embody choreography and may believe that they 'have' to have someone to copy. While allowing the student just to follow in their first class may give them the confidence to stay, in the long run you will short-change them if you don't ask them to step up and take on the movements for themselves. Like any other sense, proprioception sharpens when it's used. You will need to teach patiently, in small manageable chunks with many repetitions, and praise small gains to build your student's confidence.

Remember, too, that being a visual learner is not the same as being permanently dependent on having someone to follow. It's fine to mark postures for your student if it helps them to see the shapes, but work with the intention of having them eventually go solo.

Using imagination

If you ask a student with poor proprioception to engage a particular group of muscles, they may feel overwhelmed or incapable – and may end up reverting to compensatory patterns instead. Inviting the student to imagine engaging the muscles can feel less threatening and is more likely to offer them access to as-yet unmapped movement possibilities because they are tapping into unconscious dimensions of their mind. Imagining is a great tactic when a student knows what a muscle group is, where it is and what it should do, but does not know how to engage it. For example:

Student: I can't engage my glutes. I just can't feel them.

Teacher: That's fine. Just imagine that your glutes are engaging, picturing the muscles around your sitbones firing and stabilising, and know that in this way you are starting to build neural pathways.

'But it hurts...'

When we try out a new way of working for strength, a new approach to a posture or a new exercise, it's normal to feel sore for a day or two afterwards. Because of the nature of hypermobile tissues, the after-effects for a hypermobile student may be more dramatic and may last longer. If a student with hypermobility reports to you that they felt sore after experimenting with a different movement strategy with you, don't automatically assume that they should stop doing it, particularly if it's one that was designed to be hypermobility friendly. You may need to do some investigative work with your student to find out what sort of pain they're experiencing; whether they have done a lot of the new movement in their own practice; and if they have, how they have done it. As a hypermobile mover, it's easy to become afraid of all unfamiliar or uncomfortable sensations, because most of us have experienced many instances in which a new exercise resulted in an exacerbation of pain and dysfunction. However, excessive caution gets in the way of building strength and establishing more helpful kinetic patterns. While listening to your student and taking their concerns seriously are paramount, you may also need to explain to them that just because it hurts a bit does not necessarily mean that the new movement is deleterious and encourage them to experiment. If pain is escalating, your student may need to:

- check with you that they are doing the movement in a functional way
- stop for a few weeks, allow tissues to calm down and then try again
- do fewer repetitions
- work in a smaller range of motion
- have more time in between (do the new movement once a week rather than every day).

If none of these strategies works, or if your student is really sure that the new movement is not helping them, let it go and try something different.

'Resistant' students

How do you work with hypermobile students who insist on doing things their way? I have two hypermobile students who just won't listen when I try to explain about engaging muscles and not working for flexibility all the time. They only want to throw themselves into the splits and do extreme backbends. I know this isn't good for them. What should I do?

Callie (CT-typical yoga teacher)

One of the things I hear often from yoga teachers is that hypermobile students are resistant to being redirected towards more hypermobility-friendly ways of working. While there are definitely times when I have experienced communication fail with hypermobile practitioners, on the whole this apparently widespread lack of receptivity is unfamiliar to me. Far and away the majority of hypermobile students I come across are delighted to have found a teacher who knows something about hypermobility and are hungry for informed help and sensitive guidance. So why the discrepancy? In my experience, hypermobile students most often reject a teacher's input because from their perspective:

- Their practice is being criticised: Hypermobile students who have already worked hard to stabilise and strengthen (with varying results) may feel dispirited when a new teacher pulls them up for being 'too floppy', lacking postural integrity and the like.

- Their achievement is being brought into question: Those hypermobile students for whom yoga is a haven of success (when most sports and fitness activities have been a site of repeated failure and dread) may be sensitive to any suggestion that they are actually getting yoga 'wrong'.

- Postures that give them pleasure or physical relief are being subtracted from their practice: No one wants to feel that something they enjoy is being taken away.

- They are being asked to do something they don't know how to do: 'Engage your abdominals' may seem like a simple instruction to a CT-typical yoga teacher, but for many hypermobile people this kind of cue is a minefield of proprioceptive confusion.

- They feel that you are trying to take over: Because proprioceptive deficits often give rise to confusion about body boundaries, maintaining control over their own body may be particularly important for some

117

hypermobile people, and they may feel threatened by any suggestion that you are trying to take charge.

- They feel that you are imposing your own interpretation on what they are doing.

Jude, a CT-typical yoga teacher, brought this experience to a Hypermobility on the Yoga Mat training day:

> A woman came to my class who was obviously hypermobile. When I taught *upavishta konasana* [Open Angle Pose], she launched herself into the most extreme version possible of *samakonasana* [Equal Angle Pose/box splits], turning her legs backwards and practically pulling her hips apart. Then she looked really pleased with herself. I tried to get her back into *upavishta*, but she just wasn't interested in doing basic postures.

As I listened to Jude's story, I noticed that I was feeling triggered. Like this student, I have often been the recipient of a teacher's exasperation, judgement and projection onto my experience as a result of my hypermobility. In fact, we don't actually know why our students are doing what they're doing or what they're feeling when they do it. If we approach our hypermobile students from a place of reactivity based on our stories about them, we are very likely to meet with resistance to any of our suggestions. I invited Jude to reflect on any assumptions she might be making about this student and to consider responding to her something like this:

> Good work! You have great flexibility in this posture. Sometimes when there's a lot of natural flexibility, strength and stability can be a bit less developed, and it may be useful to add some work to create more engagement. Over the long term, this can help to guard against joint degeneration and dislocations, and can also help you to access yoga postures that require more strength. If you're interested, I can show you some hip variations that are more geared to creating engagement. You can mix these in with your flexibility work so that you have a few options in terms of how you want to practise on any given day.

Most students are going to be open to an approach like this. It's respectful of their current practice and personhood; presumes nothing about their knowledge, aims and intentions; and it feels inviting. The chances are that this is completely new information for the student.

Students are most likely to receive your input well if you:

- take time initially to ask the student about what they are doing and feeling in the posture, *listen* to their responses and offer teaching on the basis of what they are actually experiencing

- find out about the student's past practice history (if they have one) – what they have tried in relation to practising yoga with hypermobility and what the outcome was

- acknowledge that they have obviously worked hard and are already doing well

- frame your teaching as ways to build on their existing capacity – by adding more strength, stability, balance and refinement – rather than taking postures away

- work with the student collaboratively – a style that supports what they already know and adds value to how they already practise will generally be well received

- maintain a friendly and encouraging attitude, meet the student where they are and respond to questions and comments with curiosity and an open mind.

For example:

Teacher: How's this forward bend going, Freddie?

Freddie: I like it, but my sitbones sometimes hurt a bit.

Teacher: You've got great hip mobility here, and you're getting the hip flexion really well. For people who have a lot of facility in folding forwards, sitbone pain can be a result of pulling too much on the hamstrings. Sometimes the glutes then tighten up to try to act as 'brakes'. One way to work with this is by engaging the abdominals more strongly and coming slightly out of hip flexion and more into spinal flexion. Would you like to experiment with that? It may help you to create a more balanced engagement and strengthen the abdominals.

Freddie: Yes, I'd like to give it a try.

Teacher: OK, let me show you and we can see how it works for you.

Where a hypermobile student is not experiencing pain, discomfort, subluxation or other problems (in other words, they are hypermobile but they have not developed a hypermobility syndrome), it can be hard for them to understand why they need to change the way they're practising. If you have offered them a simple explanation of the benefits of working in a more hypermobility-aware way and they aren't interested…it's their practice and how they do it is their prerogative. Remember that our role as teachers is to suggest and support, not to evangelise, impose or promote a view.

Where you and your student are fundamentally out of synch, usually the student will recognise that their approach to their practice is not aligned with your intentions as a teacher and will not stick around for long. If they do wish to continue coming to your class, however, you will need to consider whether you feel comfortable in a teaching situation where you are at cross purposes with your student and – potentially – whether you feel able to go on teaching a student who is practising in a way that you consider to be high-risk. This may be a situation for referral. Sometimes a teacher with more experience or a different personality will resonate with the student and be able to work more fruitfully with them.

Seasoned practitioners with hypermobility

As a teacher – even an experienced one – it can be daunting to encounter a seasoned practitioner in your class, particularly if they are also a teacher themselves. We may doubt our own skills and ability, and feel inadequate to offer anything of value – or we may jump to the opposite pole and try to prove how knowledgeable we are, compensating for the holes in our experience by imposing rigid rules and ways of doing things.

If you're working with a long-time hypermobile practitioner for the first time, my suggestions are as follows:

- Take time to talk to the person, ask about their practice experience to date and how it has been affected by their hypermobility and find out what they'd like to receive from you. This question is very important, as it will determine how you approach your work with the student.

- Take time simply to witness the person's practice – rather than jumping in and reconfiguring it for them. Know that you may have valuable perspectives to offer…and at the same time respect their existing body of experience.

- Don't feel that you have to prove yourself or show that you know more than your student does; just be present and ready to offer anything you might have of use. You are not an authority, just a companion walking alongside your student for a short time on a much longer journey.

- Be aware that hypermobility sometimes attracts a surfeit of technical input. You may or may not be giving your experienced student something new. Enquire and offer rather than insist and impose.

Standing still and endurance

Rosemary Keer and Katherine Butler note that:

> Hypermobile individuals frequently dislike static postures and report difficulty with standing still, such as when queuing, shopping or attending exhibitions, and sitting for prolonged periods of time.[20]

With good reason. Lack of connective tissue support and hypotonicity in postural muscles combine with POTS to make for a pretty lethal cocktail when it comes to being upright and still. While it definitely is possible – and desirable – to improve muscular strength and stamina in hypermobility, this has to be done in small, manageable pieces. Framing the holding of static postures (particularly standing ones) as a feat of endurance is not helpful. Even with very good muscle strength, a hypermobile student may lack the fascial integrity to hold a standing posture for what would be a normal period of time for other students. Holding beyond their range of comfort may not increase the student's stamina but cause muscles to go into spasm, and tendons, ligaments and fascia to become inflamed and overstretched.

Sitting meditation

For many years, I struggled to create a sitting practice. While other meditators described peace, joy and ecstatic states (along with periodic trawls through the shit heap), my experience was a smorgasbord of different types of physical pain and a sort of mental white-out. Eventually, I realised that for me sitting generated low-level trauma. When you think about it objectively, it's not difficult to understand why. Sitting upright, static and without support quickly caused muscles to spasm (Ehlers-Danlos) and also made me feel dizzy and faint (POTS). The situation was compounded by autism. Autistic people generally move (or stim) in order to process experiences (see 'Stillness and stimming' in Chapter 4); forced to sit still, it wasn't long before I experienced nervous-system overload. Sitting was, for me, a small form of torture.

CT-typical yoga teachers, take note. While sitting practice may be fabulous for you, it may not be so great for your hypermobile students. While mind and body appear to me to be a kind of co-arising, we live in a culture in which mind has traditionally been hived off and elevated over body. Many yoga teachers have absorbed this hierarchical split: yoga *asana* – actually a sophisticated awareness practice in itself – is often framed as a preparation for sitting meditation (the 'real work'). Actually, there's nothing intrinsically 'present' about sitting still; indeed, awareness in movement offers access to a whole realm of embodied knowledge that may not yet be available to conscious mind.

If you include sitting meditation in your classes, make sure you offer alternative ways to access the practice. This will also help any students in your class with PTSD and complex trauma, as well those with some other mental health conditions. Options might include:

- gentle, improvised (by the student) movement in a sitting or standing position (eyes closed or eyes open)

- physical stillness in a supported restorative (perhaps semi-reclined) position, using plenty of bolsters, blankets and so on; let the student know it's fine to fidget and adjust their position as they need

- *savasana*, with supportive props if available. Don't worry if some students fall asleep. Sometimes sleeping is an intelligent response to traumatic memories that the person isn't ready to deal with yet. Sometimes it's a response to fatigue and is exactly what the person needs. In our culture, many of us are permanently tired.

Projection

Oftentimes teachers see my innate flexibility and either 'call me out' in class as an example, or just ignore me entirely as if 'I've got it right' when in reality, I neither have it right, nor should be an example for others. Rather, I'm on my own journey in discovering how to manage my range of motion and learning how to support it with adequate, complementary strength.

Elaine (yoga practitioner with HSD)

For yoga teachers, being mindful of our projections is, of course, part of the job – I've written a lot more about this in *The Yoga Teacher Mentor*.[21] For some teachers, extra care is needed in relation to hypermobile students, who may attract projections related to the teacher's own desire (conscious or not) to be flexible and may be inappropriately praised or criticised as a result.

Teachers may be unhelpfully fascinated by a student's flexibility, seeking to push them into extreme ranges of motion to 'see how far it will go'. On the other hand, I have not infrequently witnessed yoga teachers blaming hypermobile students for being flexible, floppy or unable to control their movement. This is not an attitude that teachers generally adopt towards a student who is constitutionally stiff. It's assumed that the stiff student can't help it.

It's important to remember that hypermobility is not something the student is doing; it's something they are being. There's no choice or agency involved. It's not about you, or about the student's attitude to *asana*; it's simply a genetic condition – something they were born with. If a hypermobile student consistently pushes into end range of motion, it's less likely that they are showing off, practising aggressively or flouting your suggestion that they pull back, and more likely that the furthest edge is the only one they can feel. This is physiologically driven rather than an aspect of their personality.

Heightened sensitivity

Heightened sensitivity among hypermobile students is another common trigger for projection on the part of teachers. As we will see in Chapter 4 (see 'Sensory issues'), extreme sensitivity is generally most marked among autistic hypermobile people, but those who are allistic and hypermobile are often more than usually sensitive too. Sensitivity may be both to external phenomena (textures, smells, sounds, etc.) and to sensory experience arising internally. Sensitive students are sometimes considered to be stupid, lazy, arrogant or not interested in 'improving' when in fact they are receiving an overload of sensory information, which impacts on their ability to focus on what the teacher is saying and implement any suggestions. Students who disclose interoceptive information may be labelled as hypochondriac, neurotic or dramatic when in fact they are registering somatic experience in a range that for the teacher is under the radar.

Naming hypermobility for the student

A question that often arises when I teach teachers about hypermobility is: 'If I think a student is hypermobile, should I tell them?' This is a tricky area, and there isn't a single simple answer. First off, as I've already mentioned, we need to be clear, with our students and in our own mind, that we are not diagnosticians. That said, we are movement professionals, and our knowledge and experience may put us in a better position than most GPs to identify signs of genetic hypermobility.

There are basic ways to talk about hypermobility that don't reference a medical condition. If a student is new to you, you might open a conversation by saying something like: 'I see you're very flexible, so for you most of the work is going to be on building strength.' In some cases your interaction with the student may never need to progress beyond this level. Sometimes, though, not disclosing can get in the way of working effectively with the student, and it may start to feel as if there's an elephant in the room. Where a student is struggling with pain, proprioceptive problems, difficulties with building muscle and a variety of unexplained health problems, it can be very helpful for them to know that there may be a reason for this – especially if they have consulted doctors and been dismissed or disbelieved, as all too often happens to people with a genetic hypermobility syndrome. In this case, having someone besides themselves notice their difficulties can be tremendously affirming.

If you feel that it would be beneficial to broach the subject of hypermobility with a student, choose a moment when both of you have time for a short discussion – not in the middle of class (unless you're teaching Mysore style and have the luxury of being able to work with individual students at some length). A good, neutral way in is to say, 'I'm wondering if you've considered that you may be hypermobile.' Usually the student will ask, 'What's that?', so have a quick, simple explanation ready. Be aware that 'genetic condition' spells serious pathology to many people, so be careful not to terrify your student with overly medical language and worst-case scenarios. For some with hEDS/HSD/MFS, the consequences are indeed severe and life-altering...but for others they are really not. Explain simply and without drama, and feel into how much and what kind of information your student wants to receive. For some students this will be a lot, for others little.

Students often respond to the observation that they are extremely flexible with disbelief and disavowal. They are usually not feigning modesty. Remember that while a hypermobile student may look very, very bendy to you, their felt experience is often one of stiffness and immobility. You may need to explain to the student that hypermobility isn't being able to pretzel your way into advanced postures like an Olympic gymnast and that many hypermobile people experience, pain, tightness and proprioceptive challenges that can get in the way of accessing even quite simple postures. Where 'flexible' is alien, remember that some hypermobile students will identify with feeling floppy. Have a link to the Hypermobility Syndromes

Association's website to hand for more information (www.hypermobility. org). Personal stories can be more relatable than medical descriptions. There are lots on The Ehlers-Danlos Society's website. Find them at www.ehlers-danlos.com/stories.

Joint hypermobility is a spectrum condition

Some people with joint hypermobility are wheelchair users with many life-affecting disabilities, others are professional dancers, gymnasts and circus performers. In a yoga class context, some hypermobile students will be successful at building strength and will have effective strategies for dealing with proprioceptive difficulties. These students may easily be able to enter physically challenging postures and will sail through acrobatic flows without experiencing any ill effects. Others will always struggle to create sufficient stability to move well and may be dogged by injury and chronic pain. As we saw in Chapter 1 (see 'Hypermobility compared with hypermobility syndrome'), variations in the particular genes involved may partly account for this disparity, but we don't really know definitively why joint hypermobility may manifest as a pathology for some and an asset for others.

Proficiency accrues with repetition, and if we don't show up, we don't build skills and abilities. However, it's not uncommon for senior teachers practising postures requiring Olympian strength, stamina and flexibility to argue that anyone can do the same if they just commit to daily practice. The humility inherent in this view is commendable, but it would be more accurate to say that if you are gifted with the appropriate genetic capacities and are lucky enough to have a physiology that withstands injuries of attrition, practising with dedication will eventually give you access to acrobatic sequences of *asana*. Be mindful not to evaluate *any* students, and especially hypermobile ones, on their physical performance. It's not an equal playing field and consistency is not all. What matters in a practice, in any case, is pleasure in moving, cultivation of attention and the simplicity of presence, without motive or agenda.

3

Hypermobility-Aware *Asana*: The Practicals

स्थिरसुखमासनम् ।

sthira-sukham-āsanam

Steady and easeful posture[1]

In this chapter, we will be looking at some practical techniques you can use to help your hypermobile students to access postures in safer and more biomechanically functional ways. These are suggestions – possibilities to explore – not 'rules'. It's important to be aware that no technique is going to be appropriate for all hypermobile students all of the time. Hypermobility teaching needs to be collaborative and based on feedback from the person about how particular suggestions are going for them. It's a suck-it-and-see process, through which you and the student together evolve ways of working that are helpful and effective for them, and which tend towards improvements in proprioception, gains in strength and control, lessening of fatigue and so on.

That said, I will be talking quite a bit about what you might describe as alignment in this chapter. This is not because some ways of stacking up body parts are inherently 'correct' and others are not, but because – due to limited proprioception and anomalies in childhood development – our hypermobile students often arrive at yoga with little sense of where they are placing one body part in relation to another. Sometimes they are aware that their biomechanics are, in various ways, painful and unhelpful, but are confused about how they need to change. While, for example, it is not intrinsically dangerous to allow your knee to move past your heel when you bend your leg (in fact your knee makes this movement every time you go upstairs), asking a hypermobile student to ensure that their knee is placed above (not past) their ankle in *virabhadrasana II* (Warrior II) provides them with a reference point, and may begin to signpost them out of a sort of collapsed lunge and into a stable two-legged base with muscular support. As senior yoga teacher and therapist, Jill Miller, says:

> Alignment gives us a sense of 'home base' from which we can safely navigate and explore our range of motion... Alignment can mitigate injury risk especially as practitioners frequently veer into exaggerated end ranges of motion where it is difficult to maintain strength integrity.[2]

Embodying some foundational cues also supports proprioception, providing a ground of sensing-in-body from which our hypermobile students can gradually move into feeling for themselves.

This chapter focuses on basic postures that are common to most styles of yoga practice and in the repertoire of the majority of teachers. The principles discussed can all be translated to more challenging variations as your hypermobile students develop increasing strength and control. The strategies outlined here are those that I use frequently when working with hypermobile students and are intended to give you a basic toolbox. They are by no means comprehensive. There are many approaches to moving well, and any sound principle for functional movement and structural integrity you have learnt is potentially going to be useful for hypermobile students. Many of the principles for teaching hypermobile people are also best practice for working with *all* students and so are easy to incorporate into a general group class.

Some hypermobile people have many, complex needs. Remember that it is ethical and professional – not a sign of failure – to refer if you feel out of your depth with a student. This might be to a more experienced teacher or to one with a hypermobility specialism, or it might be to an allied professional – yoga therapist, physiotherapist, Pilates teacher and the like.

Muscle engagement for beginners

When my yoga teacher asked me whether I was engaged in paschimottanasana [Straight-Legged Forward Bend], I didn't know what she was talking about. Then it slowly dawned on me! Oh, I'm meant to be using strength in yoga!

Denny (yoga teacher trainee with HSD)

Denny would not be the first hypermobile person ever to have flopped and drooped their way through a goodly number of yoga classes before the light dawned. Sometimes this is not because teachers have omitted to tell them that yoga requires muscular engagement, but because they haven't been able to translate their teachers' words into meaning. Often, for hypermobile people, flopping has been a *modus vivendi*, and the leap of understanding involved in shifting into activation is very great – and may extend beyond the physical into ways of being and doing in the world.

For many hypermobile people, static standing is in itself complex to achieve, and may also be orthostatically challenging, and it may be useful to introduce principles of engagement in a sitting or lying position. For real beginners, multiple engagements will be proprioceptively confusing and impossible to create, so stick to one engagement at a time with these students. More experienced hypermobile practitioners may be able to take on several muscle activations simultaneously – and eventually produce a fully activated posture seamlessly. The following are some ways to explore basic engagement in *dandasana* (Staff Pose).

Activated dandasana

For a lot of beginning yoga practitioners, *dandasana* seems like an opportunity for a little rest, and it's common to see hypermobile students slumped and hanging in their joints here. However, there are many possibilities for engaging muscles in this posture.

1. Cue your student to draw (or imagine drawing) their kneecaps up towards their body to activate their quadriceps. Have them place their hands on top of their thighs and feel the quads engaging as they draw the kneecaps up…and releasing as they let the kneecaps go. For many beginning hypermobile students, having this kind of palpable feedback is helpful and reassuring that their body is getting it 'right'.

2. If your student habitually hyperextends their knees (see 'Micro-bending and hyperextension' below), activating the quads will often cause this to happen big time: the backs of their knees will be pressing into the floor and their heels lifting up off the floor. They could release the hyperextension by micro-bending their knees, but this approach may create a feeling of disengagement in their legs. Instead, ask your student to keep lifting their kneecaps and at the same time press the backs of their heels firmly into the floor. Now they will feel their

hamstrings firing a little to oppose the action of the quads. Draw their attention to the backs of their legs and ask them to notice any sensation they feel there. Explain that they are feeling the 'brakes' going on to prevent their knees from locking back.

3. Ask the student to press into the floor firmly through their hands. If they have a longer torso and shorter arms, they may need blocks under their hands to do this. Check that they are neither hiking their shoulders up towards their ears (overly activating the upper trapezius muscles) nor pulling their shoulders strongly down – neutral shoulders.

4. Ask the student to draw their abdomen – from just above their pubic bone up to the little hollow where the two sets of front ribs meet – back towards their spine (*uddiyana bandha*). If this engagement isn't in place and the student is overly loose in the posterior chain, the action of the arms and collarbone may cause the ribs to flare, the lumbar spine to over-arch and the pelvis to tilt too far anteriorly (the top of the pelvis tips forwards). For more on *uddiyana bandha* *see* 'Working with *bandha*' below.

5. Ask the student to press away evenly through all four corners of their feet – ball of the foot, little toe joint, outer corner of the heel, inner corner of the heel). Have them first dorsiflex their foot (draw the foot towards the shin) and then while keeping some of the dorsiflexing action, also plantarflex (send the ball of the foot away from the shin). They should feel their instep lift and firm. Ask them to extend their toes (draw the toes towards their body) and then while keeping some of the extending action, also flex their toes (send the toes back away from their body) to create neutral positioning.

6. Cue the student out of *dandasana* and invite them to relax. Explain that this is the kind of engagement they are working towards in every posture.

Micro-bending and hyperextension

The one thing I learnt about hypermobility in my teacher training was about locked-out elbows and knees and that the student should bend them. But I've never really been sure why.

Vicky (CT-typical yoga teacher)

If you ask a random group of yoga teachers how they would work with a hypermobile student, the number one response is likely to be: 'Tell them to micro-bend their knees and elbows.' That most teachers nowadays know what hypermobility is, can identify one indicator that it's present and can suggest a way to work with it…is definitely an improvement. On the downside, the micro-bending strategy has unfortunately become something of a quick fix, with teachers not necessarily knowing why the student should micro-bend or understanding what to aim for in the larger biomechanical picture – or appreciating that not all hypermobile people present with banana legs and inside-out elbows.

In this section, we're going to look at micro-bending in a bit more detail, starting with spotting hyperextensions and understanding how they relate to genetic joint hypermobility, and going on to consider why micro-bending may be a helpful response.

What is a hyperextension?

Hyperextension occurs when the bones in a joint move beyond what is a healthy and functional angle. Many joints can hyperextend, but since we're in the territory of micro-bending here, we'll stick to discussing elbows and knees.

In a textbook arm (which doesn't exist, by the way), when the humeroulnar (humerus + ulnar) joint extends, the ligaments and fascia encapsulating the joint, together with the bone shapes of the humeral and ulnar heads, prevent the angle of the elbow from opening more than 180 degrees. When the humeroulnar joint does have the capacity to open more than 180 degrees (giving the impression that the elbow is hinging slightly backwards), this is a hyperextension. Likewise in the leg, when the tibiofemoral (tibia + femur) joint extends beyond 180 degrees, the knee is hyperextended – giving the 'swayed back' (or banana) shape coveted by ballet dancers.

Does hyperextension always indicate genetic hypermobility?

Hyperextension of the elbows is pretty common, and it's not unusual to see it in CT-typical people. Assuming that the person hasn't experienced a serious trauma to the elbow, this is usually because the heads of the humerus and ulnar are shaped in such a way that they allow for opening beyond a straight line – rather than because the joint capsule is loose or humeroulnar ligaments are lax. In my not very scientific observation, hyperextending knees tend to be slightly more indicative of hypermobility, perhaps because the joint surfaces of the knee don't interlock deeply,[3] so the shapes of the bones involved in the joint may have less of an impact on the opening angle – and any hyperextension is therefore more likely to be due to connective tissue laxity combined with muscle hypotonicity.

It's also entirely possible for a hypermobile person *not* to have hyperextending elbows or knees, or to have the knees but not the elbows, or vice versa. On the whole, however, hyperextensions in both these joints occur much more frequently in the hypermobile population than in the CT-typical one.

Why do hypermobile people hyperextend?

The obvious reason is: because we can. The majority of people can't press their knee back beyond a straight line because the tensility of ligaments and fascia, and the action of the hamstrings, quads and popliteus (a small muscle that wraps around the back of the knee and functions as a brake on hyperextension) do not allow this to happen. But there's more to it than that. If there's laxity in the structures meant to give support to the joint, the muscles have to work a lot harder to keep the joint in a neutral position... but hypermobile muscles are also generally lacking in resting muscle tone, so you could say that whereas everyone else is starting from zero when it comes to building muscle strength, a hypermobile person is starting from a negative value. It may therefore require a huge amount of effort for the hypermobile person just to maintain a joint in neutral – and they haven't actually 'done' anything yet! 'Locking back' the joint, or resting the bone heads against one another for support (hyperextension), may therefore feel like the most economical strategy in terms of energy expenditure. Bear in mind, too, that this is most likely the strategy by which the hypermobile infant first managed to sit and stand, and may be the only way of achieving these basic postures that they have neurologically mapped (for more information, see 'Early movement acquisition' in Chapter 6). In order for the person to come out of hyperextension, a number of things have to happen:

- They must become proprioceptively aware of how the joint is currently positioned and how this position needs to shift.

- They must create neuromuscular maps to turn on the muscles needed to support the new position.

- They must develop sufficient muscular strength to use the appropriate muscles effectively and consistently.

Why is hyperextension a problem?

Hypermobile students often experience hyperextended positions as stable and comfortable – whereas when they are coached into more neutral joint positions they frequently feel wobbly and 'all over the place'. So why might it be beneficial for them to shift out of their old familiar alignment?

Joint wear and tear

Suboptimal joint positions increase wear and tear of joint surfaces and may further stretch ligaments that are already overextended. Senior Iyengar yoga teacher, Roger Cole, explains:

> Hyperextension stresses the front of the knee joint surfaces and weakens the quadriceps muscles. Over time, this misalignment may create deeper hyperextension, ligament strains or tears, cartilage degeneration (including meniscus damage), and arthritis of the knee joint or kneecap. What's more, if you push the knee back with enough force, you can tear a ligament, most likely the anterior cruciate.[4]

Rosemary Keer (senior physiotherapist and hypermobility specialist) and Katherine Butler (hand therapist and hypermobility specialist) add that when hyperextended postures are sustained, 'fluid is forced out and tissue nutrition is adversely affected'.[5] Not a good scenario.

Weakening muscles

When a hypermobile person relies on 'locking back' to create support instead of turning on muscles, they create a downward spiral in which the muscles get weaker, so are utilised even less. This is why when a hypermobile student is helped out of a hyperextension, they often feel weak and unsteady, and their arms or legs may visibly shake.

Misdirected forces

When the bones are optimally aligned, they distribute forces throughout the body in a balanced way, setting up a situation in which opposing muscle groups can be equally activated – with no set of muscles straining to keep any joint in true. Orthopaedic surgeon and founder of Bandha Yoga, Roy Strong, explains that:

> If the elbows are hyperextending in Dog Pose [*adhomukhasvanasana*], then the force of the hands pushing into the mat is angled inward. Ideally this force should be directed through the long axes of the forearm bones, humerus, and shoulders and then through to the trunk and pelvis.[6]

Distortions in the movement chain

Hyperextension in one joint affects the whole kinetic chain. Rosemary Keer and Katherine Butler describe the whole-body ripple effect of hyperextension in the knees:

> with the patella [knee-cap] displaced caudally [downwards and back in the direction of the tailbone] and contact of the femoral condyles [bulges on the femoral heads] on the tibial plateau [surface of the tibia] shifted more anteriorly [forwards]…the ankle joint held in plantarflexion, producing changes in the calf muscles, and also into the hip and lumbar spine' (so that the fronts-of-hips are hyperextended and the lumbar curve is hyperflexed).[7]

No joint is an island, and excessive flexion in the lumbar region carries along the whole spine and into the neck and shoulders, while, moving downwards, body weight shifts back onto the heels. Not surprisingly, this series of adaptations can cause joint pain and excessive wear and tear.

Nervous-system dysregulation

In my experience, creating structure by stacking bone ends together is a bit like holding on to the cliff edge with your fingernails. It puts the person in fight/flight/freeze mode – whereas solid muscular support grounds and calms the nervous system and tends to reduce the adrenal response. Remember that hypermobile people are routinely producing elevated levels of adrenaline (see 'Adrenaline levels, hypermobility and PTSD' in Chapter 1), so any strategy for nervous-system regulation is one that we want to encourage them to explore.

How can the teacher help?

The first line of student–teacher enquiry here is the famous micro-bend: we guide the student to move out of hyperextension and into neutral alignment by slightly softening the overstretched side of the joint (backs of knees, inside of elbows). Some students will already be aware of their own tendency to hyperextend and will just need a reminder of what to do. For those who are new to yoga and have no idea that their knees/elbows are doing anything untoward, however, the new joint position will usually be very difficult to feel, never mind maintain, and you will probably need to use a range of tools to help them find it. These may include:

- verbal cues

- visual cues

- engagement and counter-engagement (spirals)

- hands-on guidance

- imagery.

We'll be looking at all of these approaches in more detail shortly, when we go on to consider hyperextension in a couple of specific postures.

This is a situation where the hypermobile person may not feel an immediate gain; in fact, initially they are likely to feel wobbly and insecure in the new, neutral position and may not be able to square this experience with the expressed aim of creating strength and stability. As the teacher, you will need to explain why this is so and what the longer-term benefits might be. Frame moving out of hyperextension as a process and a project, rather than a one-time correction or something you expect the student to 'get' in a single class, and reassure them that they are doing well and that what they are experiencing is normal. As a teacher, the key qualities to bring to the table here are patience, kindness, encouragement and a sense of gentle humour – to defuse any tension and prevent things from getting overly serious.

Remember that hypermobile students are vulnerable to injury if they do too much too fast, so keep hold times short. In a led group-class situation, encourage the person to come to rest in *balasana* (Child's Pose) or *savasana* (Corpse Pose), or another appropriate pausing place, after a few breaths in the new and challenging alignment.

Hyperextensions in elbows and knees are relatively easy to spot, even if you don't have a lot of experience in reading bodies and identifying movement patterns – which is probably why the micro-bend has become the go-to hypermobility solution. However, 'correcting' the hyperextension is going to be only minimally helpful (and sometimes even counterproductive) if you don't attend to how your intervention affects the whole of the person's movement chain and help them to integrate the ensuing shifts in a kinetically helpful way. As physiotherapist and senior Iyengar yoga teacher, Julie Gudmestad, explains:

> As you begin to correct your knee alignment, you may become aware that your hyperextended knees are part of a bigger posture problem. As the knees curve back, there's a tendency for the pelvis to push forward, the chest to collapse back, and the head to jut forward. These forward-and-back shifts form a system of compensation that can contribute not only to knee problems but also to lower back and neck pain.[8]

These are some of the things you want to look at in this regard:

- How is the weight now distributed through the person's body?
- Does any part of their body look contracted or pinched?
- Does any part of their body look overextended?
- Is their stance balanced and easy?
- Is any part of their body straining?

You also need to check with the person how the change feels *to them*. While you can expect some initial disorientation and floundering around in the new position, it shouldn't hurt.

Let's consider how this might look in a couple of specific postures.

Utthita trikonasana

Utthita trikonasana (Triangle Pose) presents a challenging leg situation for many hypermobile people and may be where you first spot that your student is hyperextending their knees. If you look at the front leg in *utthita trikonasana*, you want to see a straight line from the hip to the ankle, with the knee striking it. If the knee is hanging behind the line, it's hyperextending. Don't forget that your student has two legs! When working with hyperextensions in *utthita trikonasana*, it's very easy for both teacher and student to get overly focused on the front leg. However, when the front leg is hyperextending, it's likely that the back one is too, so have a look.

The following are some approaches you can use to help your student bring their legs back into neutral alignment:

- Check the person's stance – I use one of their own leg lengths as a starting point (but always modify to accommodate individual needs). It's harder to control knee hyperextensions with a longer stance, so (if anything) err on the side of stepping it in.

- Ask the person to create a slight bend (micro-bend) in their legs. 'Micro' is very hard to feel with limited proprioception, particularly when, as in a hyperextending leg, 'straight' doesn't correlate with tension in the ligaments. Most hypermobile students will initially overshoot the mark, ending up with knees in flexion, so you will usually need to utilise some additional tools.

- Use your hands to make a 'joint capsule', holding the person's knee in the neutral alignment as they move into and hold the posture. 'Move into' is a key place here. We want the student to become gradually able to feel the hyperextension happening as they initiate the entry to the posture and to be able to employ a different movement strategy. I suggest you do this first with the front knee, as for most people this is slightly easier to feel, and then with the back one.

- Put a hand on the front of the student's knee and ask them to press their knee into your palm as they enter the posture and to maintain contact as they hold. By adding your hand, you are giving the person a little more proprioceptive feedback. Do the same for the other leg.

- Ask the student to put their hand on the front of their shin and to press shin into hand to create resistance against the hyperextension.

- Ask the student to come into the posture by micro-bending and micro-straightening their legs repeatedly (without ever straightening into the locked-back position) so that the posture becomes dynamic. Coach them to find the mid-point, where both legs are in neutral alignment, and then to hold there, noticing any sensations they are aware of. This approach will usually work better with students who have a little more movement experience.

- Ask the student to notice where their weight is distributed over their feet (typically, if the student is hyperextending, it will be concentrated in their heels) and to lift it up and over the instep. In order to do this, they will need to come out of hyperextension. Invite them to imagine that their pelvis is light and buoyant and can easily float up and shift in one direction or another. Again, this approach will usually work best with students who are already fairly experienced movers.

- If you have a mirror in the room, invite the student to use it for visual feedback. Hypermobile students often don't know that they're hyperextending because the hyperextension registers proprioceptively as neutral. By using the mirror they can begin to recalibrate. Explain to the student that matching sensation to actual position involves neural remapping and is a process rather than something they can expect to be able to do immediately.

Cueing muscle activation

In a sense, all of the above suggestions involve creating muscle activation. Let's look in a little more detail at what's being activated. The front of the knee is stabilised, via the kneecap, by the four quadriceps muscles, which attach to the front of the hip (rectus femoris) and femur (the three vastus muscles), and to the tibia. The quads straighten the knee. The back of the knee is stabilised by the hamstrings, which attach to the sitbone (all three hamstrings), and femur (short head of biceps femoris), and to the tibia and fibula. The hamstrings bend the knee. If the quads are tight or overdeveloped, and the hamstrings are not strong enough to oppose their action, the quads can act to force the knee into hyperextension. If your hypermobile student is someone who can also easily hinge from the hip into a bobby-pin forward bend, suspect that their hamstrings may be loose and weak and require more activation. (The hamstrings are part of the posterior chain, which plays an important role in general stabilisation and injury prevention, and which is often underdeveloped in yoga practitioners.)

The biomechanics of the lower kinetic chain (hips, knees, ankles) are complicated, with muscles doing different jobs depending on the kind of movement involved, and – confusingly – it's also possible for hyperextension to be a result of weak quads and overactive hamstrings. This is because when the quads don't hold the front of the knee together efficiently, the hamstrings take on a role in hip extension and plantarflexion, and as a result may tend to pull the knee backwards. If your student is experiencing pain and biomechanical difficulties as a result of knee hyperextensions, refer them to a physiotherapist to have the causes properly diagnosed. As a yoga teacher, the main thing to be aware of is that the action of quads and hamstrings needs to be balanced, so you want to coach your student to activate both sets of muscles. The following is a way to do this in *utthita trikonasana*:

1. Cue the student to micro-bend their legs (if they struggle to find neutral, err on the side of too much bend rather than too little) as they imagine the muscles all around each thigh activating and drawing the femur up towards the hip socket.

2. Invite them to feel the play between front of leg (quads) and back of leg (hamstrings), noticing how the action of one counters the action of the other.

3. Cue them to find the 'sweet spot', where both muscles are balanced and the knees are in a neutral position. If necessary, give them feedback on where their legs are neutral.

4. Have them hold the position for as long as they can maintain even muscular contraction all around the thighbones, and the knees in neutral alignment – this may not be long.

If your student finds it difficult to feel their hamstrings (a common problem among us bobby-pin people), have them take the stance for *utthita trikonasana* and then, without letting their front foot actually move, try to drag it towards the back one. This will engage the hamstring and in many people will immediately counteract the hyperextension. If the knee is now too bent, cue the student to slowly engage the quadriceps to straighten the knee. Thanks to Ray Long for this suggestion.[9] Engaging opposing muscle groups (agonists and antagonists) in this way is known as 'co-contraction' or 'co-activation' – key to creating strength and stability in a hypermobile body.

The information in this section can be adapted for any standing posture that involves at least one straight leg – *parsvottanasana* (Intense Side Stretch), *ardha chandrasana* (Half-Moon Pose) and all the Warriors, as well as balancing postures such as *vrksasana* (Tree Pose) and *utthita hasta padangushtasana* (Extended Hand to Big Toe Pose).

For more on *utthita trikonasana* and sacral stability, see 'Utthita trikonasana' in the 'Triangles, side angles, twists: preserving sacroiliac joint stability' section.

Downdog

In Downdog there is potential for both elbows and knees to hyperextend, but since we've already looked at knee hyperextensions above, here we're going to focus on elbows and the upper body.

For many CT-typical yoga beginners, the main elbow issue in Downdog is *hypo*-extension, with limited mobility in the shoulders, combined with weakness in the shoulders and arms, giving rise to collapsing arms with elbows that bow outwards. The situation is often exacerbated by tightness in the posterior chain, which causes the student to pitch all their weight forwards into their shoulders and arms. The work here is to increase flexibility in the calves, hamstrings and gluteals, and to generate strength and create better flexibility in external rotation of the humerus, which will straighten the arms and rotate the insides of the elbows to face more forwards.

For beginning hypermobile students, the situation is often very different. We might typically see the knees locking back into the banana shape discussed above; hyper-flexion at the hip and hyperextension along the spine (with little or no abdominal support), as a result of which the rib cage is pressing towards the floor and the shoulder joint is effectively being pulled apart; and elbows hyperextending so that the points are angling in towards the person's midline. Whereas the CT-typical student will probably need to externally rotate the humerus in order to bring the arm into true, the hypermobile student will typically need to internally rotate it.

In this situation, clearly, many things need attention, but let's start with some ideas for helping the student to bring their elbows into a more neutral position. As you will see, some of the suggestions above for working with hyperextending knees are also appropriate for elbows.

- On the whole, it will be easier for a hypermobile student to control their limbs and find core stability in a shorter stance, so check the distance from their hands to their feet and, as with *utthita trikonasana*, err on the side of stepping it slightly in. There is an idea abroad among some yoga teachers that if the person's heels are on the floor in Downdog, their stance is too short. Presumably the thinking is that the stance should be wide enough for the person to be feeling a calf stretch and that if their heels are on the floor, their calves aren't stretching (not necessarily true). Like many hypermobile people, I have lots of calf and back-of-ankle flexibility, and it simply isn't possible for me to make Downdog long enough for my heels to float, even if this were a helpful objective. Many hypermobile people, if given heels-off as a Downdog parameter, will end up hanging from their joints in an unfeasibly long stance with no possibility of creating engagement and at high risk of shoulder injury.

- Ask the person to create a micro-bend in their elbow. Explain that when their arms are in the neutral position, the 'eyes' of their elbows (the little dents on the insides) will be looking at one another. As with knees, for most students the micro-bend will be challenging to feel, and you will usually need to use some additional tools, such as the following – discussed in more detail in '*Utthita trikonasana*' above:

    - Use your hands to stabilise the student's elbows in neutral alignment.

    - Ask the student to press their elbows out into your hands and to maintain contact.

    - Ask the student to enter the posture by micro-bending and micro-straightening their arms repeatedly, coaching them to find neutral.

    - If a mirror is available, invite the student to use it for visual feedback.

- Loop a yoga belt around the student's arms, adjust the D-ring so that the belt sits snugly just above the student's elbows when they are in neutral alignment and ask the student to press their elbows out into the belt. Students with hyperextending elbows are often used to pressing their elbows inwards to create the Downdog structure, so the belt can give them helpful feedback for generating a different action. (Check that the student is happy to use a yoga belt before offering this strategy – for people who have been restrained in the past, a belt may be triggering.)

- Thanks again to Ray Long for this suggestion. Cue the student to keep their hands steady on the floor and at the same time try to draw them in towards one another – without letting their hands actually move. Ray explains that, 'This engages the elbow flexors – the biceps and brachialis muscles – and bends the elbows to counteract hyperextension.'[10] If the student now overshoots the mark and ends up with bent arms, ask them to very gradually straighten their arms (by engaging the triceps). Give them feedback on when their arms are in neutral.

- Teach the student to spiral their arms. This is one of my favourite ways of working with hyperextending elbows because it requires the person to create a balanced engagement in both upper and lower arm. That said, if your student is new to yoga and is really struggling with proprioception, one of the suggestions above might be more appropriate.

– When first introduced to this way of working, most students will initially try to produce the upper-arm spiral from their whole shoulder, so the first step is to teach them to differentiate an isolated rotation of the humerus from whole-shoulder movement. Show the student how their whole shoulder can move forwards and backwards (and up and down). Then ask them to maintain the shoulder in neutral and just rotate the head of the humerus in the socket. Nothing else moves – only the humerus. Not everyone knows what a humerus is, so make sure your student is clear that you're referring to the big, long upper-arm bone. If necessary, use touch and gesture to map out the geography of the humerus on your own or the student's arm.

– Explain to the student that when the humerus rotates in towards the centre line of their front body it is internally rotating…and when it rotates out away from the centre line of their front body it is externally rotating. Have them explore this movement a few times, and connect it with the words, just sitting or standing (not in Downdog yet).

– Have the person kneel down and put their hands on the floor as they would for Downdog, about shoulder-width apart, fingers pointing forwards. Ask them to externally rotate the humerus, as they have just been practising, and at the same time to internally rotate the lower arm. When both actions are happening in a balanced way, the arm will be straight and fully engaged, with the elbow points facing outwards, and the 'eyes' of the elbows looking at each other.

– When the student can feel these actions while minimally weight-bearing, they are ready to try them in Downdog.

It's challenging to create and maintain a spiral engagement, so give your student lots of feedback, and explain to them that it will probably take a while to embody this new structure but, given time and practice, it will eventually become naturalised.

You can use any of the tools suggested for hyperextending knees in 'Utthita trikonasana' above to help the student create a neutral leg alignment. To help them create engagement in their shoulders, ribcage and hips, try the following:

- Stand in front of your student and lift their lower ribcage up and a little towards you (so that it is no longer pressing down towards the floor). Ask your student to create internal support by drawing the abdominal muscles back towards their spine – from just above the pubic bone up to the notch where the two sets of ribs meet at the front, but focusing particularly on engagement just below the ribs so that they feel their rib crests lifting in and up. Invite them to imagine their front ribs knitting together to create a sense of closure and stability.

- Clarify the movement intentions for the posture. Many students think that the aim in Downdog is to press their chest towards the floor – and, indeed, for someone with very limited shoulder mobility, this may sometimes be a helpful approach. With hypermobility, however, this strategy will generally put the shoulder joints under enormous stress, and a more useful objective is to lift the torso up and away from the floor, creating as much muscular engagement as possible.

- Pressing the hips backwards towards the heels is generally helpful for students with tightness in the posterior chain, but many of our hypermobile students are already overly mobilised here and will benefit from strongly engaging the abdominals to lift their centre and shift their weight up and forwards onto their hands. They will be moving into less hip flexion and more spinal flexion. This alignment may initially feel strange, but over the course of time will build abdominal and upper body strength – whereas continuing to press back into the heels will further stretch (and potentially strain) areas that are already loose and weak. For more information, see 'Forward bends, "yoga bum" and hip versus lumbar flexion' below.

Remember that making these changes is a process and a practice in itself. The time frame is usually months, or even years, not a few classes, and requires commitment and ongoing careful repetition.

For more on working with shoulders, see 'Plank, chaturanga and shoulder stability' below.

Knock-knees

Several of my hypermobile students have rolling-in knees and flat feet.
Is this part of their hypermobility. Should I be doing something about
this alignment?

Desi (CT-typical yoga teacher)

While many teachers can identify hyperextensions in locked-back knees
and make a connection with potential hypermobility, fewer may notice
and understand the possible implications of knock-knees – knees that
hyperextend medially, so that the inner seam of the leg collapses inwards
and the knee rolls in and down. Hypermobile students with this pattern may
have been W-sitters in childhood, and as a result have the capacity for a very
high degree of internal rotation of the femur at the hip, and lateral rotation
of the tibia at the knee. (For more on W-sitting, see 'The W-sit' in Chapter 6.)

Medial hyperextensions frequently occur together with over-pronating
feet (dropped arches). The technical name for this situation is pronation
distortion syndrome. Whereas the classic locked-back knee distributes body
weight back onto the heels, knock-knees direct it diagonally onto the medial
side of the instep, potentially overstretching and weakening the medial arch of
the foot. People with this kind of hyperextension may also 'turn out' their feet
from the ankle, angling them at ten to two. A two-way, mutually reinforcing
movement dynamic is happening here. In hypermobility, ligaments and
fascia designed to support the arches of the foot are often lax, and muscular
support diminished, so the foot isn't able to provide resistance against the
descending force of the tibia, therefore allowing it to drop at the ankle and
roll in at the knee. And, going from down to up, foot pronation can also give
rise to problems higher up the kinetic chain. According to the US National
Academy of Sports Medicine (NASM):

> It has been shown that excessive pronation of the foot during weight bearing
> causes altered alignment of the tibia, femur, and pelvic girdle, and can lead
> to internal rotation stresses at the lower extremity and pelvis, which may
> lead to increased strain on soft tissues (Achilles tendon, plantar fascia,
> patella tendon, IT band) and compressive forces on the joints (subtalar joint,
> patellofemoral joint, tibiofemoral joint, iliofemoral joint, and sacroiliac joint),
> which can become symptomatic. The lumbo-pelvic-hip complex alignment
> has been shown…to be directly affected by bilateral hyperpronation of the
> feet. Hyperpronation of the feet induced anterior pelvic tilt of the lumbo-
> pelvic-hip complex.[11]

In my view, it's helpful, therefore, to approach this situation both from the foot upwards and the hip downwards.

It's normal for women to be slightly more medially rotated at the hip than men. This is due to the wider female pelvis shape, which requires the femurs to angle inwards a little more. While there are individual exceptions, if you look from the back at a mixed-sex group of students in Downdog, on the whole you will be able to observe this difference.

The following are some suggestions for working with knock-knees and pronation in postures involving weight-bearing on the feet.

Parallel standing

- Ask the student to stand with their feet hip-width apart and parallel to one another – not turned in and not turned out...even a little bit. For some people, finding this position will already be proprioceptively challenging. If necessary, ask them to look at their feet to check what's actually happening, and give them verbal feedback.

- Now invite the student to become aware of the underside of each foot from the ball, under the bridge of the toes, along the lateral sole, and across the underside of the heel, and to actively press down into the floor through this lateral elongated horse-shoe shape, feeling the muscles of the feet and lower legs engage as they do so. This will usually spread their body weight more evenly across the feet, so that the instep spontaneously lifts a little. You may already see the knees start to move laterally towards alignment over the second two toes.

- Ask the student to relax their knees slightly (without fully bending them). This will take the knees out of the hyperextension at the medial side.

- Cue the student to feel the heads of the thigh bones lifting up and into the sockets. This will turn on the deep gluteals, providing stability and tending to lift the pelvis a little more upright if it has been too anteriorly tilted. Ask them to feel the outer hips firming and pressing towards each other...and the outer thighs creating the same action. Ask them to feel the inner thighs firming and drawing towards one another. Help them to find the amount of activity in the gluteals that will centre the knees in a neutral position. A student with medially rotating knees will need to err on the side of external rotation, but you're looking for a balance of both internal and external rotation, with one set of muscles offering resistance to the other, so effectively the student is both internally and externally rotating at the same time.

For most students, creating all of these actions simultaneously will initially be very hard work – and they haven't even done any 'yoga' yet. The intention is that over time, this basic engagement becomes naturalised and will carry forwards into other, more challenging postures organically. For now, keep bringing the person back to this neutral, 'switched on' standing. For stronger and more physically able students, one of the opportunities of a sun salutation (*surya namaskar*) is in the repeated return to active standing.

Samasthitihi/tadasana

All of the above applies when we bring the feet together into *samasthitihi* (Equal Standing)/*tadasana* (Mountain Pose) – two names for the same posture. Some of my apprentice and assistant teachers have learnt dogmatic approaches in teacher training as to whether the heels should be together or slightly apart in *samasthitihi*. My view is that the 'correct' position depends on how it enables the student to align themselves from the foot upwards. Having the heels together tends to generate a little more external rotation of the legs and may be helpful for students with a more knock-kneed pattern. Having the heels slightly apart tends to encourage the legs to rotate internally, and may be helpful for students whose natural orientation is for lateral rotation. Explore small shifts in foot position with your student and, together with them, notice the effects each has on their movement chain.

For some of my students with bunions, separating the heels slightly allows them to roll the big toe medially and spread it away from the second toe, so shifting out of the 'bunion' position and back towards a neutral foot.

Downdog

When you look from behind at a medially hyperextending student in Downdog, you will probably notice that their insteps are touching (or nearly touching) the floor, and their knees are falling in towards one another. Sometimes, too, their toes will be turning out. If this latter is the case, start by helping the student to line their heels up behind their mid-toes. Use the foot cues for 'Parallel standing' above to help the person activate their feet. The student will not be able to change the orientation of their knees if their knees are locked. Ask them to fully bend (not just micro-bend) their legs, letting their heels come off the floor if necessary. Kneel down behind the student and roll their knees out to line them up with their toes. Depending on your relative sizes, you may be able to place your knees on the floor between the student's heels, so that as they straighten their legs – slowly and with control, and maintaining the new neutral alignment, they can't turn their heels back inwards towards their midline. Alternatively, you could place a block (landscape for most people) between their feet.

Asking a hypermobile student to press their heels back to the floor can be a recipe for knee hyperextensions, whether the person hyperextends at the back of the knee or medially. If their feet are high off the floor, it may sometimes be helpful to place a block under each heel, so that they can ground their heels without creating hyperextension. Rather than cueing the student to stretch down towards the floor through the whole hip, knee and ankle complex, ask them to imagine only their heel dropping down towards the floor, opening up space at the junction between it and the ankle. They will be gapping the talus (and calcaneus) away from the tibia. This should enable the knee joint to remain a little soft, and shift the emphasis away from stretching gluteals, hamstrings and calves, and towards making space in the posterior foot and ankle.

Parsvottanasana and Warrior II

It's biomechanically optimal to have the knee facing in the same direction as the foot – that much is pretty obvious. Knock-kneed hypermobile students may tend to allow the bent knee in postures such as *parsvottanasana* (Intense Side Stretch) and Warrior (*virabhadrasana*) II to swing inwards. Where the knee is bent, and both knee and foot are in view of the person, bringing both back in line is relatively easy and usually takes just a verbal cue or a simple manual adjustment – and lots of repetition to embody the new pattern. If you require your students to stack the hips vertically one above the other (or to get as close to this as they can), many of them won't be able to create the desired foot–knee alignment – and this may be the least of their problems. We'll be talking more about optimal hip alignment in side-facing standing postures and sacroiliac (SI) joint health later (see 'Triangles, side angles, twists: preserving sacroiliac joint stability'). For now, just be aware that the most SI-joint friendly approach to postures oriented towards the long side of the mat is with the back toes angled slightly in, so that the femur can internally rotate a little bit and the upper hip can swing forwards and down a little. When this happens, it's easy for the front knee to face the same way as its foot.

Utthita trikonasana

Utthita trikonasana is another place where your medially rotating students may need to roll out their front knee laterally. It's not possible to reorient the knee with a straight leg, so ask the person to bend their knee, then have them align it with the second two toes of its foot, using hands-on adjustment if it's helpful. Once they have the knee facing the same way as the foot, ask them to slowly straighten their leg, keeping the alignment. This will require them to make the leg more active. As for *parsvottanasana* and Warrior II, have the back toes angled slightly in and avoid stacking the hips vertically. This will give the student a fighting chance of being in the posture without either torqueing their knee or straining their SI joints.

Strengthening external rotators

In my travels through yogaland I come across countless workshops, videos and articles about 'opening' the hips, but relatively few about strengthening them, which is vitally important for, well, all yoga practitioners, but especially hypermobile ones. The student with medially rotating knees is – almost by definition – weak in the external (or lateral) hip rotators. There are seven of these. The largest and most superficial (top layer) is gluteus maximus, which gives the rounded shape to the buttocks. Beneath gluteus maximus lies piriformis. The remaining five external rotators lie even deeper, and function mainly as stabilisers (rather than movers). These are:

- gemellus superior

- obturator externus

- gemellus inferior

- obturator internus

- quadratus femoris.

Collectively these muscles are known by the acronym GOGOQ.

There are yoga postures that strengthen the external rotators – we'll look at some in a moment – but these require complex muscle activations. If a student is weak in external rotation or finds it difficult to locate and turn on some of the muscles required, I would suggest Pilates or a slow body conditioning class (with a hypermobility-aware teacher) as a first step. These approaches include exercises to isolate the external rotators and involve the small repetitions necessary to strengthen them. If you'd like to offer your students a basic exercise to isolate and strengthen external rotation, the Clamshell is a good place to start:

1. Have your student lie on their right side, with their legs a little in front of them, one on top of the other, and their knees bent to about 90 degrees or slightly less. They can rest their head on their extended right arm or lift their shoulders up slightly and use their right hand to support their head. The left hand is placed on the floor just in front of their waist for balance. Cue the student to engage their abdominals to support the starting position – and maintain the engagement throughout.

2. Keeping their feet together and their pelvis fixed, they raise their left knee up as far as it will go without their pelvis tipping – either backwards or up towards the armpit – then lower their knee down again, and repeat. Keeping the pelvis static is important. The range of movement may be small, and that's fine. Students with wide hips may not be able to lie on their side without tipping their pelvis and will benefit from having their torso raised on some folded blankets or blocks. Have the student try the exercise with their feet pointed and toes together…and feet flexed and heels together. Invite them to notice any differences and to be aware of which variation (if any) is easier in terms of muscle activation.

3. With hypermobile students, five repetitions may initially be enough, gradually building up to ten. You can make the exercise more challenging by having the student lift both feet about 15 cm (6 inches) off the floor (à la Little Mermaid) and keep them raised as they make the clamshell movement. Their knees are still on the floor. Placing the left hand on the left hip will require the abdominals to work harder to stabilise.

4. Change to the second side.

As the student gains better control of the rotation and is more able to feel the muscles they need to activate, they can start to find it in any of the following basic yoga postures:

- *Vrksasana.* Unless your student has perfectly turned out (retroverted) hips, remind them that the intention in this posture is not to abduct their bent knee 180 degrees to their hip (few people have the skeletal structure to allow this to happen), but to feel the external rotators firing and stabilising the movement – so their knee may be well in front of their hip, and that's OK. Make sure the student keeps their pelvis fixed (rather than swinging it to one side), so that the movement comes from the femur rotating (and abducting), rather than the pelvis turning.

- *Parsvottanasana* and Warrior II. Cue your student to feel the rotation of the front leg from the buttock: gluteus maximus turning on and, beneath, the deeper rotators firing to hold the leg rotation solid and strong. Cue the student to feel the head of the femur drawing into the socket so that it is held firmly. This will also help to turn on deep rotation.

- Warrior I (with the back heel on the floor). In this posture, the back leg is the one in external rotation. As in Warrior II, cue the student to feel gluteus maximus and the deep rotators firming the hip joint. Students with a lot of internal rotation (and flexibility in the Achilles tendon area) will sometimes place their back foot at the same angle as the front one, which will not strengthen external rotation. Cue them to place the back foot with the toes turned out at about 45 degrees to a plumb line from heel to heel. Ask the student to press into the outer edge of the back foot, firming the back leg. They should feel that both legs are equally active (not that they are lunging into the front one).

- *Ardha chandrasana* (Half-Moon Pose). Make sure your student is strong and stable in the former three postures before you progress to this one. It's at the standing leg that the external rotation occurs. (In most people, the extended leg is in slight internal rotation.) In this posture, the pelvis revolves around the femoral head to create the rotation (rather than vice versa, as in the preceding postures). Invite the student to imagine space in the hip socket, so that the pelvis can easily lift up and away and turn, like a wheel, externally to the thigh bone.

- *Utkata konasana* (Goddess Pose). Make sure your student can feel and control external rotation in one hip before progressing to this posture, which requires them to find and hold active external rotation in both hip sockets. If the student's knees are falling forwards of their ankles, ask them to turn their toes slightly more in and have their feet more forward of their pelvis. Cue them to feel their pelvis pressing forwards and their knees rolling back (laterally) while they fire the external rotators, as in the two Warriors.

More challenging postures for strengthening lateral rotation include:

- Part two – leg to the side – of both *utthita hasta padangushtasana* (Extended Hand to Big Toe Pose) and *supta padangushtasana* (Supine Big Toe Pose). As for *vrksasana*, make sure the movement comes from the femur revolving and abducting in the socket, not the hips swinging (or tipping). This is the hard part and is what makes this a more difficult posture.

- *Vashistasana* (Side Plank) with the top leg raised and bound, finger to big toe.

- *Vishvamitrasana* (Friend of the Universe Pose).

Strengthening the feet

As a long-time dancer, I'm always struck by how little attention is given in yoga to the feet – such a crucial body part, with so many bones (26) and joints (33), and so many individual and collective movement possibilities. Foot strengthening is another area where I would suggest that students need to look outside yoga for comprehensive and thoroughgoing strategies. Small isolated repetitions build the strength and endurance necessary to use the feet effectively in the more complex, whole-body movements of yoga. Ballet conditioning is a treasure trove of foot and ankle exercises, and a quick search on YouTube will bring up many free resources. Working specifically with the feet makes a huge difference to a yoga practice: foot strength and resilience translates into legs, and from there all the way up through the kinetic chain.

The following are some suggestions for a basic foot strengthening and stabilising routine for hypermobile students with pronation distortion syndrome and generally weak feet. There are many more exercises that could be added – this subject is worth a book in its own right.

1. This exercise strengthens the toe flexors and the metatarsal arch. Have the student sit on the floor (or if the floor is not possible, this exercise can be done in a chair), bend their knee and dorsiflex their foot (toes move towards shins). Their heel is on the floor. Ask them to curl all five toes, slowly and with control…and then, slowly and with control, uncurl them. Make sure they don't claw their toes. They are going for

a long, balanced arc along the toes and across the top of the metatarsal arch, and engagement in the muscles on the underside. Also make sure that their big toe doesn't cross over the first toe. Crossing the toes in this way will play into the movement pattern that creates bunions in those with a genetic vulnerability – more on bunions in Chapter 4 (see 'Bunions (hallux valgus)'). If the big toe does cross, first check the student's timing. They need to synch the toes so that they all curl at the same rate. Because the big toe has its own muscle (flexor hallucis longus), whereas the other four toes all share flexor digitorum longus, this co-ordination can be challenging. If timing is not the issue, give the student a 'spacer' – ask them to put a bunched-up sock between the two toes so that they stay separated. Start with whatever number of repetitions the student can do with control, and work up to ten.

As they get stronger, students can make the exercise more challenging by wrapping a latex band (theraband) around their toes. The type of band they need is about 15 cm (6 inches) wide and roughly a metre long. (I've recommended latex bands to students for foot work and had them come back with something the size of a loop of hair ribbon – that's not the thing!) Latex bands come in different, colour-coded densities. Have your student start with the lightest one and build up slowly to the tougher, more resistant bands.

2. This exercise strengthens the toe flexors, metatarsal arch and medial arch (instep). The student starts with their foot flat on the floor. Slowly and with control, they drag their toes towards their instep, keeping the toes long and in contact with the floor. The metatarsal and medial arches dome up, but the toes don't claw. Invite the student to imagine that they are trying to pull a piece of fabric towards them with their forefoot. Repetitions are as for exercise 1. There's no latex band version of this exercise.

3. This exercise strengthens the medial arch, metatarsal arch, toe extensors and toe flexors. Set up in the same way as for exercise 1, foot dorsiflexed, heel on the floor.

    i. Keeping their heel on the floor, the student lowers the ball of their foot, together with the corresponding joints of all four smaller toes, down to the floor, keeping the medial arch firmed and lifting up and away from the floor.

    ii. Next, they lengthen their toes down onto the floor.

iii. Now they arch the metatarsals away from the floor, as in the previous exercise, as if they were trying to draw a piece of fabric towards them with their toes.

iv. Finally, they lift the foot back up into dorsiflexion.

I've set this exercise out in steps for clarity, but it's actually all one sinuous, snake-like movement. Invite the student to feel into all the tiny intrinsic muscles activating underneath the foot. Key cues are 'slow' and 'juicy'. Repetitions are as above. A latex band can be added.

4. This exercise strengthens the medial arch, metatarsal arch, toe flexors and toe extensors. This is the reverse movement of exercise 3. Set up in the same way. This time, the tips of the toes go down first (rather than the ball of the foot). The student extends and straightens their toes against the floor and from there moves back into dorsiflexion. Repetitions are as above. A latex band can be added.

5. This exercise strengthens the toe flexors. You will need a light latex band. Have the student place their foot flat on the floor, wrap the band around their big toe and draw it up into extension. Working against the resistance of the band, they flex the toe down to the floor and hold for a second or two, then repeat, working up gradually to ten repetitions. Once they have mastered the big toe, they can move on to their little toe, from there to its neighbour and so on. The big toe is easiest to isolate because, as we have already seen, it has its own flexor, whereas the four smaller toes are each flexed by a separate tendon of a single muscle. With time and practice, however, all five toes can move independently of one another.

These movements sound complicated when they're written down, but are actually quite simple. You can see a video of me doing some of them at: https://youtu.be/_DF6-_fXMpI. Please be aware that it was made for my Mysore students and is not professionally produced – clearly! You can see in the video that my right big toe is very mobile and is crossing over the second toe. I've been working on synchronising the movement of big toe with smaller toes. Ballet dancer/teacher Kathryn Morgan also has a video of the first four exercises, plus a few more, at: https://youtu.be/JVvMrGMujxY. Finally, if you're doing flex and point latex band exercises, I recommend watching Episode 2 of Lisa Howell's 'Safe Dance Practice Series', 'Theraband Exercises'. You can find it at: https://youtu.be/MirGTEsvE1A.

While standard yoga postures aren't the first resort for basic foot work, once your student has some stability in their insteps, and a proprioceptive awareness of different foot articulations and of biomechanically helpful foot placements in standing, there are opportunities for further strengthening the insteps and countering pronation in *asana*. We've already discussed activation of the feet in parallel standing and *samasthitihi/tadasana*. The following are a few more postures where your hypermobile students can work on foot strength and stabilisation.

Padangushtasana and 'trigger finger' postures

Yoga offers us a variety of opportunities for binding the big toe with the first two fingers and the thumb – in *padangushtasana*, *hasta* and *supta padangushtasana*, *ubhaya padangushtasana* (Both Feet and Thumbs Pose), *vashistasana* with leg raise... For simplicity, I'm going to focus on *padangushtasana* here, but the same principles apply to any posture that involves catching the big toe with trigger fingers. Your student can bend their knees a little if necessary to reach their toes. If they're struggling with a lot of posterior chain tightness at present, leave this exploration for later.

Have your student come to parallel standing, fold forward and take hold of their big toes with trigger fingers. The first two fingers slide between the big toe and the first toe, and the thumb is wrapped above and around the big toe. (Students sometimes get the grip the back-to-front, creating a less efficient position for their shoulders.) Ask them to actively lift the toe away from the floor – so that it is in extension. Invite them to notice their instep lifting and firming. Now ask them to resist the pulling-up action of their fingers with their big toe, by pressing the toe back into the floor, while maintaining the finger grip. They are engaging the big toe flexors. The student has created a movement and a counter-movement and should now feel the inner side of their foot and their big toe fully engaged.

In postures where the leg is raised, for example *hasta padangushtasana*, the student can also experiment with dorsiflexing their foot...plantarflexing their foot...dorsiflexing...plantarflexing...reducing and refining the alternate movements until they are both dorsiflexing and plantarflexing at the same time, and so creating full engagement.

Plank

Hypermobile students with medially hyperextending knees on standing will often reproduce this pattern in Plank (*phalakasana*), with their knees rolling in and their heels either dropping in towards their midline (for more on why this might be, see 'Lateral Tibial Torsion' in Chapter 6) or tipping out laterally. Check that your student's feet are placed not wider than their hips. A slightly narrower placement can be easier to control. Ask your student to engage their gluteals strongly, feeling the femurs drawing up into the sockets. The resulting external rotation will roll their knees laterally so that their kneecaps face directly down towards the floor, or at least are moving more in that direction. Ask your student to stack up their heels over the balls of their feet, feeling all five metatarsals equally on the floor and a dynamic engagement along the centre of their back leg from heel to sitbones...and from sitbones to heel. You can add a yoga belt looped around the student's ankles for proprioceptive feedback. If they tend to drop their heels towards their midline, ask your student to press their heels into the belt. If they tend to drop their heels out laterally, ask them to keep their heels in contact with the belt without pressing into it.

If your student's heels tend to fall in towards their midline, once they have changed their basic alignment back to neutral and stabilised there, you can increase the demand of the posture in terms of strength by adding a latex band tied into a loop around their ankles/heels. This will add resistance as they press their heels out into the band. Remember not to overtax your hypermobile student by adding too much too soon.

A standard cue for Plank is to press the heels back. While this is not an unhelpful suggestion in general, students with a lot of ankle mobility may end up with their heels excessively dorsiflexed in response, so ask them to keep their heels actively pressing away *and* simultaneously pitching a little forward, so that they don't go to the limit of their possible dorsiflexion and their heels are aligned over the balls of their feet. Alternatively, have them set up with their feet to the wall, so that they can press their heels into the wall to feel the neutral position.

Typically, a hypermobile student in Plank will allow their toes to be pressed passively into extension – against the floor – by the force of their own weight under gravity. Have them actively resist the floor by pressing into it through their toes (they are creating some toe flexion within the toe extension). If the angle between their toes and the top of their foot is less than 90 degrees, their toes are hyperextending, and they may benefit from creating more toe flexion. Metatarsal pain, due to overstretching ligaments, tendons and fascia; can be the long-term consequence of weight-bearing on hyperextending toes.

Chaturanga

If your student medially rotates their knees in Plank, they probably will in *chaturanga dandasana* (Four-Legged Staff Pose) too, and you can offer the same explorations with them here as in Plank. It can take a very long time for a hypermobile student to be able to practise *chaturanga* in a safe and stable way – more on this later (see 'Plank, *chaturanga* and shoulder stability'). If your student has not yet reached this stage, work on some of the component actions of the posture instead, and leave the explorations above for later.

Dandasana

We have already explored the foot action in *dandasana* at the beginning of this chapter (see 'Activated *dandasana*'). In this posture, the feet are placed as if in standing, but the student is, of course, sitting, so there is an opportunity for them to create a fully lifted and engaged instep without the added challenge of weight-bearing.

Updog

When the knees medially rotate, the heels may also fall out to the side (sickle) in Updog (*urdhvamukhasvanasana*). Since the student can't see their feet in this position, and may not be receiving the relevant proprioceptive information, it can be particularly hard for them to know what's happening, and they will usually need teacher feedback. A manual adjustment is often helpful here. Once the heels are in line, ask the student to press down firmly into the floor through the tops of their toes, at the same time drawing the femurs into the sockets. You should see that as well as their heels aligning, their legs engage and their pelvis lifts away from the floor. If there is any excessive lumbar extension it will spread more evenly along their whole spine. For more on lumbar extension in Updog, see 'Updog, Cobra and sun salutations' below.

Plank, *chaturanga* and shoulder stability

I have several hypermobile students in my class who droop towards the floor in Plank and collapse down into chaturanga with their elbows pointing out to the sides. However I cue them, they're weak and wobbly.

Jana (CT-typical yoga teacher)

The majority of hypermobile yoga beginners who show up in vinyasa-type classes are in no way physically prepared for the demands of Plank and (especially) *chaturanga dandasana*. Yet most often they are immediately launched into a series of fast-paced sun salutations, with little or no explanation of how they should be producing the required movements. This is a recipe for shoulder strains, subluxations and injuries. The shoulder is the most mobile joint in the body (and the most commonly dislocated), with a shallow socket, a loose joint capsule and only very limited interface between the humerus and scapula. What beginning hypermobile students need initially in order to support – not compromise – shoulder joint health is upper body strengthening and stabilising in less loaded postures, with lots of time to find the necessary actions to create the shapes in functional ways.

Let's have a look at the major muscular mechanisms for creating shoulder stability and consider some ways we can approach strengthening them.

Rotator cuff

The rotator cuff is made up of four muscles. Starting from the top, on the upper scapula, and working down, these are:

- supraspinatus (raises the arm)

- infraspinatus (externally rotates the arm)

- teres minor (externally rotates the arm)

- subscapularis (internally rotates the arm).

These go under the handy, top-to-bottom mnemonic SITS.

The rotator cuff muscles play an important role in creating arm movement and also in ensuring glenohumeral (humerus in socket) stability, surrounding the head of the humerus like a supportive cuff – hence the name. Ideally, they allow the humerus to rotate evenly in the socket, without subluxating or dislocating. So synonymous is this muscle group with injury that I have had students tell me, 'I have a rotator cuff,' in response to an enquiry about their shoulder pain. Needless to say, they'd be in a bit of a pickle if they *didn't* have a rotator cuff! In my experience, major causes of rotator cuff issues in yoga are:

- practising weight-bearing-on-the-arms postures that the person doesn't have the strength to sustain

- overdoing the amount and frequency of weight-bearing-on-the-arms postures.

Once upon a time, I did a whole ashtanga vinyasa series every day – until my right rotator cuff, shoulder and much of the upper right side of my back went into a very painful spasm. The spasm released after a few weeks, but the shoulder has taken years to rehabilitate. Now I practise ashtanga three times a week and usually only half a series at a time. Whereas previously my shoulders were constantly overstressed, sore and irritated, at this level of endurance it has been possible for them slowly to gain strength.

Strengthening supraspinatus

Supraspinatus is engaged when we bring the arms up from the sides towards overhead. Supraspinatus initiates this action, abducting the arm from 0 to 15 degrees,[12] after which the deltoids take over, so from the point of view of rotator cuff strengthening, ask your student to focus on the beginning phase of the arm raise, lifting only a little and lowering down a few times. If your student is just sort of wafting their arms up, obviously they're going to get less out of this important movement than if they slow it right down and seek resistance.

Students can work on consciously engaging and strengthening supraspinatus whenever they bring their arms out and up, for example in *ekam* inhale (the first movement in the ashtanga vinyasa sun salutation), Warrior II, *utkatasana* (Chair Pose), Tree Pose with arms overhead and any seated forward bends in which the arms are raised up from the sides before the fold forwards. For the maximum benefit, cue your student to allow their shoulders to rise naturally as their arms go up. While we don't want them to pull their shoulders up to their ears, overusing the upper part of trapezius, drawing the shoulders forcefully down (as often cued in yoga classes) prevents the shoulder from working in an organic way and actually makes rotator cuff injury more likely.

Note that if the student brings their hands to prayer position and up, they are not using supraspinatus. That doesn't mean that the prayer position version is the 'wrong' way to bring arms up or that it isn't beneficial in other ways – just that they aren't using supraspinatus.

Strengthening infraspinatus and teres minor

These two muscles work in concert to externally rotate the humerus. My favourite way to activate them is to lie on my back with my arms bent, fingers pointing at the ceiling, upper arms in close to my sides and then rotate my arms out laterally (to the sides), so the backs of my hands are moving towards the floor. I often hold for a while and then do a few small repetitions, lifting a few inches and lowering again. Make sure the action originates in the shoulders, cueing the student to draw their rib crests firmly in and engage their abdominal muscles. Their lumbar spine shouldn't be participating in the action.

Infraspinatus and teres minor are also working to externally rotate the arm in the supraspinatus postures above. To emphasise the infra and teres action, have the student start with their arms down, palms facing into their sides (medially rotated). Before they start to bring their arms up, ask them to rotate their arms *slowly* outwards (laterally) from the shoulder – not just the elbow – so that their palms face forwards. They should feel a contraction underneath the shoulder blade, where infraspinatus originates. Remind them to maintain abdominal engagement so that their rib crests don't flare and their lower back does not flex excessively.

Once your student has some familiarity with, and strength in, the action of external rotation, they could try practising it in *gomukhasana* (Cow Face Pose). This is an *asana* that many hypermobile people initially approach with spaghetti arms – lots of flexibility, little engagement – so the task here is helping them to actively turn on infraspinatus and teres minor to create the movement. If they can access the posture easily, ask them to externally rotate…and then also create a little internal rotation: movement + counter-movement = engagement.

Strengthening subscapularis

If you're an ashtanga vinyasa practitioner, you already do many of the internal rotations that strengthen subscapularis: *parsvottanasana* (Intense Side Stretch), binding the *Marichi* postures (Sage Marichi Poses), binding *supta kurmasana* (Sleeping Turtle Pose) and so on.

Your students can strengthen subscapularis in reverse prayer position. It doesn't matter whether or not they can get into the full monty. Ask them to bring their hands down by their sides and to feel their collarbones lifting and opening from the centre outwards. Keeping this feeling of collarbone opening – i.e. not rounding their back and caving their chest, but isolating the movement in the shoulder joint, they begin the internal rotation by moving the thumb side of their arms in towards their body. Have them move the thumb side in and then out again a few times, feeling the movement coming from the shoulder, not just from the elbow, and keeping their arms active. They will feel subscapularis engaging deep in the armpit.

If they are able to go further into the posture, they can start to take their hands behind them and up their back, maintaining the movement in their shoulders and not dropping their shoulders and caving their chest. If their shoulder blades start to wing (the medial edge of the shoulder blade lifts up high off their back), they have gone too far.

Serratus anterior and the rhomboids (protract/retract)

In order for your student to be able to produce Plank and *chaturanga* and to be able to transition between them, they need to understand – in their body, not just theoretically – the actions of protraction and retraction of the scapular, or shoulder blade. Key to creating protraction and retraction are serratus anterior and the rhomboids respectively. We're going to be looking at each of these actions separately and then considering how they fit together in sun salutations.

Serratus anterior/protract

Many of our hypermobile students, even – and perhaps especially – those with quite a bit of yoga experience, are very weak in protraction. These are often the students who cave their chest towards the floor in Downdog. We've already talked a bit about the elbows in this scenario above – see 'Downdog' in the 'Micro-bending and hyperextension' section). Yoga teacher, Meagan McCrary, says:

> Having once been heavily immersed in the Anusara yoga method, I spent my first six years of *asana* practice 'melting my heart'. I took pride in my ability to soften (or rather collapse) the place between my shoulder blades – creating the deepest trench possible along my thoracic spine – when in reality I was just playing into and relying on my hypermobility. I experienced a profound shift in both my practice and understanding of *asana* when someone taught me how to protract my shoulder blades in preparation for handstand.[13]

If one or both of your student's shoulder blades wings in protraction postures – a common scenario among hypermobile yoga practitioners – it's likely that they are weak in serratus anterior. The approaches to protraction below will help your student to lift their ribcage up into their shoulder blades... and draw their shoulder blades (particularly the medial edge) down onto their back.

In protraction, serratus anterior engages to rotate the shoulder blades upwards and draw them around the ribs, away from the spine. Another way to view this latter movement is as abduction. Serratus attaches to the inside (medial) edge of the scapula, not on top but underneath, and to ribs one to nine, at the side of the ribcage – roughly where your arms rest when they're by your sides. When serratus engages, the action can be felt in the side ribs, as well as under the shoulder blades.

To help your student identify and strengthen protraction, have them come onto all fours. Make sure their knees are well padded. (Kneeling postures can be particularly uncomfortable for Ehlers-Danlos people with very elastic skin – the effect is a bit like a friction burn – so don't keep them in this position for ages.) Check that their shoulders are over their wrists, and their knees under their hips. Ask them to press firmly down into the floor through active hands as they arc their body up and away from the floor, drawing their abdominals towards their spine and lifting the lower ribs in. They are in Cat Pose (*marjaryasana*): protraction. Invite them to notice their side ribs firming and their shoulder blades drawing laterally around their ribs.

Once your student feels strong and supported in the basic Cat, they can change it up a little by raising one hand, then the other: kneading Cat.

Your student can also practise shoulder blade protraction by doing Plank against the wall. Ask them to come to parallel standing, arm's length away from the wall. Have them place their palms on the wall and press into it firmly. If they cannot press into flexed wrists, have them walk in a bit, bend their elbows to 90 degrees and press their forearms and palms into the wall. Hypermobile students will often move into spinal extension when they press into the wall, tipping their ribcage back off its axis. Cue them to maintain a neutral spine by engaging the abdominal muscles. A manual adjustment can be helpful here. Standing behind your student, place your thumbs on the back of their lower ribcage, fingers on their rib crests, and gently but firmly tilt their ribcage forwards into neutral, supporting it there if necessary to help your student feel the position.

The closer to the wall, the easier it is to protract, so start your student close in and have them gradually walk their feet out as their ability to hold steady, with their shoulder blades and ribcage well supported, increases. From the wall, they can transition to hands on a table…on a pile of blocks… and finally on the floor. Practising on stairs is a good way to make a graduated downward transition over a period of time. If you have access to the big wedge-shaped piece of gym equipment we used to call a cheeseboard at school, even better. Explain to your student that they are looking to find the action of the Cat in their Plank: pushing away from the floor and drawing their front body in towards their spine, as they abduct their shoulder blades around their ribcage.

The clue to this posture is in the name: it should look like a Plank, not a hammock. The required engagement can be very difficult for hypermobile students to feel. Manually lifting the student's ribcage in and up, away from the floor, can help them to feel the position they're aiming for. If possible, have the student do the posture side on to a mirror, so they can see how what they're feeling corresponds with the shape they're making.

If your student has wrist issues, they can work with their forearms on the floor. The effect in the shoulders and torso will be the same.

Rhomboids/retract

The rhomboids lie beneath the trapezius, attaching the medial edge of the scapular, on the underside, and to vertebrae C7 to T5. They engage to downwardly rotate and retract the shoulder blades – or hug them in towards the spine. Another way to view this latter movement is as adduction. We have already seen how our students can experience their shoulder blades protracting in Cat Pose; they can feel shoulder blade retraction in Cow Pose (*bitilasana*). Hypermobile students tend to drop passively towards the floor in this posture, so cue them to maintain abdominal engagement as they arc, feeling their shoulder blades drawing together and fighting shy of their maximum range of motion.

While protraction is a key action for Plank, *chaturanga dandasana* requires retraction. That said, if your student is an over-retractor and very flexible in this action (this is the chest-to-the-floor-in-Downdog student), cue them to find a little protraction within their retraction, so they are rounding slightly up and away from the floor, rather than sinking right down between their shoulder blades, like a slack washing line suspended from the twin poles of their humeral heads.

Just as your student can practise Plank/protraction against a wall, so they can also practise *chaturanga*/retraction. Have your student come to parallel standing with their back to the wall and their elbows bent to 90 degrees. Ask them to press the backs of their arms firmly into the wall to find retraction.

Once they can feel retraction in this movement, have them turn to face the wall, a little more than their own forearm's length away, elbows bent to 90 degrees, palms on the wall. Have them press firmly into the wall through their hands, as they attempt to lower their chest through their arms. The intention is to feel the shoulder blades retracting and the shoulders firming rather than to bring the chest flat to the wall.

Placing hands and elbows

In general, for *chaturanga*, your student's elbows need to be about the same width as their shoulders (this is optimal for the glenohumeral joint in most people) and at a right angle, not less. This means that their hands will not be under their shoulders – but exactly where they are placed will depend on the proportions of the individual student (length of humerus/length of torso).

When aligned in this way, a student (like me) with long arms and a short body may have their hands close to their waist, and elbows grazing their hips when they lower down – challenging for the weight-bearing required in this posture. However, these are proportions that you will see often among hypermobile people with a Marfan habitus. A student with short arms and a long body will have their hands by the upper part of their ribcage – much less strength required, but it may be harder for this student to maintain a lifted (not sagging) spine.

In *chaturanga dandasana*, the latissimus dorsi should engage to draw the elbows in line with the shoulders. However, it's common to see hypermobile students who are weak in *chaturanga* allowing their elbows to flare out. This positioning allows the humeral heads to drop forwards of the body and the chest to concave. Your student can start to explore hand positioning on the wall:

- In wall *chaturanga*, ask your student to stick their elbows out laterally and notice how their humeral heads fall forward and their chest collapses.

- Now have them draw their elbows in towards their sides, noticing how the humeral head is lined up with (not dropped below) their body, and their sternum feels light and lifted.

'Hug your elbows into your sides' is a common cue for *chaturanga*, and for many hypermobile students this action is helpful. However, we also need to pay attention to individual physiologies and movement patterns. For students with wide shoulders and a tapered ribcage, hugging their elbows into their sides may bring the elbows narrower than the shoulders, placing strain on both the shoulder girdle and the elbows. Even without this body type, it's possible to overuse the latissimus dorsi, drawing the elbows inside the line of the hands and shoulders – a.k.a. squeezing the elbows in too far medially. My own shoulder problems were partly created by this pattern. Given the length of my arms, I have found it helpful in my own practice to take my hands a little wider than my shoulders in *chaturanga*, so that I'm using proportionately more pectoral strength when I lower down. The aim is still to have the elbows in line with the hands, not winging out.

Protecting the biceps tendons

It's pretty common for hypermobile vinyasa practitioners to experience biceps tendonitis – strain or micro-tearing of the biceps tendons – felt as a persistent dull ache at the front of the shoulders. If you look at the alignment of these students on the wall, you will often see that their hands are under or close to their shoulders rather than by the side of their ribcage – a position that makes it difficult not to hunch the shoulders. If you have them lower down from plank to *chaturanga* on the wall, you may notice that their shoulders round in towards their chest and rise towards their ears. Have them take the optimal *chaturanga* position on the wall – upper and lower arms at a right angle to one another – and press into the wall with their hands, strongly retracting their shoulder blades and lifting their shoulders open and down their back. If this is painful, your student may need to take a break from all *chaturanga* work for a while in order to let the tendons heal.

Once your student can hold this alignment close to the wall – without pain – they can begin to step out a little, eventually progressing onto a table or pile of blocks, as in Plank. *Chaturanga* on the floor is the final progression. Don't rush to get there. There are no shortcuts in strengthening work.

Preparing for sun salutations

The basic work of Plank to *chaturanga*/protract to retract in a vinyasa-style sun salutation also happens in Cat to Cow, and these postures can always be substituted if you have a busy class with not much time to work one to one. Make sure that your hypermobile student understands how to create the actions of the shoulder blades and how to engage their ribcage and abdominal muscles. Students often think that if they go on doing difficult postures badly, they will eventually get good at them – whereas actually in most cases they just get injured. It's always better for your student to practise preparatory movements that they can produce in a biomechanically functional way than to persevere with versions of postures that are inappropriately difficult. This is especially the case when the student is hypermobile.

Sun salutations on the wall

If a hypermobile student does not yet have the muscular integrity for sun salutations on the floor, it may be beneficial for them to work with the wall. Removing most of the load of their own body weight can make it easier for them to find and turn on the required muscles, and the wall offers some additional proprioceptive feedback. This version of the sun salutation involves a bit of stepping forwards and back to adjust stance, so it's not quite as smooth as the classic version on the floor. It looks something like the following. You can make adaptations for individual needs. I've included the ashtanga vinyasa Sanskrit counts; if you're not working within the ashtanga system, you can ignore these:

1. *Samasthitihi*: student stands just far enough away from the wall that they can fold forwards without hitting their head! Invite them to feel their feet rooting down into the floor, the inner seam of their legs engaging, their front body lifting into their back body, their chest opening while at the same time their lower rib crests draw in and down, their waist lengthening, the top of their head lifting towards the ceiling. The feeling is of being drawn both downwards through the feet and upwards through the crown.

2. *Ekam* inhale: student raises their arms, giving attention to muscular engagement and creating resistance.

3. *Dve* exhale: student folds forward. If your student has very limited mobility in the posterior chain, they can fold to hip height (or a little higher), hands on the wall, bending their knees as necessary. Otherwise, your student can fold fully to the floor in the usual way, 'bobby-pin' students maintaining lots of abdominal engagement so that they do not flex only from the hip.

4. *Trini* inhale: student moves into a small spinal extension (easy, non-weight-bearing shoulder blade retraction).

5. *Chatvari* exhale: student steps the appropriate distance from the wall for their current shoulder strength and stability in Plank/*chaturanga*. This is the position where they can both protract and retract their shoulders and can lower into wall *chaturanga* without any scapula winging. From the protracted plank position, they lower into the retracted *chaturanga* position. Cue them to find the Cat movement (protract) in their Plank, and the Cow movement (retract) in their *chaturanga*.

6. *Pancha* inhale: student straightens arms, arcing up and away from the wall (spinal extension, shoulder blade retraction). This is wall Updog.

7. *Shat* exhale: student steps away from the wall for Downdog. Whereas students who are very mobile in the posterior chain might want to press their chest to the floor (retraction), cue them to lift their centre up and shift their weight forwards, more onto their hands, pushing the floor away with their hands and feeling serratus anterior engage (protraction). The limited-posterior-mobility student can do Downdog with their hands on the wall. This student will usually benefit from finding shoulder blade retraction in the posture.

8. *Sapta* inhale: student arches into a little spinal extension and shoulder blade retraction. In a regular sun salutation they would also step or jump their feet to their hands here, but if they do that when working with the wall they won't have space to fold forwards in step 9, so have them just adjust their position if necessary.

9. *Ashtau* exhale: student folds over their legs (hip flexion, spinal flexion, shoulder protraction). 'Bobby-pin' students once again shift the flexion more into their spine, by strongly engaging the abdominal muscles. The Downdog-on-the-wall student keeps their hands on the wall and finds as much hip flexion as possible, bending their knees as necessary.

10. *Nava* inhale: student brings arms up overhead as they return to standing.

11. Exhale, *samasthitihi*: student returns to starting position.

If you have a large group class, I suggest initially teaching the wall sun salutation to everyone. Even very able practitioners will be challenged by it if they are required to really work at the shoulder blade protraction/retraction element and at creating engagement throughout. For these students, you can frame the exercise as a preparatory tune-up for the full *surya namaskar*. Those students who will benefit more from working on the wall can continue to do so while you move the stronger members of your class onto the floor for the remaining sun salutations.

If your teaching situation allows it, have students transition from the wall onto a table top, pile of blocks or staircase once they are able to protract and retract solidly and consistently against the wall. Being on the floor is a huge hike in terms of strength required relative to working against the wall, and having intermediate options can be very helpful.

Transitioning to the floor

Unless they have worked their way down a staircase or handy ramp, most hypermobile students will need to begin sun salutations on the floor on their hands and knees. Hypermobile students often feel that weakness in their arms is what prevents them from lowering into *chaturanga* – and Plank/ *chaturanga* manoeuvres do, of course, take strength in the biceps and triceps – but much more significant, especially for this student group, is shoulder and core body engagement. Emphasise for your student that the most important thing is not how far down they can lower but how well they can maintain this engagement. Initially, have them lower down only 2 cm (1 inch) or so, making sure they don't flare their ribs and arch their lower back. At first, they will probably need your help to know if this is happening, and verbal and hands-on cues to bring them back into engagement. Progress slowly into a deeper knee *chaturanga*, and only when the student can consistently graze the floor with control proceed up onto feet – where you need to repeat the same process, starting by lowering down only a very little.

Rather than seeing Plank to *chaturanga* to Updog (or back to Plank) as a series of things they do with their arms, it will usually help your students to think about initiating the movements with protraction and retraction – things they do with their back and shoulders. Then there's much more integral support and centre-body strength available.

Push-ups

Plank to *chaturanga* (into Updog) is sometimes described as a yoga push-up, but in fact the pushing up part is missing from this series of actions, and students who do a lot of vinyasa without any kind of cross training are often imbalanced in this regard. At least half the vinyasa in my own practice now consists of Plank to *chaturanga* to Plank. Then, from Plank, I roll over my feet into Updog. This way I am also training the press back up from retraction (*chaturanga*) into protraction (Plank). This is hard. Even my very strong, long-term and CT-typical students have needed time to develop the strength required to push back up. From serious shoulder breakdown to being able to do this series of movements strongly and consistently on my knees, lowering right down to touch the floor, has taken me about four years. I'm currently transitioning onto my feet. I anticipate it may take a couple more years to be able to do this comfortably and consistently throughout a short (i.e. not three hours) and measured practice. These are the kinds of timescales often involved when we are working with hypermobile students. Slow and steady is better than overshooting and having to return to 'go'. Fortunately, yoga is about process rather than destination.

A word on the ribcage

My shoulder repatterning and *chaturanga* recovery was initiated by working with the Thoracic Ring Approach™ (TRA), which I mentioned in Chapter 1 (see 'Scoliosis'). Dr Linda-Joy Lee, the physiotherapist who created TRA explains that:

> Thoracic Ring Approach™ techniques employ palpation points and forces applied around the anterior, lateral and posterior ribcage to assess and treat the rings in an integrated, 3-dimensional way that assesses connections between the thoracic spine and the ribcage, as well as the connections between neighbouring thoracic rings, and between the rings and other regions of the body.[14]

TRA is a gentle method that helped me enormously with neural mapping and enabled me to create more balanced engagement in the thoracic area. The shoulder blades cannot function well on a structure that lacks the stability to hold its form and offer appropriate resistance. If your hypermobile student's ribcage is like a collapsed accordion (mine was), there's no way they are going to be able to create a strong and comfortable *chaturanga*. In this case, TRA might be a helpful intervention for them to explore. There is a list of physiotherapists trained to offer TRA here: https://ljlee.ca/connecttherapy-certified-practitioners.

Allow the shoulders to rise

> *I can't get my students to pull their shoulders down and straighten their arms in Downdog. What am I doing wrong?*

Carolyn (yoga teacher with HSD)

If your student has a ballet background or has been taught by certain old-school yoga teachers, they may have been told to pull their shoulders down in flexion – i.e. when they raise their arms relative to their torso (or their torso relative to their arms), for example in *ekam* inhale, Downdog, Warrior I, Handstands (*adho mukha vrksasana*) and *urdhva dhanurasana* (Upward-Facing Bow Pose). In fact, as Julie Gudmestad explains, 'It's actually a kinesiological law that the scapula must rotate upward for the shoulder to flex.'[15] When students try to keep their shoulders down away from their ears, they are most often forced to bend their elbows to accommodate the shoulder flexion. I see this quite often in Downdog. Now, on the other hand, we don't want our students to hike their shoulders hard up to their ears, overusing the upper trapezius. The upward rotation of the shoulder blades comes from the action of serratus anterior, and can be felt as the lift starting in the sides of the ribcage. There is a sensation of not just the shoulder, but the whole ribcage lifting, expanding and rotating upwards. Serratus strongly stabilises the shoulder blades, and when it isn't allowed to participate in shoulder flexion postures (because the shoulders are pulled down), the integrity of the shoulder joint is put at risk, potentially leading to strains, sprains and dislocations. This is so for all our students, but for those who already have genetic shoulder instability, the risk of injury is far greater.

To explore this movement, invite your student to tune into their breath. For hypermobile people with significant orthostatic issues, it will be most comfortable to do this lying or sitting. In a standing position they are likely to feel faint and find it more difficult to breathe. Any time we work with breath, the first step is to make sure that the student is able to breathe abdominally in a natural way. If they are unable to do this at present, don't go any further. Assuming that your student has an easy abdominal breath, invite them to deepen it, taking the inhalation from their belly up into their ribcage, giving particular attention to filling the side and back ribcage. If your student routinely works with *bandhas*, they can use them here.

Now have your student come to parallel standing, or to *samasthitihi/ tadasana*, or to sitting upright in a chair. Give them a few moments to re-establish their breath. Cue the student to bring their arms up, from the side, on an in-breath, as they do so feeling the ribcage expand and the shoulder blades riding on the ribcage, like a boat on a wave. Invite them to allow the movement of the ribcage and shoulder blades to carry the arms. There is a sense of a great turning, like a cartwheel.

Once your student has found this movement in standing/sitting, they can begin to explore it in:

- Warrior I, *utkatasana* and other arms-up standing postures

- seated forward bends starting with arms overhead

- weight-bearing on their arms in Downdog.

Forward bends, 'yoga bum' and hip versus lumbar flexion

Several of my hypermobile students are complaining of a sharp sitbone pain. I'm a vinyasa flow teacher, and I've heard that there can be too much forward bending in vinyasa yoga and that this can lead to problems, but I'm not sure what I should be doing differently.

Fran (yoga teacher with hEDS)

With the current fashion for sun salutations and flow forms based on vinyasa, yoga has become very heavy on forward bending. While not all hypermobile people have extreme facility in forward folds, for those who are very flexible in the lower posterior chain, this kind of practice can be a recipe for disaster – unless it is modified for posterior stability and muscular strength. What we are looking for in a forward bend is a balanced action of hips and spine. Yoga anatomist and ashtanga vinyasa teacher David Keil suggests that, 'an ideal or complete forward bend, where the chest is on the thighs, is the result of approximately two-thirds movement at the hip joint and one-third movement at the spine'.[16]

Hip bone shapes and forward folding

Just because a student has connective tissue laxity, it doesn't mean that they have the capacity to produce extreme versions of every yoga posture. No matter how accommodating the soft tissue structures, if the bone shapes do not allow for the necessary degree of articulation, the more crazy-flexible presentations of the posture will not be possible.

In forward bends, the orientation of the ilia (hip bones) makes a significant difference to how we are able to fold forwards. If the ilia angle more medially, so that the upper rim of the hip bone is pointing somewhat forwards (rather than out to the sides), the ilia will compress with the femurs before the belly comes to rest on the thighs. This person will never have a flat forward bend, no matter how much they stretch their hamstrings and loosen their posterior chain. If, on the other hand, the ilia are oriented more laterally, so that they present as pretty flat on to the front, the pelvis has the capacity to close on the femurs like a book. Assuming no other limiting factors, the person with this pelvis will be able to lie flat on their thighs.

Sideways-oriented ilia also predispose to easy squatting with feet together and flat on the floor, even where the person is not spectacularly flexible in connective tissue terms. For students with forward-orientated hips, this position will be impossible – although they may be able to squat well with their feet hip-width apart, perhaps with both legs and feet turned out laterally or with their heels on a block. This is because when their feet and legs are zipped up at the inner seam, the forward-slanting ilia bump into the femurs – just as they do in the forward bend, before the person can sit low enough to create the squat. This will be the case even if your student has connective tissue laxity.[17]

Students with limited hip flexion

It's common for CT-typical yoga beginners to arrive in class with very tight hamstrings and glutes, and little if any hip flexion. They may also appear hunched in the upper back, with round shoulders and chest collapsed in on itself. Yoga teachers are often surprised to learn that some hypermobile people also present with this pattern. This student group in mind, I'm going to start by addressing some of the ways that as teachers we can help the limited-hip-flexion person (hypermobile or not) to find their capacity for hip flexion, taking *paschimottanasana* (Straight-Legged Forward Bend) as an example – although most of these strategies can be adapted to any forward fold where the legs are straight. Since most yoga teacher training still operates on the premise that the teacher's chief task in *asana* is to increase flexibility in tight people, some of these strategies may already be familiar to you.

Why is limited hip flexion a problem?

When we are unable to flex forward from the hip (or tilt the pelvis anteriorly), we compensate by using the spine. Flexing the spine is a normal movement that a healthy human being should be able to do with no problem. Difficulties arise when flexion is overused as a movement strategy or is the only one the person knows or has access to. As Bonny Bainbridge Cohen (founder of the Body-Mind Centering® approach to somatics) observes, 'There are no wrong postures – only positions we have forgotten to come out of.'[18]

In modern Western culture, many people do overuse spinal flexion, as a result of activities like sitting at a desk, looking at a screen and driving a car. Habitually flexing in this way can lead to lower back pain and lumbar disk issues, such as herniation (when the covering of the disk frays or breaks, allowing the liquid centre of the disk to leak out). Over the course of a lifetime of living in a gravitational field, excessive spinal flexion can result in kyphosis, in which the upper back becomes abnormally rounded.

Working with too little hip flexion

The following are some approaches to try with students who have difficulty in accessing forward hip flexion (anterior pelvic tilt).

BLOCK AND TACKLE

The first recourse of most yoga teachers when encountering a student with limited hip flexion is to have them sit on the edge of a yoga block and ask them to bend their knees, so releasing the hamstrings and enabling the pelvis to tilt forwards. This is not a bad strategy – I use it with students quite a lot myself. However, there are some considerations to be aware of here for the sitbone attachments of the hamstrings – we'll be looking at these in a moment (see 'Yoga bum').

ROTATE THE PELVIS

Often when a student has become accustomed to bending forwards from the spine, they have lost the internal map for hip flexion. You can help them to rediscover it by offering hands-on guidance. In this adjustment, you use the hipbones as a pair of handles. The intention is to turn the pelvis, tipping it forwards into flexion.

1. Ask the student if they would like some help, and check that they are happy for you to use physical adjustment.

2. Kneel behind the student and place your hands around their hipbones. Your fingers will be at the front of their pelvis, around the iliac crest. Your thumbs will be at the back of their pelvis, roughly parallel with your first finger.

3. Use your hands to rotate the whole pelvis evenly forwards towards the femurs. The student will often want to bow forward into spinal flexion, so cue them to stay in neutral spine or slight spinal extension, bending their knees if necessary to achieve this. When you give this cue, your student may continue to round their back and instead lift their chin up, shortening the back of their neck. Ask them to lower their chin to neutral (not right into their chest) and help them once again to find spinal extension. The intention is to introduce (or reintroduce) them to the sensation of hips (rather than spine) flexing.

Sometimes there will be no visible movement in the pelvis as a result of the adjustment – but you are still helping the person to remap hip flexion proprioceptively. Sometimes there will be a dramatic tipping of the pelvis towards the femurs. Often, this is because the action of your hands has cued the student to relax tense hip flexors...

RELAX THE HIP FLEXORS

When a person habitually folds forwards from the spine, they frequently recruit not only the abdominal muscles to do so, but also the hip flexors. This is actually counterproductive; in order for the forward bend to happen more from the hips, the hip flexors need to relax. For some people, finding the capacity to switch off the hip flexors and allow the hips to hinge passively is a movement revelation. You can cue the student to relax their hip flexors, but initially they are unlikely to know how to do this and will need some hands-on guidance. Placing your fingers at the front of the person's hips and inviting them to soften there can be helpful – as can the adjustment above.

LIFT THE PELVIS UP AND OVER

Rather than viewing the forward bend as a hinge formed by the femurs and pelvis, invite the student to imagine the pelvis lifting up and rotating around the femoral heads, with plenty of space in the hip sockets. Thanks to David Keil for this suggestion. David explains that this subtle shift, 'can change our intention as well as the sensation that we seek in our forward bends'.[19]

FIND THE BACKBEND IN YOUR FORWARD BEND

Give the student a belt to loop around their feet. Ask them to bend their knees until they have some extension (arch) in their back and to take hold of the ends of the belt. Typically, as soon as the student takes hold of the belt, they will default to spinal flexion, with their chest caved, and will try to pull themselves down towards their legs. Pause them. Bring them back into spinal extension. Ask the student to use the belt to pull *away from* (not towards) their legs, so that they are opening their chest. Make sure their knees are bent enough that it's possible for them to create this action. Point out to the student how their pelvis is now tilting forwards – so that their belly is moving closer to their thighs (rather than their chin to their knees). At first, you will probably have to adjust the student repeatedly back into spinal extension. As they begin to develop an extension pattern over time, they can gradually begin to straighten their legs a little more.

Make sure that the student's feet stay dorsiflexed – as they would be if the student was standing on them. If the student is tight in the posterior chain, their feet may start to turn out when they fold forwards. You can help them to maintain the foot position by giving them a block. They place the soles of their feet on the block, loop the belt around it and hold the ends of the belt with their hands. As they fold forwards, they aim to keep their feet in contact with the block and parallel to one another.

SPREAD THE SITBONES AND LIFT THE TAIL

Students with limited capacity to forward fold are sometimes gripping their buttocks or tight in the pelvic floor (see 'Pelvic floor dysfunction' in Chapter 4). This can be a long-standing response to fear, so when you work with this pattern, be slow and sensitive, and refer to a trauma specialist if it becomes clear that the student is dealing with something more than a movement habit. Invite the student to spread their buttocks laterally (out to the sides). They can do this with their hands to get the feeling. As they fold forwards, cue them to keep the buttocks soft and spreading away from each other and to imagine their tail lifting up and lengthening towards the sky. This can create a feeling of more space in the pelvis and help to initiate the anterior tilt.

Students with excessive hip flexion

Whereas the majority of beginning CT-typical students (and some hypermobile students) will arrive in a yoga class with limited hip flexion, more typically hypermobile students will present with excessive hip flexion. The techniques described above – those which are most usually offered in a yoga class – are going to be exactly what these people don't need, and are calculated to put their biomechanics even more out of whack, by further mobilising a lower posterior chain that is already weak and lax.

The person with excessive hip flexion will generally approach a forward bend with their spine in extension and abdominals disengaged – so that they are backbending into their forward bend. Yoga therapist Doug Keller calls this pattern, 'the swan dive'.[20] As we saw above, this might be a useful strategy for a student who approaches a forward bend in spinal flexion, but the excessive-hip-flexion student is already overdoing spinal extension.

Why is excessive hip flexion a problem?

Like flexing the spine, extending it is a normal movement and is not in itself problematic. However, a number of problems may arise when spinal flexion is overused as a movement strategy over a long period of time.

SPONDYLOLISTHESIS

Doug Keller explains that when a person folds forwards in excessive spinal extension, the multifidi (tiny intervertebral muscles whose role is to stabilise the spine) are placed in a position where they are very limited in their capacity to function, leaving the spine reliant predominantly on ligaments for stabilisation. This is definitely not an optimal situation for anyone, but if the person is hypermobile, and their ligaments are lax, they are at high risk of injury. Doug explains that:

> It's especially down around the sacrum and L5 that...the multifidi...are much thicker and stronger, and they have a specific job to do there. Because of the tilt of these vertebrae and the sacrum, there's much more of a tendency for the vertebrae to slide forward... This is called spondylolisthesis, which is a condition that causes narrowing or pinching of the spinal cord. It can even fracture the processes of the vertebrae at the back and can cause a significant amount of back pain.[21]

As we saw in Chapter 1, spondylolisthesis is more common among hypermobile people (see 'Spondylolisthesis'). For more on working with this condition in a yoga class, see 'Spondylolisthesis' in Chapter 4.

'YOGA BUM'

> *It felt as if my sitting bones had become sharp. Just sitting was painful, and folding forward (which I'd always been able to do really easily) was excruciating.*
>
> Casey (yoga practitioner with HSD)

'Yoga bum' (or 'yoga butt' as it's known on the other side of the pond), manifests as intense pain in the sitbones that is made worse by sitting (especially for long periods), bending forwards and sometimes also by walking. 'Yoga bum' is obviously not a technical term, and there are a few possible medical causes marching under this general banner:

- Proximal hamstring tendinopathy. The proximal hamstring tendon attaches to the ischial tuberosity (sitbone). If the tendon is repeatedly pulled away from the sitbone – as in forward bending, *hanumanasana* (Front Splits), *parsvottanasana* and the like – it becomes sore and inflamed, and may sustain micro-tears. The same situation can result if a student suddenly increases the amount of forward-bending practices they do (especially if they are erratic and tend to lapse and then overdo), or from general overuse and overloading, which does not allow time for rest and routine repair. Physiotherapist Kara Murphy explains:

> Research shows tendons take 24 hours to adapt to a load. Without sufficient recovery time, the tendon structure can become impaired.[22]

- Gluteal tendinopathy. The same situation can occur with the tendons of the gluteus muscles.

- Tightness and spasming of the coccygeus. The coccygeus is a pelvic floor muscle that attaches to the coccyx together with the very lowest part of the sacrum, and to the ischium. While this syndrome might better be categorised as a pelvic floor dysfunction (see 'Pelvic floor dysfunction' in Chapter 4), it does cause sitbone pain on folding forwards and can play into the tendinopathies above.

The primary series of ashtanga vinyasa, with its many forward bends, is notorious for causing yoga bum. This is one reason why, at the half-primary-series point, and sometimes even before, I now tend to teach my ashtanga students some modified second-series backbends, rather than adding in yet more primary series forward folds.

Aside from making sure the student is not engaging in an excessive amount of forward bending, the main way to work with 'yoga bum' is to help the student to change their flexion pattern. We're going to talk about that now.

Working with too much hip flexion

Students who hinge at the hip with excessive facility are generally underusing abdominals and gluteals, and the main strategies for helping them towards more balance are geared towards engagement and strengthening here.

ANTERIORLY ROTATE THE PELVIS

Whereas when we adjust a spinal-flexion student in a forward bend, we want to use our hands to help them to tip their pelvis anteriorly, with a spinal-extension student, we want to use our hands to create resistance against forward tilt, so compelling the lumbar spine to flex a little, which in turn will switch on muscular support in the abdomen.

Place your hands in the same position as you did for the 'Rotate the pelvis' adjustment in the 'Working with too little hip flexion' section above. This time, rather than tipping the pelvis forward, you're going to pull the hip points at the front of the pelvis back towards you (posterior tilt). Pelvic hyper-flexers have often been pancaked onto their legs one time too many by ill-informed teachers, so it may be helpful to explain to the student that you are going to draw them back and away from their edge (not push them further into it). Students often express a sense of relief after receiving this adjustment – not only because they haven't been pancaked, but also because they experience a sense of release in the lumbar area.

LUMBAR FLEXION FIRST

As a lifelong bobby pin who has experienced a lot of sitbone tendinitis in my time, I've found this principle a game changer in my own practice. Think about what your very tight students look like when they forward bend. You're going to cue your hyperextension student to embody something of that pattern. Ask the person to keep their pelvis upright and imagine that their lower back is pressing backwards, while they draw their belly back towards their spine. Then, as they keep this engagement, cue them to start pitching forwards from the ribcage, now allowing some flexion also to happen from the hip. Your student will probably feel as if they are rounding their back – they are slightly, and this is A Good Thing (for this particular student). To the casual observer, though, their forward bend may not look all that different from before.

It will take a while for most students to integrate this new flexion-first pattern. However, they may immediately notice a slight lessening in any current sitbone pain. This is because the pull on the hamstrings and gluteal tendons has been reduced. Over time, practising in this way (along with active strengthening in practices outside yoga) will allow the hamstring and/or gluteal tendons to calm down and repair.

FIRM THE HIP POINTS

This is a suggestion I've adopted from Doug Keller. What I like about it is the delicious sense of containment it provides in the pelvis. Your hypermobile students, on the whole, are going to love feeling contained.

Have your student place their fingers around the front of their hips. They will be resting on the anterior superior iliac spine (ASIS) – or ridge around the front of each ilium. The most prominent place on the ASIS is the front hip point. Now have them move their thumbs around their sacrum to find the most prominent points on the posterior superior iliac spine (PSIS). These are two bony protuberances, two or three finger-widths away from their spine and are usually easy to locate. Once the student is familiar with all four hip points, ask them to imagine the hip points at the front drawing towards one another. This will firm the lower abdomen. At the same time, ask them to imagine the hip points at the back also drawing towards one another. This will stabilise the sacrum. Doug notes:

> This is a different action from tucking the pelvis or scooping the tail bone, and it's actually more effective for working with the spine than trying to scoop the tail bone, which often runs into a conflict between the sacrum and the lumbar spine. This is much more integrative.[23]

I can vouch for the very different feeling and intention of the hip point action from tucking or scooping. Please don't ask your student to do either of those.

Doug adds a further action, which he describes as, 'drawing the pit of the abdomen in and up…just above the pubic bone, like you're zipping up your pants'.[24] In other words, *uddiyana bandha* – more about this later (see 'Working with *bandha*').

STRENGTHENING THE GLUTEALS

Consider this story from well-known online fitness coach (and hypermobile person), Caroline Jordan:

> As a dancer, the yoga studio always felt like home to me. It was a place I found community, got in touch with my body, relaxed my mind, and pressed the re-set button… I would take class one to three times per week and often include postures in the morning and evening. Forward folds and hip openers were my favourite… But after several years of yoga-euphoria, something changed. First my practice plateaued. And then it started to hurt. I started to have hip pain and contributed [sic] it to tight muscles from my love of running, spinning, and group fitness. So I stopped all other activity and did only yoga thinking it would help. Yoga is the 'safe' form of exercise right? The opposite happened. It got worse.[25]

When Caroline sought professional help, she learnt that her lower posterior chain was weak and loose; in other words, by focusing on forward bending she had overstretched her hamstrings and glutes at the expense of strengthening them – a common syndrome among dancers, yoga practitioners and hypermobile people.

There are three pairs of gluteals. The largest is the outer layer, gluteus maximus, which extends the hip (lengthens the front of the hip and carries the leg out and up behind) and laterally (externally) rotates the hip. In the middle is gluteus medius, which stabilises the hip in weight-bearing by abducting the thigh. When your student transfers their weight into their standing leg for a balance, they are recruiting gluteus medius. This same action happens repeatedly as we transfer our weight in walking. The deepest gluteal is gluteus minimus, which abducts, medially (internally) rotates and flexes the hip – through the latter two actions opposing and balancing gluteus medius. When a student habitually hyperextends their knees and swings their pelvis forward (as described in 'Distortions in the movement chain' above), the glutes, which should be providing support in standing, are not able to fire properly, so students with this standing pattern are particularly likely to be entering your class with a longstanding weakness in this area.

Where we mostly recruit the gluteals in a yoga practice is in backbends (geared for strength rather than super-extensibility), so as a teacher you want to make sure you're offering your hypermobile students plenty of low Bridges (*setu bandha sarvangasana*) and Locusts (*shalabhasana*). Other helpful glute-building postures are *utkatasana*, Warriors II and III, and *utkata konasana*. However, we also want to help our students to create some resistance in their glutes when they are actually in a forward bend.

- Ask your student to sit in *dandasana*. Have them internally rotate their legs slightly (so that their knees roll a little towards their midline) and fold forwards. In this position the glutes are turned off and offer no resistance to pelvic flexion (the forward bend).

- Now ask your student to slightly externally rotate their legs – but at the same time resist by internally rotating, so that their legs actually remain in a neutral position. The student's legs will be fully active at this point. Ask them to fold forwards. They won't be able to fold as far into the forward bend as they may be used to – which is what we want for this student group. We're looking for more engagement and less flopping and diving.

It's important to be clear with our students that practising *only* yoga will lead them further out of kilter in terms of the flexibility/strength + stability equation in the posterior chain. As Caroline Jordan says:

> While yoga involves some body weight strength postures, it is not enough to balance out the muscles. To build real-world strength, you have to use real-world resistance.[26]

Squats, dead lifts and kettle bells figured largely in Caroline's recovery. Three years on, she is back on her yoga mat, doing essentially the same yoga practice, but in a radically different way. And she hasn't dropped the strength work. If you're hypermobile, this kind of regular conditioning needs to be a habit for life.

BENDING THE KNEES

Whereas bending the knees is often a useful strategy for students who otherwise are unable to flex at the hip with their legs extended – it's not always the most helpful approach for students who are experiencing sitbone pain as a result of excessive capacity for hip flexion. David Keil explains:

> Because the hamstrings are two-joint muscles, changing the position at one of the two joints (the hip or the knee) changes the end of the muscles that will receive more force from the actual stretch. When you bend your knees in a forward bend, you add more force to the end of the hamstrings that connects to the sitbones.[27]

Of course, we don't want our hypermobile students to lock back their knees (so overstretching and weakening the hamstrings), but keeping knees in a neutral engaged position and working for strength and stability in the ways suggested above may be the most beneficial way to practise in the long term.

BEND AND STRETCH

However, there's more than one way to shuck peas. In my own practice, I've found it helpful to enter standing forward bends with a little bit of bend and stretch into straight legs. This feels to me more juicy and less aggressive to the hamstring tendons and other myofascia in the sitbone area than moving straight into full knee extension. Some of my hypermobile students have liked this approach in *prasarita padottanasana* (Wide-Legged Forward Bend) too. When working with all students, and especially hypermobile ones, there's always an element of trying on different approaches to see. Check in with your student to find out what worked and what didn't, help them to join up any dots where a pattern has now become apparent and if they need permission to drop unhelpful strategies, offer it.

Hip stabilisation, backbends and finding the glutes

I've been trying for literally years to strengthen weak but tight glutes.

Paul (yoga teacher with HSD)

Many hypermobile yoga practitioners I talk to report finding it very difficult to feel and activate their gluteal muscles. Speaking for myself, I know that certain areas of my glutes fire really well…and other areas are less easy to connect with, weak and hypertonic – a difficult combination to strengthen. A painful dislocation/subluxation of my right femur last year provided a challenging but very useful glute activation intensive, and I have now learnt to plug the head of my femur into the socket, using what feel to me like 'deep glutes' – more on this later (see 'Backbends').

According to Shirley Sahrmann, hip instability may be part of a movement impairment syndrome in which the tensor fascia lata (TFL), another important hip stabiliser, takes over the work of gluteus medius.[28] The person with this syndrome will experience tightness in the lateral hip and down the lateral side of the leg, where TFL morphs into the iliotibial (IT) band. Why might many hypermobile people have a dominant TFL? The actions of gluteus medius are hip extension, abduction and external rotation (think of a ballet dancer in *attitude en arrière*). The actions of TFL are hip flexion, abduction and internal rotation. If you try these movements on, you may end up sitting in a wide-legged *virasana* (Hero Pose). As we will see in Chapter 6, many hypermobile children habitually sit in a feet-turned-out version of this posture known as the W-position: TFL activated, gluteus medius mostly switched off. Remember the hypermobile students with the knock-knees and pronating feet? Here they are again (if you don't remember them, see 'Knock-knees' above).

As we have seen, students with back-of-the-knee hyperextensions may also have hypotonic glutes, sometimes observable as a flattening of these usually convex muscles. Doug Keller explains that when the knees are locked back and the weight is shifted onto the heels in standing, the hamstrings tighten and it's difficult to recruit the gluteals[29] – try this standing posture and see. Now roll your weight forwards over your mid-foot and notice how the glutes start to switch on.

To help your student feel their glutes firing and stabilising, have them come to parallel standing.

1. Ask your student to cup their buttock cheeks with their hands and shift their knees into a neutral position, so that they are neither rolling in nor locked back, and their weight is over the mid-foot. They should feel some initial firming in the glutes.

2. Either continuing with their hands on their buttocks if the feedback is useful or bringing their arms down by their sides, cue them to feel their hips drawing in towards the midline of their body.

3. Continuing to draw in their outer hips in this way, ask them to feel as if they are lifting up out of their hips. As they do this, they should feel the transverse abdominis – the deep *mula/uddiyana bandha* muscles just above the pubic bone – firm and engage (for more on these, see 'Working with *bandha*' below). There's a sense here, too, of the sides drawing in towards the middle.

In my experience, when hypermobile students 'can't feel' an action, they are sometimes expecting a big red arrow and an unmistakable sensation. In reality, the physical feelings that go with new engagements are often very subtle, especially at first when the muscles required are still relatively weak. As the muscles begin to strengthen, the sensations of engagement also become more obvious. For now, invite your student to trust whatever sensation they *can* feel, no matter how small, uncertain or intermittent. Developing proprioception is always a bit like groping in the dark at the beginning, but if we can tolerate being unsure for a while, gradually some light begins to dawn.

Backbends

I have a very hypermobile student with an incredibly mobile spine. Is it OK for her to be going into so much spinal extension? She isn't feeling any discomfort. Should she be using her glutes for support? Or is that harmful?

Jez (CT-typical yoga teacher)

Preternatural spinal extension is sometimes seen as synonymous with joint hypermobility. It's not unusual for students who fully meet the criteria for a hypermobility syndrome to declare that they cannot be hypermobile because they're 'not good at backbends'. In fact, just as not all hypermobile people can easily fold like a bobby pin, not all of us have the spine of a cobra. Connective tissue flexibility is just one factor that plays into whether a person has facility in spinal extension, along with age, conditioning, bone shapes and so on.

You might think that the more extreme the backbend the hypermobile person can produce, the more likely they are to experience pain and injury; however, I have not personally noticed a correlation here.[30] What does seem to be important is the degree of strength and control the person has in the movements required, as well as their capacity to discern, and willingness to respect, their own edge.

The great gluteal controversy

If you think yoga teachers are a happy band of love-bunnies, you probably haven't introduced the topic of gluteal engagement in backbends into a yoga teacher gathering yet. Nothing is more likely to factionalise and divide. As Roger Cole explains:

> Some teachers are 'Grippers', who urge their students to contract the gluteals as hard as they can; others are 'Soft Pedalers', who try to sell their students the idea that they must always keep the muscles completely relaxed; and still others are 'Peacemakers', who try to find some compromise between the two.[31]

The glute we are mainly talking about here is gluteus maximus, which, as we have seen, has roles in both hip extension and lateral (or external) rotation of the femur. Extension is what happens to the hip in postures such as *kapotasana* (Pigeon Pose) and *urdhva dhanurasana* (Upward-Facing Bow Pose), in which the fronts of the hips lengthen and stretch. We've already discussed external rotation of the femur. When the knees are turned out at ten to two, the legs are externally rotated. While we do want our students to extend their hips in backbends, we don't want them to externally rotate their femurs. Why? Because muscles don't activate in isolation. When glute max is turned on, so are the deeper external rotators, such as piriformis. When these rotators engage, and the feet and legs turn out, the arch in the lower back increases, causing instability both in the lumbar region and at the front of the hip socket. Not great for anybody, but particularly undesirable for our hypermobile students.

When it comes to backbends, then, in which we want to extend the hips and at the same time internally rotate the femurs so that the legs stay parallel to one another, the extension + lateral rotation combination of gluteal actions is seen by some as presenting a dilemma. In terms of hypermobility teaching, in which we are always looking to switch on both the primary action and the counter-action (or co-contract), it seems to me to present a perfect opportunity for strengthening and engagement.

It's mostly the upper portion of the glutes, above the sitbones and down the sides of the buttock cheeks (along the knicker line), that externally rotates the femurs, whereas the lower portion, underneath the sitbones abducts the hips. If your student focuses on engaging in this 'under-sits' area, they will not only be preferentially creating hip abduction with gluteus max, but will also be engaging the hamstrings to assist in the backbend. I think about this action as firming the head of the thigh bone up into the socket. If your student is a bobby-pin forward bender, this action will also help to strengthen loose, weak glutes and hamstrings and make them more resilient against injury. The opposing action comes from the adductors, the inside thighs, which do what it says on the tin, adduct the femurs, or draw them in towards one another. The adductors also prevent the legs from rolling out laterally.

Students who are very turned out, or laterally rotated, at the hip (either naturally, due to the shapes of the bones in their hips, or because of ballet training, or both), will need to work particularly hard on the adduction part of this pair of actions. Placing a block between their feet in supine backbends, such as *setu bandha* and *urdhva dhanurasana* can help to train the foot position. The student's task is to keep the entire inside edge of their foot against the block throughout the backbend. For most people, I place the block portrait in *setu bandha* and landscape in *urdhva D*. Explain to the student that the action they are seeking actually comes not from their feet but from their inside thighs and that they are aiming to line up knee, heel and toes with the hip (or as close to as possible). Your student can also use a light-weight brick, landscape, between their knees. Knock-kneed, or internally rotated, students will be able to put more energy into gluteal engagement, but these students, too, will benefit from working also for inner thigh adduction.

According to Roger Cole:

> Soft Pedalers are quick to point out that contracting the glutes can make it impossible for highly flexible yogis to move completely into the deepest backbends. For a maximal backbend, the pelvis has to tilt backward. When you tighten your gluteus maximus, it tilts your pelvis back at first, but when it reaches full contraction, it forms a hard lump of muscle that sits between the back of the pelvis and the back of the thigh. In extreme backbends, this lump physically blocks the pelvis from tilting back any farther, so a flexible practitioner can't extend to his or her full capacity.[32]

If you've read this far, you won't be surprised to know that in my view having stabilising muscles engaged and offering support is much more important for highly flexible yogis than being able to extend to their full capacity. Indeed, the intention of stabilisation is that it allows us to expand into the full range of our functional mobility while preventing us from jamming bones into extreme ranges of motion.

Updog, Cobra and sun salutations

Updog is a basic component of the vinyasa-style sun salutation. In this posture, the palms and tops of feet are the weight-bearers; the arms are straight; the hips are off the floor; and the entire body from the feet to the top of the head forms a long, upward-swooping arc. In the more curly, curvy and mobility-orientated Sivananda sun salutation, the Updog slot is filled by *bhujangasana* (Cobra Pose), a position in which the arms are bent and the pubic bone is on the floor, creating a shorter, tauter spinal extension, in which the thrust of the arch is angled more into the lower back. While it is possible – and desirable – to create Cobra in a more rather than less engaged way, on the whole this posture is more about flexibility and less about strength than Updog. I therefore do not suggest it as a vinyasa modification for beginning hypermobile students. Bear in mind that in a vinyasa practice, the *chaturanga*–Updog–Downdog sequence recurs frequently as a kind of reset between postures. The emphasis here therefore needs to be on stabilisation and neutral alignment. (In the Sivananda system, the sun salutation happens a few times near the beginning of the practice and is not repeated again.) Many beginning students confuse Updog with Cobra, and it's worth taking time to point out that these are two distinct postures and explain the main differences.

In my experience, when a hypermobile student is having difficulty producing Updog within a sun salutation, they are most often overwhelmed by all the different movements and have no idea what they're actually meant to be doing, so the first line of action is to extrapolate the posture and explain the actions. This can be offered as a teaching focus for a whole class. Most people will appreciate knowing how to squeeze more juice out of the pose. The following are some things to look at.

- Hypermobile practitioners frequently roll out their arms laterally, pressing the eyes of their elbows forwards in Updog. This arm alignment generates a lot of shoulder blade retraction, and many students equate this shoulder-blades-retracting sensation with creating a 'deep' backbend. Try cueing your student to find some medial arm rotation within the lateral, so that they keep the eyes of their elbows facing one another and their arms and shoulders engaged as they press down through their hands and lift their chest up and forwards through their arms. Invite them to notice where the work is now happening in their back. In my experience, this approach creates a stronger, stabler and more balanced backbend.

- For most students, straightening the arms will lift the pubic bone off the floor. Explain to the student that this is an action they are looking for. Invite them to firm the area just under their sitbones, drawing the femurs strongly into the sockets. This will engage gluteus maximus in stabilising and activate the upper hamstrings. As they do this, invite them to notice the fronts of their hips lengthening.

- If your student's Updog looks collapsed, clarify for them that the intention of this posture is to create a long, stable arc, with the shoulders pressing down through the arms into the hands, the hands and tops of the feet pressing firmly into the floor, the belly drawing strongly in towards the spine and the pubic bone lifting up clear away.

- If your student's heels are collapsing out laterally, cue them to draw their heels in. You may have to adjust their feet manually so that they can feel this position. You may also see the heels in and the toes shifted out laterally. Cue the student to draw the forefoot in, in line with the heel. They are looking to make an unbroken line from each sitbone down through the knee, ankle, heel and toes.

- Cue your student to press down through the tops of their toes and notice how this lifts them up and away from the floor, and spreads the extension out of the lower back and more evenly through the spine.

Students who cannot yet fully manage the logistics of the sun salutation may end up in Updog with their toes tucked under. This foot position is not ideal because it tends to shift the extension more into the lumbar spine. If your student cannot roll over their feet, have them lower to the floor and untuck their toes before lifting into Updog. Sometimes the issue is not strength but has to do with the way the student is organising themselves longwise in terms of arm position relative to torso and to feet. How they can most optimally place themselves will depend on their individual proportions – length of legs, arms and torso – and is something you will need to explore with each student individually.

Practising Updog with a brick under each hand may enable beginning students with short arms to access the lift off the floor and opening in the shoulders and chest.

Backbends for strength

We tend to think of backbends in yoga as mobilisers; however, when practised small, low and with repetitions, they can also be gold-standard strengtheners of the posterior chain – crucial for many of our hypermobile students. The following are a few suggestions for gearing backbend practice to creating strength and stability. For maximum effect, be sure to include both repetitions (for strengthening fast-twitch muscle fibres) and isometric holds (for strengthening slow-twitch – endurance – muscle fibres). There are many more variations on this theme. Feel free to explore, adapt, adopt and invent.

SHALABHASANA

It's not possible to get a lot of range of motion out of *shalabhasana*, which makes it a great place to start hypermobile students who are stuck on ratcheting themselves up into extreme spinal extensions without attention to muscular support. Cue your student to:

- engage strongly just underneath the sitbones, firming the femurs into the sockets, to activate gluteus maximus and the hamstrings, particularly around the attachment

- draw their inside thighs in towards each other to activate the adductors (and oppose the externally rotating action of gluteus maximus)

- lengthen the fronts of their hips

- retract their shoulder blades and open their chest.

Your student's feet may be barely 2 cm (1 inch) off the floor. This is fine. What we're looking for here is not height but engagement.

You can change it up by having the student do the following things:

- Extend their arms out in front of them on the floor. Lift their right arm and left leg and hold...then their left arm and right leg and hold. Repeat a few times. This movement can develop into 'swimming', in which they alternate both movements rapidly, like a cartoon swimmer.

- Extend their arms out in front of them on the floor, lift up the arms, head and shoulders (like Superman), then lower down...and lift up their legs. They can do repetitions of each individual movement and/ or alternate both. As a grand finale, have them lift up arms, shoulders and legs all at the same time. Here, too, they can do a few lower-and-lift repetitions.

- Repeat the above with the hands behind the head...and the arms extended out to the sides.

- With the arms bent and forehead resting on their hands, lift and lower their legs several times. They can do single legs and/or both together.

- With the arms bent and forehead resting on their hands, bend their right leg into a 90-degree angle, slowly and with control…and slowly and with control lower it to the floor again. Repeat several times and then do the left side. This exercise strengthens the hamstrings. Your student will get the most out of it if they keep their working foot flexed.

HALF-COBRA

Your student can do Half-Cobra Pose (*ardha bhujangasana*) on their forearms or on their palms with their elbows bent and raised a little off the floor. If they choose the latter variation, make sure they don't lift up too high. Remind them that in this exercise they are working for strength, not extension. Have them lift their head, shoulders and chest and then lower down flat to the floor several times. You can also introduce a brief hold at the top of the posture. Cue your student to engage the deep glutes and hamstrings and to press down through their forearms or palms.

You can make the posture harder by having your student lift up into the forearms-down version of Half-Cobra and then raise their right arm off the floor, hold for a few moments, replace and raise the left arm. This is surprisingly challenging.

BRIDGE

In this version of Bridge, the intention is not to lift high up away from the floor, opening the chest and raising the hips – and, indeed, this will be impossible in some of the variations – but to create a lower, stronger structure.

Have your student set up in the usual way. Cue them to place their upper arms on the floor and bend their elbows, so that their fingertips are facing the ceiling (robot arms). They initiate the posture by squeezing their upper arms into their sides and at the same time pressing them strongly down into the floor…while also pressing strongly down into the floor through their feet. As they lift up, cue them to keep all these actions switched on, making sure that:

- their elbows don't drift outwards

- their knees stay in line with their hips

- their feet stay parallel

- the balls of their feet stay fully engaged with the floor.

Have your student lift and lower several times, adding a hold at the apex of the Bridge if you like, always emphasising that the focus here is on stability and engagement rather than height. You can change it up by having the student lift into the Bridge position and:

- raise their right leg up to the ceiling and then down to the floor. Alternate legs, or repeat a few times and then change to the left leg

- raise their right leg up to the ceiling. Keeping the leg raised, lower the bridge down to the floor and then lift back up again. Alternate legs, or repeat a few times and then change to the left. You can also introduce small pulses, up and down, in the Bridge, with the leg raised.

Remember not to overtax your hypermobile student. They will get more benefit out of doing a basic version of one of these variations twice with control than from floundering through several with some muscle groups switched off and others compensating.

Creating a symmetrical arc

Hypermobile students who have trained for flexibility, for example in contortion, may have been taught to lever into the junction between the lumbar and thoracic spine (or any other part of their spine where they naturally 'hinge'). In *urdhva dhanurasana* for example, they may shunt their body weight from their feet and hips hard into the most flexible spot. Not surprisingly, the long-term result is often pain – accompanied by an understandable reluctance to do backbends any more. These students may have no idea that there are other more helpful ways to approach spinal extension – or that yoga is not about creating infinitely more flexibility in places that are already overstretched, but may be about creating strength, structure and a sense of greater security in the body.

Generally, the intention with students who approach backbends in this way is to create a more even distribution of force, with a longer and more symmetrical arc. I also want to make sure that they are fully stabilised, so I might cue them to engage their shoulders and hips (in any of the ways I have already described), perhaps walking their feet out (rather than in), so that they can focus on strength. It may be useful to help your student shift the apex of their backbend so that it is no longer at the most flexible point in their spine but at a tighter spot. You can do this by having them rock their weight from hands to hips into different parts of their spine. Your student can also practise 'push-ups' in this position, lowering their head to the floor, slowly and with control, and lifting back up again into the Bow, slowly and with control – and without walking their feet in. This isn't about creating more flexibility.

Triangles, side angles, twists: preserving sacroiliac joint stability

I have a hypermobile student who says she needs to mobilise her SI joint. Am I right to think this is not a good idea. She sometimes experiences a clunk in the joint. That doesn't sound like a good thing to me.

Jayne (yoga teacher with hEDS)

The science of anatomy is far less cut and dried than some yoga teacher trainings would lead us to believe, and few anatomical structures have been the subject of more controversy over the years than the sacroiliac (SI) joint. David Keil points out that, 'Most of what we *know* about the SI joint, and therefore, most of the discussion in the yoga community about the SI joint (what to do with it, and what not to do with it) is not based on data that has measured what the SI joint does *in yoga postures*'.[33] The information in this section is based on what I, my hypermobile students and other senior yoga teachers who are well grounded in anatomy and physiology have found to be true and useful in personal practice and teaching. As with any yoga teaching you are offered, I suggest that you try it out on yourself and with your students, and adopt and adapt as necessary. In this section, I'm going to be discussing how we can present some frequently practised – and potentially risky – postures in such a way as to avoid creating SI joint dysfunction among vulnerable hypermobile students. In Chapter 4, we'll be considering how to work with students who are already experiencing SI joint subluxation and/ or pain (see 'Sacroiliac joint problems').

Given that hypermobile people experience global joint laxity, it will be no surprise to learn that instability of the SI joint is particularly common among this group. The female pelvis is inherently less stable than the male version, being shorter and broader and providing less contact between the sacrum and the ilia, and therefore more vulnerable to dysfunction – and pregnancy and childbirth, during which sacral movement naturally increases, can cause further destabilisation in the long term. Skeletal asymmetry, such as leg length difference, may exert further force on the SI joints, acting to pull them out of true.

The SI joint is made up of the sacrum and the two ilia, which are bound together by multiple, strong, dense ligaments. Its major function is to provide stability on standing. Physiotherapist and Iyengar yoga teacher, Judith Lasater, describes this mechanism: 'The sacrum bone wedges down into the pelvic joints due to the weight of the trunk—similar to the way a padlock closes.'[34]

Nevertheless, the SI joints do allow for a small amount of movement, enabling the sacrum to nod forwards (nutation) and backwards (counternutation) on a transverse axis. This movement is not to be confused with the tilting of the whole pelvis forwards (anterior) and backwards (posterior); nutation and counternutation involve only the sacrum, in isolation within the pelvis. This sacral motion is essential to ease in sitting, walking and moving between sitting and standing.

Donna Farhi explains that the spine (and head) and the two femurs (and lower legs) act as strong levers on the SI joint.[35] This leverage can be used to create strength (through small repetitions of movement, isometric work and so on), or – less helpfully – to pry the joint apart (through long, passive, loaded stretches). As Donna explains, 'Many yoga postures cantilever the spine off the pelvis.'[36] Where a student is CT-typical and has good core body strength, it's possible that this movement will not interfere with healthy SI joint function; where they are hypermobile, weak and very focused on extensibility, however, it can create serious instability.

So which postures may potentially present risks to the SI joint and how can we approach them in a way that best protects integrity here?

Utthita trikonasana

In *utthita trikonasana*, the spine acts as a lever on the SI joint, with the head adding weight at the extreme end, where leverage is most powerful. Does this mean that *utthita trikonasana* is dangerous and should be excised from our classroom repertoire? No, of course not, but care needs to be taken over how your students – especially the hypermobile ones – set up and practise this posture.

As I mentioned above, I generally suggest that students step out one of their own leg lengths for *utthita trikonasana*. This stride can then be modified a little according to individual anatomy. Hypermobile students sometimes step out very long because they 'can't feel the stretch' in a more useable stride. In this case, I suggest you reframe the intention of the posture for them, explaining that the concern here is with muscular engagement rather than stretching. On the other hand, students who are aware of their own hypermobility, and seeking to find a sense of control, sometimes step their feet in…and in…ending up with a stance that is so short it doesn't actually allow room for the posture. In this case, I suggest you gently ease the student out into a more feasible stride.

As a starting point, have your student line their front heel up with their back instep. This, again, is a little modifiable for individual needs. Have them turn their back-foot toes in a little, so that their femur is slightly internally rotated – this may be different from the foot position they have previously learnt. The toes of their front foot are pointing directly forwards. Check that their knees are neither locking back nor rolling in – see 'Utthita trikonasana' in the 'Micro-bending and hyperextension' section above.

Rather than attempting to stack one ilium above the other, as they may have been taught in other classes, your student is going to allow their upper ilium to pitch slightly forward of the lower one. The slight internal rotation of the back thigh bone will facilitate this. When they make this movement, most hypermobile students will also arch their spine into extension. Cue them instead to draw their front body strongly into their back body, especially right below the ribcage, to create mild spinal flexion, abdominal muscles engaged. This action sometimes causes the student to collapse their upper shoulder towards the floor. If so, adjust or cue them to open their chest, lifting the top shoulder up and back – without losing the abdominal engagement or shifting the foundation of legs and hips. Check that their underneath hip, at the iliofemoral joint (top of the leg), hasn't swung back behind its ankle. If it has, adjust it forwards so that there is a plumb line from ankle to hip socket. This placement will be unfamiliar to many students, and you may have to help them repeatedly back into it.

Some of the teachers I mentor have been taught that in *utthita trikonasana* there should be no weight in the front hand. This may be OK if the student is strong and super-solid in the SI joints, but for most practitioners, and especially hypermobile ones, this is a rather risky proposition in the long term. I suggest you have your student hold onto their leg with their front hand. This provides support for the far end of the spinal lever, so that the spine is not hanging from the pelvis, and so mitigates its SI-joint-levering effect. Some students will be holding their foot/ankle, others their shin. The 'correct' hand placement is the one that enables them to maintain the posture with structure and integrity; further down the leg is not better. They can now press into their hand to create lift away from the floor, feeling their lower shoulder stabilise and continuing to engage core support. If your student tends to lock back their knees, make sure that they are not using their hand to push the front knee into hyperextension but are resisting through the leg – see 'Utthita trikonasana' in the 'Micro-bending and hyperextension' section above.

Ultimately, it's the individual student's skeleton (shape of the head of the femur and of the acetabulum) that determines how close they can bring their side torso down towards their leg (and hand towards foot). In an effort to achieve 'the full posture', once they have reached the limit of iliofemoral motion, hypermobile practitioners may look for more movement by levering the ilium away from the sacrum (because, unlike most CT-typical practitioners, they can). Emphasise that in this posture we are looking to preserve a generous angle between the torso and the front thigh, and that the idea is to create a sense of solidity – not to sag the torso down towards the leg.

Check that your student's head is not drooping. A head that hangs off the neck adds further weight to the spinal lever. Many hypermobile students have chronic neck pain from the ongoing fatigue of supporting the weight of their head. If this is the case for your student, limit the hold time to one they can actually sustain, and experiment with different head positions. Looking to the upper hand is only one possibility. Your student can also look forwards or down (shifting the position of their whole head, not just their eyes). They can also keep their head in motion if holding it static tends to create muscle spasm.

Utthita trikonasana strengthens the glutes and external rotators, so if practised in this way, for SI joint integrity, it can help to support the SI joints in the longer term.

Utthita parsvakonasana

The same basic principles can be applied to *parsvakonasana*. Make sure that your student has something to press their front arm into to mitigate against spinal leverage – forearm on bent leg, hand on the floor or hand on a block or brick.

Twists – moving all in one piece

When students fix their hips and twist their spine, they exert a lot of force on their SI joints, and in the worst-case scenario, may literally wrench them apart. In sitting twists, for example *marichi* posture (Sage Marichi Pose) C/D, the situation is exacerbated if they use an arm as a lever to create the twist. Cue your student to move their pelvis as a single unit, allowing the sitbones to shift on the floor. The twist is facilitated not by the arm but by abdominal engagement – lifting in and up – front body into back body – with the transverse abdominals, and rotating with the obliques. This is not to say all arm action is outlawed but that it's safer for the SI joints if the arms aren't driving the twist. Once the twist has been established from the core body, the bind can happen in a less SI-joint-risky way.

The same principles apply in standing twists, such as *parivrrta trikonasana* (Revolved Triangle) and *parivrrta parsvakonasana* (Revolved Intense Side Stretch). Traditionally, in many schools of yoga, students have been taught to fix their hips in these postures and twist only in the upper body. In fact, allowing the hips to shift, as a single unit, so that the whole torso participates in the twist, is less likely to compromise SI joint integrity for most people.

Janusirsasana

Janusirsasana (Head to Knee Pose) can be practised as a seated twist, with the bent knee abducted wide to the side and the spine pivoting towards the extended leg. If you've read this far, you can probably already see the potential flash point here for students with excessive mobility in the SI joints, the abducted knee and twisting spine acting together potentially to lever apart the SI joint on the bent-knee side. Bear in mind, too, that the SI joints are already more open (and therefore more vulnerable) in a sitting position – remember how the weight of the trunk wedges the sacrum firmly in between the ilia on standing?

To make *janusirsasana* more SI-joint friendly, have your student place their extended leg in line with its hip (not wider). Ask them to create adduction in their bent leg by pressing its foot into the extended thigh. In other words, they are decreasing the angle between bent knee and extended leg. Check that their legs and feet are engaged, and also invite them to firm their hip points (see 'Firm the hip points'). Cue them to create abdominal engagement by lifting their front body strongly in towards their back body. As they begin to flex forwards, the bent-leg hip shifts backwards as little as possible. The student's nose is pointing not towards the centre of their extended leg, but towards its inner seam. They are in a forward bend, rather than a twist.

Working with *bandha*

I've been to classes where I've been told to use bandha, but I've never really been taught how to do this. I'm hypermobile and so are some of my students, and I've heard that bandha can be good for hypermobility.

Eric (yoga teacher with hEDS)

The *bandha* system is a vast and complex study and a lifelong embodied exploration, and it's outside the scope of this book to introduce and explain it in detail. If you're not familiar with *bandha* and would like to be, I suggest that you seek out an experienced teacher, and practise over a period of time before introducing this work to students. That said, many of you reading this chapter will have a background in styles based on the ashtanga vinyasa system, to which the practice of *bandha* is basic and intrinsic – and foundational for practising postures in a safe and engaged way.

Bandha can be practised as a *kriya* (cleansing practice), independently from *asana*; however, in this chapter I'm going to be discussing the application of *bandha* to *asana*.[37] Because this is a book about hypermobility, we will mostly be concerned with the role of *bandha* in creating biomechanical stability; however, I will also be touching on the energetic aspects of *bandha* and how to include these in a way that is helpful (rather than overwhelming) for sensitive hypermobile systems.

Defining bandha

When it comes to *bandha*, most yoga teachers are aware of the big three: *mula* (pelvic floor, or root), *uddiyana* (abdominal, or 'flying up') and *jalandhara* (throat). However, *bandhas* can be created all over the body, in the hands and feet; the armpits; and in the backs of the knees and the insides of the elbows for those who tend to hyperextend here. I view *bandha* as an interconnected web of internal engagements that creates structural integrity throughout the body, joining together what might otherwise feel like disparate body parts. Whereas more alignment-based systems, such as Iyengar, tend to stack body parts up from the floor, in *bandha*-based practices, engagement starts from the centre body and emanates outwards to the peripheries. In the best-case scenario, peripheral *bandha*, in hands and feet, loops back into the centre, creating a self-reinforcing cycle.

One of the reasons that vinyasa and other ashtanga-based styles may be high-risk for hypermobile people in group classes is that *bandha* is quite often not taught as a foundational skill in these ashtanga-derived forms. As a result, students may be practising rapid series of physically challenging postures without having developed the biomechanical structure to support them. While perhaps it can be assumed that CT-typical students walk through the door with basic structural integrity established, this is often not the case for our hypermobile students.

Teaching bandha

When I'm working with a beginning student, or teaching a class that includes beginners, I teach *bandha* before I introduce any movement. In most cases, I initially teach *mula* and *uddiyana* – because these two *bandhas* are central to creating stability in the core body. Some people will naturally also create *jalandhara* when the lower two *bandhas* activate. It's great if this happens, but personally I don't usually teach *jalandhara* in a first session – it's just too much information for most students.

When we're working with *mula* and *uddiyana bandha*, we're also modifying breath. The capacity for a natural, relaxed abdominal (diaphragmatic) breath is therefore a prerequisite for the practice of *bandha*, and I always start by guiding the student into 'regular' breath first. This is because:

- I want to be sure that they have an easy, established abdominal breath

- I want them to begin the exploration of *bandha* feeling safe and relaxed

- I want to establish abdominal breath as home base.

If your student does not have an easy, naturally occurring abdominal breath, their primary need is for work that facilitates the re-emergence of diaphragmatic breathing. There are many reasons that normal breathing patterns might be disrupted, but the most common one I come across is unresolved trauma. In this case, referral to a body-based trauma specialist would be ideal. Definitely don't push on through with *bandha* or other breath work. You will only be compounding the student's difficulties and may further compromise nervous-system dysregulation.

I generally have the student lie down for introductory *bandha* work – practising new breathing techniques in an upright position can be challenging for those with orthostatic issues. However, if your student feels vulnerable in this position, it's fine to work seated. Whichever position they are in, invite them either to let their eyes close, or to bring them into soft focus, allowing their attention to drop inside.

The following is an example of how I might cue *mula* and *uddiyana bandha*. It isn't a script. Every teacher has their own language and their own voice, and I definitely recommend that you approach the teaching of *bandha* – like all teaching – in your own authentic style. This will always communicate best. However, if there are images or phrases that work for you, please feel free to adopt and adapt.

Take some time to settle into the floor/into your seat... Notice any sensations present in your body... Notice your breath...becoming aware of your belly rising as you inhale...and falling as you exhale... You can put your hands on your belly to feel this movement if you like.

Take a moment to connect internally with your tailbone... Your tailbone is at one end of your pelvic floor. At the other end is your pubic bone. Take some time also to connect with your pubic bone... Your deep pelvic floor muscles are like a figure eight, with the top of the eight at your tailbone and the bottom of the eight at your pubic bone. The mid-point between your tailbone and your pubic bone is also the mid-point of the deep pelvic floor muscles, where the 'eight' crosses over – just behind the vaginal opening or the root of the penis. To create *mula bandha*, gently lift this mid-point up and in towards your central body. Allow your buttocks to relax, isolating the movement in the pelvic floor, and letting go of any urge to grip. The effect is like pulling on a drawstring. You will feel your entire pelvic floor lift up and your tailbone draw slightly in. Notice how you can pull the pelvic floor tightly up...and you can very subtly engage here...or you can just imagine the lift... Feeling into the different possibilities, find a degree of engagement that feels about right for you now.

Now take your attention to the front of your body and notice how, just above your pubic bone, there is already a feeling of drawing in towards the centre line as a result of the engagement of *mula bandha* (lifting the pelvic floor). You are feeling the transverse abdominis muscles engaging. Starting here, at the pubic bone, begin to zip the central line of your belly back towards your spine, all the way up to the little dip between your two rib crests. This is *uddiyana bandha*. If you have *uddiyana bandha* fully engaged, your belly will no longer be rising and falling with your breath (or only very slightly), and your breath will be in your ribcage...so now your ribcage is expanding with your in-breath...and falling away with your out-breath. If you like, you can put your hands on your ribcage to feel the movement. This way of breathing may be a little counter-intuitive at first, because usually the belly rises when we inhale. In this breath, we are deliberately drawing the lower belly back as we inhale, and keeping it lifted in and up throughout the breath cycle.

Begin to slow your in-breath down and expand it...breathing into your sides and back...as well as your chest. You are aiming, eventually, to fill your whole ribcage, up to the top of your shoulder blades at the back and your collarbone at the front. You may feel your collarbone rising as you reach the top of your in-breath. If this much opening isn't happening today, that's fine. Just be with what you can sustain. There is work involved in creating this breath, but stop short of straining.

Now, rather than collapsing into your out-breath, see if you can keep the lift of the chest you have created with your in-breath, as if your whole ribcage falls slowly away from your collarbone, in a controlled way. Notice how your rib crests draw down and in towards one another at the bottom of the exhale. See if you can maintain a little of this engagement as you start your next inhalation, so that you send the breath higher up into your ribcage, towards the top of your lungs, and into your sides and back, rather than just filling the rib crests.

- Another way to introduce *mula bandha* is to have your student breathe a regular abdominal breath. Invite them to notice how at the very end of their out-breath their pelvic floor naturally lifts a little. Invite them to maintain that slight engagement as they inhale – without gripping or straining.

- *Mula bandha* is sometimes cued as a lift of the anus. This movement actually pulls the pelvic floor out of kilter. We're aiming to lift the perineum – the crossing point of the figure eight.

- Feeling sexual sensations during the practice of *mula bandha* is completely normal – and just another experience to include in awareness. It can be helpful to mention this, in a clear, matter-of-fact way, avoiding euphemisms. For some students, such sensations may be pleasurable; for others, work with *mula bandha* may bring up traumatic memories of sexual encounters or of childbirth. If you sense that this is occurring, put *mula bandha* work on hold. A trauma specialist with a somatic approach would be a good referral.

- Another way to introduce *uddiyana bandha* is to have your student direct their in-breath into the kidney area of their back, feeling the lower ribs expand and flatten into the floor, and the belly draw in and somewhat back towards the spine.

- An *uddiyana* cue that works well for some hypermobile students (I've used it throughout this book) is 'draw your front body towards your back body' (abdominal region towards spine).

- Beginning students often need feedback on whether their belly is rising as they inhale (in other words, whether they are have shifted into thoracic breath or are still breathing diaphragmatically). Ask them if it's OK for you to place a hand on their belly. Even if you have already established at the outset that touch is welcome, let your student know what you are about to do. If they are in a state of deep somatic attention, they may be startled by sudden, unexpected touch. Hold your hand just slightly above the point of the student's maximum exhale. Ask them to inhale without letting their belly touch your hand.

Once your student has *uddiyana* in place, you can also place your hands at the sides of their ribcage and ask them to breathe into your hands to help them to find expansion here.

- For students who have a basic understanding of *bandha* and capacity to engage it, I sometimes describe the breath as a wave form:

  Offer your attention to your pelvic floor... Notice the next impulse to inhale arising here... Feel the in-breath travelling up your back... fanning out into the two sides of your ribcage... and cresting over your shoulders... where it falls away on the out-breath, your front ribs and rib crests dropping in... and the breath descending... until it ebbs away at your pelvic floor... and the new breath begins to unfurl.

- With more experienced students or in settings where I have more time, I sometimes explain the movement of the diaphragm and the role of the abdominal muscles in changing it. For example:

  The diaphragm is a large, strong muscle that attaches to your lower ribs, forming a kind of muscular seal over the bottom of your ribcage. When you are breathing a normal relaxed breath, your diaphragm domes down on the inhalation, making space for the lungs to fill and pushing the abdominal organs down and up. It is this movement of the organs that is felt as your belly rising when you breathe in. Your diaphragm domes back up under your ribcage on the exhalation. When we engage *uddiyana bandha*, we restrict the downward movement of the diaphragm, causing the ribcage to expand to create the in-breath instead.

When you have finished the exploration, invite your student to open their eyes and slowly come up to sitting, and take some time to check in verbally. What was their experience like? Is there anything they'd like to ask? Was anything strange/confusing/unclear? If necessary, reassure the student that *bandha* practice is challenging and takes a while to establish. You are not expecting them to 'get it' in a single class.

Explain to your student that the intention is to maintain this engagement that they have established lying down – *mula bandha* (pelvic floor) and *uddiyana bandha* (belly) – throughout *asana* practice. Students sometimes think *bandha* practice is something they do at the beginning of class and then drop. You may need to clarify this again and again. I have had several students only really 'hear' this information months – and even a couple of years – into practice.

Too tight/too loose

Hypermobile students will often present as obviously weak and disengaged in the core body, and they may report difficulties related to hypotonicity in the pelvic floor. One of the complexities of hypermobility work, however, is that where the person is inherently weak and hypotonic, work for strength may create indiscriminate gripping, clenching and muscle spasm, rather than a smooth effective contractile force. With this in mind, it's important to introduce *bandha* as a subtle art, and offer lots of opportunities for somatic exploration. Inviting your student to imagine the *bandha* rather than actually engage it can help to mitigate against over-engagement. They should not feel that they are hanging on for dear life!

We'll be discussing hypo- and hypertonic pelvic floor in more detail in Chapter 4: 'Pelvic floor dysfunction'.

Bandhas, hypermobility and energy

Working with *bandha* is a powerful energy practice and can generate a lot of adrenaline. When *bandha* is engaged in tandem with physically challenging *asana* work, this is generally a good thing – especially in the context of a sedentary culture that presents many nervous-system challenges but few opportunities to diffuse the resulting sympathetic response in natural, physical ways. In the best case scenario, strong *asana* practice coupled with *bandha* is like taking a racehorse out for a gallop. It primes the nervous system to fire appropriately in response to the demand for physical effort... and to drop easily back into parasympathetic mode once that demand has been met.[38]

If you are incorporating *bandha* into a vigorous flowing class, it's very important to allow sufficient time for, and attention to, the important parasympathetic stage of the practice. If this substantial grounding is not present, students may walk out the door feeling high, hyper or wired – and later crash into irritability or depression. This kind of over-activation can be especially problematic for hypermobile students, in whom adrenaline levels are already chronically elevated. The following are a few suggestions for helping all your students, and especially the hypermobile ones, to move through sympathetic arousal and back to rest and relax.

- In an activating class, it's all too easy for the teacher also to get caught up in the adrenalising process. Make sure you stand outside. You are the container, not a participant, and it's your job to keep the class energetically anchored. It's particularly easy to get carried away if you do the class with your students or demonstrate most of the postures. Mark, witness, explain verbally, clarify and adjust. This will not only allow your students space to feel and emerge postures for themselves, but will also free you up to do the important work of teaching. If you have hypermobile students in your class, you will need to be available to offer individual help and feedback.

- Allow plenty of time to bring the class slowly down at the end. This is a section of practice you definitely don't want to skimp on. Shoehorning in a final challenging backbend and leaving only two minutes for *savasana* is a recipe for nervous-system dysregulation. Forward bends tend to down-regulate the nervous system, as does slower seated and lying work. Include a few energetically quieting postures as you warm down to final relaxation.

- As a rule of thumb, if you're teaching a 90-minute class, give your students at least ten minutes in *savasana*. Remember to articulate the possibility of sitting or moving gently, or of keeping eyes open if this helps the student to stay present and relax. It may be helpful to explain why this phase of practice is important and talk briefly about how the nervous system works.

- Traditionally, *bandha* has been associated with raising *kundalini* energy and as such often connotes (either consciously or not) an upwards and outwards movement. If a student is finding it difficult to ground themselves (or is feeling depleted by practice), invite them to conceptualise the movement of energy not as an upwards whoosh, but as a cycling around, from their belly up towards their head, and then back down around to their feet and up their legs. You can also invite your students to feel their energy dropping down in *savasana*, into their feet or into their contact points with the floor. The focus needs to be on grounding.

- Vigorous, flowing *asana* is designed to energise and was never intended as an evening practice; nevertheless, in the current culture evening is when the majority of fast, challenging classes take place. If your student is 'up' after the class and unable to sleep, suggest that they try shifting their energetic practice to the morning, and save the evenings for restorative work. For many sensitive hypermobile systems, this will work much better.

- Make sure that when your students come to rest in *savasana* at the end of practice, they have fully released all *bandha* and are breathing abdominally. This is very important. You could say something like:

> Let your breath drop back down into your belly…allowing your belly to completely soften…so you are no longer managing your breath… Notice your belly once again rising as you breath in…and falling as you breathe out… Allow your pelvic floor to completely soften… letting *mula bandha* dissolve away…

Working in active range

Many yoga postures can be practised in either active or passive range – or a bit of both. For example, if you are entering *vrksasana*, you can either pick one leg up with your hands and place it against the opposite inside thigh (passive), or you can have the leg do its own work by lifting it into place hands-free (active). It probably won't get anything like as close to your groin, so you'll be experiencing less passive stretch…but recruiting a lot more strength and mobilising in a way that you can actually control. In dynamic yoga styles, in which we are usually working in a mixture of active and passive range, you can help your hypermobile students to lean into strength building by having them work actively in places where they might be more accustomed to passive range. There are myriad ways to adapt yoga postures to make them more active. The following are a few suggestions.

Janusirsasana legs

Start with your student sitting on the floor, as usual for *janusirsasana*. Cue them to bend their right knee and – without using their hands – draw the thigh in towards their chest, maintaining this position for a few breaths. You can add some repetitions of this movement. Now have them find the external rotation, turning the femur out externally at the socket, leg still raised, holding in this position for a couple of breaths. Again, you can add some repetitions here: leg raised, parallel to external rotation. Now ask your student to bring their flexed leg to the floor, foot to their inner thigh. Their foot may be lower down their leg than when they place it in position manually. Change to the left side.

If your student has the facility, they can try this approach with *ardha padmasana* (Half-Lotus Pose) – very challenging! If your student has retroverted hips (sockets and femur necks that angle straight out to the side rather than forwards), with practice they may be able to achieve a hands-free Lotus (*padmasana*).

Cobra

Start with your student lying prone, as usual for Cobra. Cue them to place their hands roughly beside their shoulders, just off the floor, and lift their head, shoulders and chest up – by retracting the shoulder blades and strongly engaging the back flexors, glutes and hamstrings. Your student can lift up and hold for a few breaths and/or lift up and down a few times.

Natarajasana

This exercise, a variation on *natarajasana* (Dancer Pose) rather than the classic form, is as much about balance as strength. Your student starts in parallel standing. Cue them to raise their right leg up behind them, knee bent, and tip forward at the hip, lifting their back leg up higher as they go, into a *natarajasana*-like position (or a turned-in ballet *attitude*). As they tip, they bring their hands up towards their shoulders (as for Cobra above) to counterbalance. They are in hip extension (no external rotation) and knee flexion on the right side. Have them repeat a few times, tipping forwards and back upright (with and without holds), then do the left side.

Hasta padangushtasana

Start with your student in *samasthitihi/tadasana*. Keeping both their legs in parallel and hands on hips, have them bend their right leg and draw the thigh in towards their chest. They can repeat this movement a few times. Then have them draw the thigh in (the hands still on their hips) and straighten their leg. They can repeat this bending and straightening movement a few times. Then – without using their hands – have them bend their knee in towards their chest and externally rotate their right femur so that their knee travels out towards the side. Make sure their pelvis stays neutral and it's the femur that does the movement. They can repeat this movement a few times. Change to the left side.

You can also have your student lift their right leg from *samasthitihi/ tadasana* straight up, steadily and with control, as high as they can without tilting their pelvis posteriorly, hold for a breath or two, lower and repeat.

* * *

My colleague, Sophie Cleere, has many more ideas for adding active movement into a yoga practice. You can find some of them on her Instagram account @sophiecleere. As ever, be conservative when introducing strength-building exercises to hypermobile students. While it may be evident that stability and control is what the student needs, it's very easy to overwhelm the hypermobile proprioceptive and muscular systems, creating tightness and spasm rather than useable strength. Little is better.

Working with resistance bands

Another way to incorporate more strength building for hypermobile students in your classes is to add latex resistance bands. These come in all sorts of shapes and sizes, but the type I described in 'Strengthening the feet' above is a good all-purpose option. I suggest you buy your latex on the roll from a physiotherapy supplier and cut it to the required length. This will be much cheaper than buying individual bands. As I mentioned above, latex bands come in different, colour-coded densities. When you're working with a hypermobile student, begin with the lightest band and the least resistance – unless you know they already have good strength, stamina and co-ordination.

Working against a band offers more proprioceptive feedback. This can be very helpful for those floppy hypermobile students who just cannot seem to work out how to engage and co-contract muscles. A note of caution: just like light weights, latex bands can be overtaxing for some hypermobile people. Where a muscle is tight and weak, and hard to fire, lying on the floor and playing with tiny movements, including some holds, may be the best way to start to open up a conversation with it. The support of the floor eliminates the complex and fatiguing global activations required for standing, and does away with any orthostatic issues. As always, explore the possibilities together with your student and find out what works for them.

There are many ways to use resistance bands in a standard yoga class. The following are a few suggestions to get you started.

Downdog

This Downdog variation helps to activate and strengthen the posterior chain. Tie the band into a loop. It's going to go around your student's legs at calf height and needs to offer a little resistance when they are in parallel standing. Have your student step into the belt and walk back into Downdog – keeping the tension in the band and moving slowly and steadily. Have them raise their right leg about 30 cm (6 inches) off the floor, and lower it down again almost but not quite to the floor. If your student can go a little higher with control, that's fine, but this is not a toes-to-the-ceiling variation; the foot doesn't go above hip height. Repeat a few times. Now, have your student lift their right leg about 30 cm (6 inches) off the floor and abduct it (take it out to the side). Again, this is a smallish movement. You could introduce some little hip circles here, both clockwise and counter-clockwise. Then do the left side.

Utthita trikonasana

Have your student set up for *utthita trikonasana* with their right foot front and standing on the band. They hold the other end of the band in their right hand. Ask them to bring their right arm up, slowly and with control, into the usual *utthita trikonasana* position. Your student can do repetitions of the whole arm movement or small repetitions:

- in the initiation phase of the arm movement, raising their arm just a little and then lowering it

- or at the apex of the arm movement, coming just out of the finishing arm position and then moving back into it (but make sure your student is not working in hyperextension)

- or in mid-range.

They can also do small arm circles.

If part of the movement feels fatiguing or restricted, that's a good place to explore – sensitively. Be conservative about the number of repetitions. If your student experiences shoulder pain – and especially if, over time, it worsens – try losing the band and having them work just with the weight of their own arm. Having had the experience of external resistance may enable them now to create the movement independently.

Myofascial release with a small massage ball or Thumbby™ could be a good complement to this work (see 'Myofascial release (MFR)' in Chapter 7). As always, if your student really needs therapeutic help, refer appropriately.

Ekam, inhale

Have your student come to parallel standing (or *samasthitihi*/*tadasana* if they prefer). Tie the band into a loop and place it around their forearms. It should be tense when their arms are shoulder-width apart. On an in-breath, have them raise their arms overhead (coming up the front), going slowly and keeping even tension in the band. Then, on an out-breath, have them bring their arms down, again slowly and keeping even tension. Make sure that:

- their ribcage is involved in the arm raise, lifting and expanding as their arms go up

- their abdominal muscles stay active, preventing the rib crests from flaring and the lumbar spine from arching

- their shoulders lift slightly towards the apex of the movement.

Here, too, your student can do small repetitions at different points in the arc of the larger movement.

✷ ✷ ✷

If you'd like to explore work with resistance bands further, yoga teacher Laurel Beversdorf has several resources, including an online course. You can find these at: https://laurelbeversdorf.com.

Adjustment: speaking in hands

I wrote in *The Yoga Teacher Mentor*:

> When we talk about adjusting, what tends to arise in the popular yoga mind is an image of a teacher manipulating a student's body – often quite forcefully – into a particular predetermined shape. This is really the dark side of adjustment.[39]

Unfortunately, many hypermobile students have experienced the dark side, and some have sustained physical (and emotional) trauma as a result. While no one is likely to gain from being forcibly 'pretzelled', hypermobile students are particularly vulnerable to tears, dislocations and injuries of attrition resulting from too much force applied to fragile tissues. At the same time, perhaps no student group is more likely to benefit from sensitive, consensual hands-on work than hypermobile practitioners.

As I write this chapter, the yoga world is in a storm of discussion about when and how it is appropriate to physically adjust students and what is best practice in terms of eliciting genuine consent for touch. Some teachers have tried to remove themselves from the fray by making a policy decision never to touch any of their students at all. This seems to me wrong-headed. If a teacher verbally abuses a student, do we conclude that therefore teachers shouldn't speak to their students? Of course not. To do so would be to deny our students a fundamental element in the teaching–learning process. It's also important to be aware that not touching students is in itself a decision happening within the relational field. It's not possible to opt out here; all choices create effects. In my view, what we actually need as teachers is a level of comfort in understanding and negotiating touch as a subtle and multivalent language, with the potential both to harm and to help. My colleague, Soleil Hepner (C-IAYT), who trains Phoenix Rising yoga therapists, comments:

> I believe it's important to have training in all levels of touch (self-touch, to low touch, to other touch, to more supported 'high' touch) so that we can make informed choice as to what is 'right' – a.k.a. wise in the moment – whether for ourselves or for others (clients/students). We all have our lenses as to what we will and will not do around touch, and that's based on what we've been taught/told (per our licence perhaps), as well as what we've experienced. I've trained yoga therapists for years in the many facets of touch and have found that my students (many are talk therapists) come in with beliefs of right/ wrong without having experienced the touch of connection (versus the touch of fixing). It's been eye-opening (maybe that's 'arm-opening') for many to be able to discern what is appropriate in each moment.[40]

Interestingly, a recent survey of 931 students and teachers by Jenny Rawlings and Travis Pollen shows that whereas teachers on the whole have become much more conservative about offering adjustments, yoga students on the whole still tend to appreciate hands-on work:

> Whereas 74 per cent of students 'like' and 'strongly like' receiving touch in yoga, only 19 per cent of yoga teachers reported offering touch 'always' or

'often'. And only 10 per cent of students dislike being touched, yet nearly half of teachers offer touch 'rarely' or 'never'.[41]

Seeking consent and adjusting collaboratively

As I mentioned in Chapter 2 (see 'Adjustment'), the majority of hypermobile students are not averse to every adjustment all the time, but they need to know what kind of assistance is being proposed and to have an opportunity to negotiate, assess and potentially make adaptations. I personally am most likely to accept an adjustment if:

- the teacher is curious about my experience and respects what I already know about my body

- they listen openly to what I say and ask clarifying questions

- they offer what they know and suggest how they may be able to help without dismissing, contradicting or imposing

- they invite ongoing feedback about the adjustment and are willing to act on it – stop/go more slowly/do less/etc.

- their intention in adjusting is not to crank me further into end range of motion.

An adjustment is – or should be – a collaborative endeavour, in which the teacher elicits information from the student about how things are working for them, listens and proceeds accordingly. It should never be something the teacher does to the student and which the student passively receives – or endures. This is poor practice in work with any student and is highly likely to cause injury when the student is hypermobile.

Tuning in to the tissues

I used to launch into adjusting my students – I'm an ashtanga teacher and it was just the way things were always done. Now I go much more slowly and pay attention to what I'm feeling through physical contact with the student.

Bill (CT-typical yoga teacher)

For a teacher placing a hand on a student's body, the first priority is to feel into the tissues. If the teacher is skilled and experienced, they will (or should) know pretty immediately how dense and resistant – or elastic and fragile – are the myofascial structures they're working with. When I teach apprentices and assistant teachers, they're sometimes surprised to learn that if a student's body stretches easily, the teacher should be very careful about adjusting it. The tendency in some schools has been to 'move it as far as it will go', and if it goes a very long way, to see if it will go a bit further. In fact, if we press very 'soft' bodies into end of range, or offer them strong resistance that they cannot meet, the risk of injury is high. Mobile, elastic tissues need a careful, light touch.

How can adjustment help?

While adjustment as forced manipulation is never going to be advisable for a hypermobile student, skilful, sensitive and appropriate touch can be a good choice as a teaching tool for this student group. The following are some reasons for opting to work with physical contact:

- All of our hypermobile students will by definition be experiencing some degree of proprioceptive deficit, a significant number will actually be dyspraxic and still others may have delays in verbal processing (not necessarily evident to you as teacher). For these students, particularly if they are relatively new to embodied practice, translating verbal cues into physical movement can be challenging. Guiding sensitively with hands, feet or other appropriate and agreed body parts allows the student opportunities to take in information through tactile and kinaesthetic channels, in ways that may be more readily assimilable.

- Skilful hands-on work, in which body speaks directly to body without the need for complex cognitive translation, can enable movement mapping and enhance proprioceptive development.

- In this chapter, we have already touched on some ways you can use your own body to provide resistance for your student – for example, having them press a hyperextending knee into your hand in order to find muscular engagement and neutral placement. Here, too, the tactile and kinaesthetic dimensions of the interaction increase proprioceptive feedback, expanding resources for your student and potentially making it easier for them to embody the new information.

- Hypermobile students frequently find it very difficult to feel and engage specific muscle groups. Putting a hand on the muscle that needs to fire can give the student the proprioceptive information they need to activate it.

- An adjustment that holds the shape of the posture for the student can enable them to feel into the form and begin to find the neuromuscular pathways to create it for themselves. Remember that when we're working with hypermobile students, the desired shape will often involve a smaller range of motion and a greater degree of muscular engagement.

- Hypermobile students have often experienced adjustments that were dangerous and injurious and not attuned to their tissues. Offering sensitive and supportive touch – that isn't designed to stretch them, take them 'deeper' or manoeuvre them into position – can reassure the student that your intention is to create safety and can help to build trust, founded on experience rather than blind faith.

For more on touch and adjustments, see 'Touch' in Chapter 2. For a more detailed discussion of the ethics and purpose of adjusting, see my book *The Yoga Teacher Mentor*.[42]

Working with isolations

While a trend in the movement world lately has been towards working with complex movements, involving a variety of different muscle activations – on the basis that naturally arising movement never relies on isolating a single muscle – this may not always be the best approach for hypermobile people. Specialist hypermobility physiotherapists, Rosemary Keer and Jane Simmonds, note:

> Research has demonstrated that specific, isolated, low level, skilled stabilisation training is preferable to non-isolated functional exercise and can restore the timing of activation of postural muscles to near-normal levels [in hypermobile patients]. These changes can occur relatively quickly with instruction and practice, can lead to brain pathway reorganisation and motor learning and be transferred to functional activities.[43]

This chimes with my experience of working therapeutically with my own kinetic chains and with those of hypermobile students. One reason that isolations often work better for us may lie in the non-standard movement acquisition patterns of hypermobile infants, in which some developmental stages have typically been skipped and key patterns of muscle activation therefore not primed (for more information see 'Early movement acquisition' in Chapter 6). It's therefore not feasible to expect a hypermobile person to be able automatically to produce a 'natural' (i.e. functional) sequence of regular movements in the way that most CT-typical people can. Add to this proprioceptive deficits and hypotonicity, and it's easy to see how being asked to perform apparently simple (not simple) movement tasks can overwhelm the hypermobile system, causing it to default to familiar maladaptive patterns instead.

Most yoga postures involve complex combinations of muscle activations, and in the vinyasa forms these are strung together into even more complex skeins of movement. Unless your hypermobile student already has a lot of movement training under their belt, they stand little chance of being able to produce these choreographies in biomechanically functional ways. There are many isolations you can include in a general yoga class to create competency in core muscle activations so that your hypermobile students have the building blocks in place to tackle more complex movement. In this chapter, we have already looked at how to isolate hip stabilisation muscles (see 'Hip stabilisation, backbends and finding the glutes') and shoulder blade protraction and retraction (see 'Plank, *chaturanga* and shoulder stability'), and most of the active-range movement repetitions involve isolation (see 'Working in active range'). The following are a few more examples of simple isolations to explore:

- Sitting or standing, have your student draw a circle with one shoulder...and then the other. Repeat a few times and then reverse the circle.

- Sitting or standing, have your student bend their arms, keeping their elbows into their sides, and flex and then extend their forearms (biceps curls). Repeat a few times. They can also do one arm at a time.

- Sitting, working leg extended, have your student circle one ankle... and then the other, making sure their leg does not rotate at the knee or hip. Repeat a few times and then change sides.

- In *samasthitihi/tadasana* or parallel standing, and with arms by their sides, have your student bend their knees into an *utkatasana* position and then straighten back to standing. Repeat a few times.

Isolations are intended to be performed as repetitions, slowly, carefully and with attention. As always, start with a few and build up gradually. Bear in mind that the number of repetitions your CT-typical students can do may never be optimal for those with hypermobility, even with a lot of practice. Encourage hypermobile students to trust the information of their own experience.

✳ ✳ ✳

The challenge of hypermobility work is that while there are approaches that are definitely more rather than less likely to be helpful to this student group, there is no absolute how-to or complete step-by-step guide. These are students who need targeted work and require detailed and knowledgeable help to embody it. Rosemary Keer and Katherine Butler explain that:

> Generic exercises do not work [with hypermobile patients] without good instruction and practice, because invariably an individual will 'take the path of least resistance'... Or if they have been in pain, long-standing compensatory strategies may inhibit weaker, less dominant or 'forgotten' muscles.[44]

This is why having on-board an experienced and hypermobility-aware physiotherapist – not one who just rolls out the standard rehab – can be invaluable. Keer and Butler say:

> It is important that an assessment highlights an individual's muscle imbalance and corrects it. It may be appropriate to use manual therapy to inhibit overactive muscles and facilitate under-active ones.[45]

In other words, you can't just throw the approaches in this book at your hypermobile students and hope for the best, and you are unlikely to make much impact in a busy class where you have little time to break things down and explain. However, in settings where you are able to work slowly with your hypermobile student, build up a relationship of trust, experiment with different approaches and incorporate the work of other professionals, together you can make significant gains.

4

Working with Commonly Co-occurring Conditions

We covered hypermobility on my teacher training, but I wasn't prepared for the complexity of the issues of hypermobile people actually turning up in my class. There is so much more to it than lots of flexibility.

Jasmine (CT-typical yoga teacher)

Often, what is problematic for hypermobile students in a yoga class is less joint hypermobility *per se* and more those issues and conditions that it commonly goes hand in hand with. Because genetic hypermobility is multi-systemic, the range of potential comorbidities is vast, and it's way beyond the capacity of this book to cover all of them. It's also beyond the scope of this book to offer a full rehab programme for every condition. What I am going to offer in this chapter is some pointers for working in a helpful and positive way with those co-occurring conditions that show up in yoga classes frequently.

In an ideal world, this chapter would be intended for situations in which a condition has already been formally diagnosed. However, it can be extremely difficult to access and receive diagnosis not only for the hypermobility syndromes themselves (Ehlers-Danlos Support UK's 2019 #timetodiagnosis campaign came up with figures ranging into decades[1]) but also for some of the conditions that commonly accompany them. Hypermobile people frequently appear on the surface to be fit and well, and often baffle specialists with their diverse and extensive array of adjunctive symptoms. Students with hypermobility may be self-diagnosed with co-occurring conditions, or mystified and struggling with symptoms they don't understand. If you strongly suspect that a student may have a particular condition, it can be helpful to suggest to them that you *think* this may be the case, while being clear that you are not a diagnostician and that they should do their own research and seek confirmation from an appropriate professional.

The approaches in this section are all gentle, suitable for inclusion in a general yoga class and highly unlikely to cause any harm. However, if you are trying out a suggestion from this book and it's aggravating the person's issue – stop! If possible, refer them to a yoga teacher with experience in hypermobility work or to an appropriate professional for further investigation and advice.

Autism

As we saw in Chapter 1, there is a significant crossover between the joint hypermobility syndromes and autism, and it's highly likely that a good proportion of your hypermobile students will also be autistic, either diagnosed or not. Even where they fall outside the autistic spectrum, many hypermobile people are highly sensitive and anxious and may have some traits typical of autism. When we're working with hypermobility, it's therefore very helpful to have an awareness of the processing and communication styles of autistic people. This can help to minimise any conflict and enable you to meet the needs of these students more appropriately.

There is sometimes an assumption among allistic yoga teachers that autistic people are a rare and exotic species, seldom spotted outside special needs settings. This is not the case. We are living, working, parenting and participating in communities everywhere and are very likely to be routinely present in any group class you run. However, because there is still a huge amount of stigma and misunderstanding surrounding autism, a lot of autistic people remain in the closet, so you may not be aware of who your autistic students, friends and colleagues are.

The needs of autistic students in a general yoga class is a huge subject and warrants a book in its own right. The following are a few suggestions for working in ways that will make your classes more accessible to the majority of autistic students. However, as the saying goes, 'If you've met one autistic person...you've met one autistic person.' We wouldn't expect all our allistic students to have the same needs in a yoga class, and neither will every autistic person who walks through the door, so if you're not sure how to approach working with a particular autistic person, here's my number one suggestion...

Ask the expert

Fortunately, any time you're teaching an autistic student you already have an expert in the class. Your student knows all about what will help them to participate fully and absorb your teaching. Use this resource. Ask them what they would like to get out of practising yoga and how you can best include and enable them.

Bear in mind that many autistic people find writing easier than speaking, and it may work better for them to email to you any suggestions, thoughts and needs relating to their experience in your class (but check with the individual student; if they're also dyslexic, an email exchange may be difficult for them). Be aware that an email from an autistic person may be long. This isn't because we're needy, selfish or want to monopolise you. For us, everything is connected, and it can be hard to stop writing before all the details have been fully explained. On the one hand, this means that you will gain a very full picture of your student's experience of practising with you (how often do we wish our allistic students would give us a bit more detail?!); on the other hand, it can be easy to get into a situation where your student is overwhelming you with information and taking up a lot of your time. It's a good idea to set out some boundaries at the outset around when and how you will respond to emails. For example:

> I will read and briefly acknowledge all the emails you send me, but cannot answer in detail. Know that even if I don't enter into discussion with you in writing, I'm taking in everything you tell me and allowing it to inform how I work with you – and we can clarify in the class.

Acknowledge different neurologies

A quick and easy way to make your classes more autism-inclusive is to refer to neurological variations routinely in the course of your teaching. Allowing your own neurotypicality (if you are NT) and the neurodifference of any openly autistic or otherwise neurodivergent students to be on the table in a clear and simple way – just like your respective ages and genders – opens up the channels for conversation and makes space for everyone to be who they are. For example:

> For those of us in the class who are neurotypical, it may be comfortable to sit in stillness. Feel free to keep some part of your body in gentle motion if you are autistic, have ADHD or need to be in movement for some other reason.

Respectful humour can also be a way of honouring and including differences:

> I see some of you autistic people are already planning on researching this subject in depth! Please bring any interesting information you discover back to the class for the rest of us to enjoy!

Be cautious of using irony – autistic people sometimes take statements at face value and may totally not get it or may be confused about whether you're serious or not – and make sure that you value the particular strengths your autistic students bring to the group as a whole.

Sensory issues

> *I have organic essential oil in a diffuser at my classes. Most of my students love this, but last week a student said it made them feel nauseous and asked me if I could stop using it.*
>
> Bella (allistic and CT-typical yoga teacher)

Most autistic people are hypersensitive to some or all of: texture, smell, sight, sound and taste – and even those hypermobile people who fall off-spectrum may have heightened sensitivity in some of these areas. 'Sensitive' here doesn't mean highly emotionally reactive (although being bombarded with, for example, a nauseating smell might understandably also provoke an intense secondary emotional reaction); it refers to an acuity of senses beyond what the neurotypical population routinely experiences. Autistic motivational speaker and consultant, Mitchell LaBerge, says:

> I went to an Ear, Nose and Throat doctor to get an audiogram…to see what my level of hearing really was. It show[ed] that my hearing was very sensitive, like a person with superhuman hearing.[2]

If you want your autistic students to be able to concentrate and process well, make the environment as clear, quiet and unfussy as possible. Sensory triggers may include:

- fluorescent lights
- electronic screens
- humming and buzzing electrical equipment – and 'silent' electrical equipment (some autistic people can hear electricity)

- music

- general background noise

- incense

- scented cleaning products in the room

- scented laundry products on your own and other students' clothes

- synthetic carpet.

Sensory triggers can be very individual, so check in with autistic students about what might be bothering them. Remember, just because you can't see/hear/smell it, doesn't mean it isn't unbearably intrusive for someone else.

Pratyahara
Sensory sensitivity has obvious ramifications for the practice of *pratyahara* (withdrawal of the senses), in which we cultivate the capacity to notice our sensory experience without running after it like a dog after a sausage. Some autistic people find it helpful to practise disidentifying from sensory experience – but keep in mind that few practitioners could remain non-reactive to the sound of a pneumatic drill a few feet away or the stench of a blocked toilet, and that this may be the level of sensory input our autistic students are being called upon to disregard. Difficulty with staying present and undistracted may tell us more about the acuity of the person's senses than their spiritual attainment.

Verbal processing issues
Many autistic people experience difficulties with producing and processing speech. Some of us can understand speech (when distractions are few) but not produce it ourselves, others can communicate by typing (independently or with assistance), a third group, to which I belong, may appear – and actually be – highly articulate and yet is compensating for verbal processing delays and difficulties. Even if your autistic student appears to have no problem with speaking and understanding speech, check in with them about their needs in this area anyway. Being able to create an impression of competence does not mean that the person is processing spoken language at normal speed and with the expected ease, or that they can do so in every context. Particularly if they are tired, stressed, overwhelmed by environmental static (other people

talking in the background, strong smells, visual distractions) or bombarded with a lot of speech, they may be struggling to keep up and pass for 'normal'.

As we have already seen, proprioceptive deficits make it difficult for hypermobile people to embody complicated verbal cues; for a student who is also dealing with verbal processing challenges, a long string of spoken instructions will be doubly impermeable. Accessing language may also be more difficult for an autistic person who is absorbed in somatic process – we don't operate well on two channels. I experience this as a kind of verbal drift or as some words not being in the right boxes. If I'm asked a question, I may stumble over words and say whatever comes into my head to fill the requirement for speech (even if the result has little relationship with what I'm actually thinking or feeling). Your speech will be most digestible in this situation if you:

- keep language spare, simple and precise

- speak slowly, with pauses

- wait until the person has come out of the posture to talk to them – they can always go back into it again to try out your movement cue.

Touch

We have already discussed touch in relation to hypermobility in Chapter 2 (see 'Touch') and Chapter 3 (see 'Adjustment: speaking in hands'). When you are negotiating touch with a student who is also autistic, be aware that they may have tactile sensitivities. For some autistic people, any kind of physical contact produces sensory overwhelm and they may not want to be touched at all – not even a friendly pat on the arm in the course of conversation; others are happy to be touched in particular ways but not in others; some of us are distinctly touchy-feely. Light, floaty touch is unpleasant to some autistic people, while firm touch may feel pleasantly containing and offer a sense of body boundary – but always check with the individual: it may be different for them.

Social sense

Autistic people are not mad keen on small talk, and on the whole would rather just get down to business. Unlike most of your neurotypical students, we are not social natives and struggle to learn, retain and see the point of complex etiquette – although some of us become consummate actors, able to fake social competence by running memorised scripts. Where we have acquired a wide repertoire of scripts and agility at juggling them, our social skills may appear quite sophisticated, but don't be fooled – we are not using social language spontaneously. Don't be offended if your autistic student forgets to greet you or doesn't smile when you expect it. The chances are they're not upset or angry with you but have forgotten that these kinds of behaviours are significant in neurotypical relationships, or are too overwhelmed in the moment to produce them.

On the whole, an autistic student may be relating less to what you are saying and more to who you are being, and will prefer you to drop professional masks and dissolve social surfaces – while maintaining appropriate student–teacher boundaries. Autistic people are generally honest and straightforward to a fault, and thrive best with teachers who are likewise.

Affective empathy

Contrary to the popular stereotype, a quick scan through the literature produced by actual autistic people[3] demonstrates that autism often enhances the capacity for affective empathy, described by autistic writer, Helen Wallace-Iles, as, 'an unconscious, automatic response allowing you to feel what other people (and other living beings) are feeling'.[4] This kind of empathic receptivity can be intense and overwhelming, giving rise to a response pattern known as 'hyper-empathy'. Helen explains:

> Hyper-empathic people find that even the thought of anyone or anything suffering causes them intense emotional, psychological and often physical pain. They can be highly sensitive to any changes in atmospheres, picking up on the slightest tension between people, and becoming more and more upset as they anticipate things escalating.[5]

An autistic student may be a telegraph for the unspoken – acutely sensitive to what you are feeling but not saying, and cognizant of any discrepancy, particularly where feelings are suppressed or denied. This can create an unbearable amount of emotional static for the autistic person, and may make relationship with you untenable – so be especially diligent in taking care of your own emotional well-being if you are working with an autistic student.

Eye contact

Withholding eye contact is often read by neurotypical people as a sign of shyness, submission or deviousness. I've even been told, 'I thought you weren't looking at me because you didn't like me.' For the majority of people on the spectrum, however, sustained eye contact is physically painful. Some words I've heard autistic people use to describe eye gazing are 'agonising', 'like broken glass in your eyes' and – when eye contact is forced – 'cruel'. Many of us have learnt to fake neuro-normative gaze, but that doesn't mean we like it.

It appears to be as instinctive for allistic people to seek out and hold eye contact as it is for autistic people not to, and this can be a hard habit to break. But if you possibly can, remember not to look directly into autistic eyes: it hurts! And offer alternatives to any exercises that prescribe eye gazing, for example:

- sitting quietly side by side

- making some gentle body contact (if both partners want it)

- sensing the energy of your partner without touching them.

Eye contact may be bonding for allistic people, but it's more likely to make autistic students feel angry and compromised.

Detail

I've had a series of very strange queries from a possible new student. She has asked me what people wear in the class, whether there are fan heaters in the room, where the toilets are in the building... I'm getting really fed up with her never-ending questions. Why does she need to know these things?

Jacey (allistic and CT-typical yoga teacher)

God, going to a new place, to do a new activity – or even the same activity with a different teacher – is so scary! So much is unknown. I usually have several false starts before I manage to actually make it there.

Danni (autistic yoga practitioner with hEDS)

If you visit a site advertising an event by and for autistic people, one of the first things you will probably notice is how much detail is included about the venue, timings and content. Most autistic people find unpredictability difficult to deal with and need a sense of reliable structure. An autistic person attending a yoga class for the first time is likely to be less anxious and more able to integrate the teaching if it has been outlined for them in advance what's going to happen when, and what the intention is. They may also need to know what the venue looks like, how they access the yoga room, what they will see when they open the door and so on. New-agey advice such as, 'Let go of expectations', 'Be open to the unknown' and 'Go with the flow' is not helpful for autistic students, who may be struggling with overwhelming amounts of fear and in need of secure handholds in order to make it through your door.

Honouring the structure

If you have shared the structure for a class or workshop with your autistic student, don't change it without negotiation or explanation. Unexpected deviations from the plan are difficult for us to deal with and may completely derail us. Don't vary times without plenty of prior warning either. Most autistic people are punctilious about practical boundaries. We will uphold them exactly and will expect you to do likewise. If you tell your autistic student the workshop will finish at 6pm but you run over to 6.15pm, they may be scared, confused or angry with you for not honouring the agreement about timing, and you may lose their trust.

Stillness and stimming

> I have a student who just won't keep still in restorative postures or savasana. She is constantly fidgeting, moving a bit, adjusting her position. I find it really disconcerting and worry that it will distract the other students.

> Molly (allistic and CT-typical yoga teacher)

Most autistic people stim. A stim is something like a repetitive fidget – finger rubbing, hair twirling, face stroking, ankle circling. The word 'stim' is derived from 'stimulating' and was obviously coined by a neurotypical person, as it's a complete misnomer – good god, the last thing an autistic person wants is *more* stimulation! In fact stimming helps autistic people to calm down and self-regulate, to process the rolling boil of thoughts, feelings and sense impressions, and stay reasonably focused.

Many yoga teachers regard sitting still as intrinsic to meditation and paying attention. However, this is a false equivalence. Being in movement *helps* not only autistic people, but also those with some other forms of neurodifference, and many people with PTSD and developmental trauma, to stay present and cultivate internal space. Cai, an autistic yoga practitioner with hEDS, explains:

> *It helps me a lot to rock rhythmically if I have to sit 'still', for example for a short meditation. I'm a lot calmer – and staying in movement means that my back muscles are less likely to lock up.*

You can make your teaching generally more inclusive by giving permission for small movements in traditionally static situations. For example:

> In final relaxation you may find that your body slows to complete stillness, or some peripheral movement may continue, perhaps in your fingers or feet, or maybe elsewhere in your body. The intention is to be as relaxed as possible, while maintaining a thread of attention. Let your body feel into how it needs to be to foster this state of being.

For more on stillness and stimming, see 'Stimming, shifting and fidgeting' in Chapter 5.

The 'difficult' student

I've talked a bit about 'difficult' hypermobile students in Chapter 2, and written in detail about reframing challenging relationships with students (including those with hypermobility and autism) in *The Yoga Teacher Mentor*,[6] so I'm going revisit the subject just briefly here.

Whereas allistic people generally have the capacity to absorb the 'rules' by a sort of social osmosis, autistic people are impaired (to differing degrees) in this regard and will often need to have them made explicit. By 'rules' I'm referring to a set of unspoken behaviours and responses that have particular significance to neurotypical people and which are required in neurotypical culture to keep everyone feeling happy and congruent with the group. Neurotypical people tend to be reactive to any breaches in the 'rules', ascribing to them meanings that may perhaps be present when an allistic person has committed the offence, but are rarely intended when the offender is autistic. In a yoga class context, this may lead to autistic students being branded as rude, disruptive, disrespectful and the like…when actually we are just getting on with things in the best way we know how.

Where an infringement of protocol is happening, my suggestion is that you assume the best intentions on the part of your student and name – in an open, friendly way – what needs to happen. For example:

> I love it when people are curious about yoga and have lots of questions. We're moving into a part of the class now which is about being quiet and reflecting inwards – being with what we already know – so I'm going to ask you all to let the questions fall away for a while and come to silence.

Or:

> It usually works best to have your mat facing this way. Then you can see me, and follow my visual cues, and I can see what you're doing and will know if I need to come and help you. How will that be for you? Would it be OK to turn the mat around?

It can be a lot easier to make allowances when you know a student is autistic. It's when the student is not identified as such and is doing their best to 'pass' as neurotypical that misunderstandings with allistic teachers tend to occur. (Autistic teachers will generally recognise another autistic student immediately, whether or not the student themselves is aware of their autism – we call this 'autdar'.) As teachers, we don't know why our students are doing what they're doing or being how they're being. They may be dealing with intense levels of stress, mental illness, pain or neurodifference, and a wise, sane and grounded teacher will cultivate an open mind. Offering kindness and compassion, while maintaining the necessary boundaries for safety and group cohesion, is in my view the way to go here.

Bunions (hallux valgus)

Yoga therapist Doug Keller describes a bunion as a zigzag of the big toe and first metatarsal: 'The big toe "zigs" in toward the other toes, while the metatarsal "zags" out, causing irritation and eventually calcification at the head of the metatarsal.'[7] You don't have to be hypermobile to develop bunions, but they are more common among hypermobile people – generally those in whom the forefoot and metatarsal arch collapse (overly pronate) on weight-bearing.[8] Because bunions destabilise the foot, they may play into hyperextending knee patterns, with the person locking their knee in order to create compensatory stability.

The big toe has its own abductor, abductor hallucis, which runs down the inner ankle and along the inner heel and inner medial arch to the big toe. When abductor hallucis is weak and lax, it's unable to resist the action of its antagonist, adductor hallucis, which, as you might expect, adducts the big toe towards the smaller toes. When a student frequently wears shoes, particularly tight and narrow ones, and seldom stretches their toes, all the toe adductors may be tight and constricted and the toes pinched together. If this is the case, they may find it helpful to use a toe spacer at night. You can buy these from yoga and dance shops, but the little device designed to separate your toes for painting your nails will work just as well. This will stretch out the toe adductors while your student sleeps.

Stretching is only part of the picture though. Your student will also need to strengthen their feet. We looked at how knock-knees play into overly pronating feet in Chapter 3 (see 'Knock-knees'), and considered some ways to work with this pattern. This information will be helpful for students with bunions. Indeed, if you just look at your student's big toes and don't address what's happening with their knees and hips, you are unlikely to make much change. Likewise, if you focus on leg alignment but neglect to strengthen the feet, any improvement is likely to be limited.

The following are some ways to prevent bunions from forming in the first place and, potentially, to halt or even reverse the progress of existing bunions. The degree to which this is possible depends on the amount of bony alteration that has taken place. Work will always be more effective in the early stages of joint change.

Big toe abduction

Have your student sit on the floor or in a chair with their foot flat on the floor. First, ask them to use their fingers to stretch the big toe medially away from its neighbour. They can also interlace their fingers between their toes for a five-toe adductor stretch.

Now, without hands, and keeping the mound of their big toe firmly on the floor and the lateral side of their foot also grounded, have them move their big toe away from the second toe, hold (if possible), relax and repeat. This is a difficult movement requiring subtle proprioceptive mapping, so if initially neither you nor your student can see much happening, don't worry. Just imagining the movement will help your student to create the necessary neurological connections. Given patience and practice, movement will be possible. Invite your student to notice how their medial arch lifts as their big toe abducts.

Activating the inner (medial) foot

Have your student sit as above. Ask them to lift their big toe, while keeping the mound of the toe grounded. Check that their foot stays in a neutral position, neither inverted nor everted. Invite them to notice the medial arch of their foot lifting. Now ask them to place their big toe down on the floor while maintaining the lift in the medial arch. This is the activation they need to find in their foot on standing. Have them lift and lower their big toe a few times, and then change sides.

Once your student is able to activate the arch from their big toe, Doug Keller suggests they try this:

> Sit on the floor or on a chair with your knees bent and your feet parallel. Lift all of your toes while keeping the balls of your toes and your inner heel grounded. See how much you can lift your arch, not just from the ball of the big toe, but also from the centre of the sole in front of the heel.[9]

As someone who does over-pronate, I love this feeling. Invite your student to notice how the foot action translates all the way up the leg and into the pelvic floor, where they will also feel some activation. The soles of the feet and the pelvic floor have a synergistic relationship.

Once your student can feel these activations in sitting, they can give them a try standing. Obviously this is a lot harder, as the medial arch now has to support their body weight. Cue them to press the big toe mounds and the inner heels into the floor to maintain the arch while they reach out through the big toes. Doug suggests, 'as if you're trying to extend [the big toe] forward to push a button as it comes down' rather than 'just pressing the tip of your toe down into the floor, which just scrunches the toe'.[10] This action of the big toe activates abductor hallucis.

Activating the outer (lateral) foot

Have your student start sitting as above. This time ask them to raise all their toes and then extend their little toe down to the floor. Invite them to notice their lateral foot and outer shin activating.

✳ ✳ ✳

For more foot exercises, see 'Strengthening the feet' in Chapter 3.

Working in asana

Once your student understands the basics of foot engagement, they can start to use them in *asana*. Pretty much any active yoga posture, standing, sitting or lying, offers an opportunity to work on foot strengthening and stabilisation. As Doug says, 'The fundamental poses of *hatha* yoga provide an opportunity for a complete workout for your feet that is highly effective for preventing, slowing, and even halting the progress of bunions.'[11] It's all in the how rather than the what. The same sequence of postures that promotes healthy foot biomechanics can also reinforce unhelpful foot habits if practised without awareness. As a teacher, it's therefore important to give your student frequent and consistent feedback, as they will easily lapse back into the old and familiar. Make sure your student comes out of postures and rests when they are too tired to maintain the new foot patterns. This is important for all students, but particularly so for those who are hypermobile. The following are some places in commonly practised *asana* where your student can work on foot alignment:

- *Dandasana* (Staff Pose). Check that your student maintains equal length along both sides of their heel and presses the ball of their foot slightly away. Make sure that their instep lifts and their foot does not invert or evert. They may find it helpful to practise this posture with their feet against a wall or against a block (they loop a belt around the block and place the ends under their hands).

- Downdog (*adhomukhasvanasana*). Cue your student to keep both sides of each heel evenly on the floor and extend equally through lateral and medial foot, lengthening and abducting the big and little toes. They can use a couple of blocks if their heels are not on the floor.

- Warrior (*virabhadrasana*) II and *parsvottanasana* (Intense Side Stretch). Make sure your student doesn't shift into a lunge, with their front knee jutting beyond its ankle. (This orientation tends towards stretch, and places more pressure on the front foot, while de-emphasising strength and engagement through the back leg and stretching the back foot towards pronation – whereas we're looking for a strong square base that gives both feet the best possible chance.) Ask them to press through both big toe mounds to lift their insteps, while lengthening away through the big and little toes, making sure that there is equal weight through both lateral and medial sides of the heels, and the central column of each foot is engaged.

- Warrior III (*virabhadrasana III*) and *ardha chandrasana* (Half-Moon Pose). One-legged postures increase the demand on the standing foot and are more advanced variations. Introduce them only when your student is proficient at maintaining toe space and medial arch when standing two-legged.

- *Vrksasana* (Tree Pose): This is another more challenging one-legged variation for finding foot activation while balancing. Make sure your student is maintaining the same foot alignment and stability as when standing on two feet.

Chiari malformation Type I (CMI)

As we saw in Chapter 1, CMI is a condition in which the brain stem and spinal cord are compressed, disrupting the flow of cerebrospinal fluid. Excessive mobility of the head and neck may play a role here. For more information, see 'Chiari malformation Type I (CMI)' in Chapter 1.

The Mayfield Chiari Center advises that those with CMI maintain fitness, and suggests yoga as a low-impact activity which, 'can help stretch and tone muscles, improve balance and reduce stress'.[12] The most common symptom of CMI is a headache that feels like intense pressure in the back of the head.[13] This can be triggered by vigorous exercise and by bending over,[14] so energetic yoga practice and head-down postures are best avoided.

On the whole, we want to offer the CMI student opportunities to strengthen their neck without overtaxing it, so I suggest interspersing upright postures with supine ones, in which the neck can rest. Many hypermobile people – with or without CMI – feel as if their head is too heavy to support, and neck pain is a frequent occurrence, so this approach will be helpful to all your hypermobile students. You can also offer specific neck-strengthening exercises. This one will strengthen the upper thoracic extensors and the deep cervical flexors:

- Have your student stand with their back to a wall, heels about 6 cm (3 inches) away, and their spine against the wall.

- Cue them to engage their abdominal muscles and lengthen their upper back as they draw their head and shoulders back until they touch the wall (or as close as they can get). Make sure your student's chin is down, in a neutral position, not tipped up. Their head will be pressed directly back, rather than tilted up. Have them hold their head in this position for about five seconds. Repeat three times. If your student's neck is stronger, go for five repetitions. Gradually work up to ten. When your student has mastered the movement, they can do it away from the wall, including it, for example in *dandasana*.

Once your student has some basic neck strength and an awareness of their own neck–shoulder–chest alignment, *ardha bhujangasana* (Half-Cobra Pose) can be another helpful neck strengthener. Again, check that your student's head is not tipped back, their chin is a little dropped and the back of their neck is long. Your student can lift up and hold for a few seconds, and also do lift and lower repetitions. Make sure they don't hold to the point where they are straining. This will be counterproductive.

A gentle restorative practice will be beneficial for all the usual nervous-system reasons – especially if your student is in too much discomfort or too deconditioned for more active work. Hypermobile clients with CMI who I have worked with as a yoga therapist have found some relief from gentle tractioning of the base of the skull away from the neck to create a feeling of length in the spine.

Chronic Fatigue Syndrome/ME

As we saw in Chapter 1, the relationship between general fatigue and Chronic Fatigue Syndrome is kind of ramped up and with bells on (see 'Chronic Fatigue Syndrome'). Alison, a CT-typical yoga teacher with CFS explains:

> It is a very different thing from feeling run down... When someone has CFS they simply can't do the energetic things that most of us take for granted – and doing so can lead to significant crashes and a worsening of the condition. Before I was diagnosed with CFS I tended to try to push through things and was a great believer in exercise being a way to shift fatigue. But now it's crystal clear to me that doing too much has a massive effect on me. I can end up feeling wiped out and having palpitations for most of the day after doing an extra brisk walk in the morning – even if it's a walk that I'm usually comfortable doing at a slower pace.[15]

My own CFS was triggered by chickenpox – but rooted in years of driving myself through exhaustion, sensory overload, inappropriate work situations and so on. (For more on my experiences of CFS, see 'Autism and neurodifference' in Chapter 1.) For me, the two definitive experiences of CFS – that make it different from routine fatigue – are:

- rest makes no impact on the fatigue: you go to bed exhausted...and wake up equally exhausted

- overshooting your edge by the tiniest increment can cause a relapse.

For example, towards the end of my recovery, I was slowly working towards being able to swim a kilometre once again (30 lengths in my local pool). I was feeling almost normal and had worked back up to 28 lengths. So near and yet so far! I decided to push it. I did 30. And I was immediately thrust back into the wearisome fatigue, palpitations, breathlessness...and all the rest. It took a fortnight of rest and slow rehabilitation to work myself back up to the 28-length mark again.

CFS symptoms fluctuate, and if you're having a good day, it can be very easy to overdo it, only to end up prostrate the next. To some extent, this kind of oscillation is unavoidable, but when extreme and unmanaged, it tends to perpetuate the fatigue state. Neilon, a CT-typical yoga teacher with CFS, says:

> *It's important to try and avoid the boom and bust. When I'm feeling reasonably well I have to be super-aware of not doing too much – especially things that feel good, like swimming in the sea. The refinement of awareness that we train in yoga really comes into play here. It's important to find the subtle cues that indicate when we are getting to the end of a sensible amount of energy to use, before there's an overshoot.*[16]

Recovery is possible, even with co-existing hypermobility (I recovered), but is slow and cumulative, and many periods of relapse are a given – and part of the process. For me, resolving immune system issues was key, so that I wasn't constantly being depleted by an endless series of viruses, as was changing my work situation and coming to understand that my body was not an indestructible machine, but a sensitive organism that needed good food, supplementation, plenty of rest and appropriate care-taking. For some people, CFS intersects with childhood trauma, and recovery will also require specialist embodied work to deal with the long-term effects of trauma on the nervous system.

A person in the acute phase of CFS is not going to be able to leave their house to go to a yoga class; this is a student you will be teaching one to one in their own home. For bedridden and very debilitated students, Donna Owens' book, *Yoga, my Bed and ME* is a helpful source of easy postures that will not overstimulate.[17] For those sufficiently recovered to be able to access a group class, an appropriate practice is still going to be gentle and restorative. The following are some general suggestions, applicable to both home and class settings:

- As fit and healthy yoga teachers and practitioners, it can be easy for us to forget how much energy goes into practising even a very simple *asana*. We may also underestimate the amount of energy required to engage in social interactions, fulfil the expectations for behaviour in a public space and deal with the ensuing emotions. Know that just having you in the room or being in your class may take a student with CFS to the edge of their capacity. In this situation, an hour of supported *savasana* (Corpse Pose) might be an ideal practice.

- Any progression needs to be slow, slow, slow, and always erring on the side of less when you're not sure. Lucy, a CT-typical yoga teacher (with no personal experience of CFS), says:

  > I had a student with chronic fatigue in my class. I must admit that afterwards he told me he had a flare-up the next day. My class is very gentle. I guess I underestimated just how slowly he needed to go and how much rest he needed.

  If you're the kind of teacher who likes to push people to do a little more: don't! This approach is not appropriate with students recovering from CFS – or for those with hypermobility, for that matter.

- There are many ways to do an embodied practice that don't involve moving. Fully supported restorative postures, in which the student can rest for 20 minutes or more, are a great resource, as is yoga nidra. Just resting and breathing, within a dedicated space, can be a fantastic practice for a student who is very depleted.

- If the student is up to it, gentle mobilisation in a lying or sitting position can help with general aches and pains. Allow plenty of time for rising from lying to sitting, to avoid exacerbating any orthostatic symptoms. In my experience, POTS is often present but undiagnosed in CFS – in hindsight, I can see that it played a significant role in my own chronic fatigue.

- Frame yoga practice as nurturing and restoring rather than as exercise. Donna Owens suggests thinking of yoga, 'as your time, quiet and peaceful, warm and cosy, time between you and your body, healing and renewing, breathing and calming'.[18]

- People with CFS are often, understandably, desperate to recover – I know I was – and this can dominate their thinking. Framing yoga practice as time simply to be with what is, rather than trying to change things, can offer huge relief. This shift in orientation from doing to accepting and surrendering can in itself be a key element in recovery.

Fibromyalgia (FM)

As I mentioned in Chapter 1 (see 'Fibromyalgia (FM)'), it's very common for people with joint hypermobility to be diagnosed with FM while their hypermobility is not spotted. Fibromyalgia is given as a diagnosis when no physiological cause can be found for the person's symptoms. If, however, they have genetic hypermobility, their symptoms do have a cause and, in my view, the fibromyalgia diagnosis is superseded. When a hypermobile student also has an FM diagnosis, I work with them as someone whose hypermobility is currently producing a lot of joint pain, sleep disorder, brain fog, fatigue and so on, so general recommendations would be to offer:

- easy basic *asana* with an emphasis on creating structure and stability
- plenty of opportunities for rest and relaxation
- invitations to offer awareness to embodied experience
- yoga nidra
- education about how the nervous system works and how it can become 'stuck' out of kilter.

FM is often diagnosed as a pair with Chronic Fatigue Syndrome. If this is the case, the suggestions for working with CFS above are also appropriate.

Labral tears of the hip

For me, having a labral tear, it has been useful to really warm up the hip well with movement and to change my expectation of the range of motion that is healthy for me now – this is mostly a mental challenge! I have found strengthening the muscles around the hip reduces my pain. I now add lots of other exercises and weight training to work on glute, hamstring and quad strength, and this has probably had the most positive impact.

Joelle (yoga teacher with HSD)[19]

The labrum is a fibrous cartilage lining of the acetabulum, which extends and adds stability to the joint, helping to manage joint forces and limiting excessive movement. The most common type of labral tear is at the front of the hip, where lack of blood vessels may create greater vulnerability. Posterior tears happen less frequently and are associated with movements that stress the back of the hip joints such as squats.[20] Laxity of the hip joint and/or hip dysplasia (in which an open, shallow acetabulum allows the femoral head to slip out of place) may predispose to labral tears.[21] According to dance physiotherapist, Lisa Howell, a further risk factor is absence or early loss (in utero) of the ligamentum teres, a small ligament, once considered redundant, now recognised as playing a role in femoral blood supply, which attaches from the head of the femur to the acetabulum. Lisa says:

> It seems that if this [ligament] is ruptured very early on, it doesn't cause too many problems, but the head of the femur is smaller, and there is a normal-sized hip socket. This means there's a lot more movement. The person can go into extreme hip positions quite easily without feeling like they're risking breaking anything or tearing anything.[22]

Not surprisingly, labral tears are more common among those with Ehlers-Danlos,[23] and I think we can reasonably extrapolate this prevalence to all forms of joint hypermobility.

The most common sign of a labral tear is a pinching feeling in the hip, often around the inside thigh or groin, when the joint is in a certain position (which position depends on the location of the tear). There may also be deep joint pain and pain at the back of the hip. Popping, snapping and clicking are also common,[24] as is (increased) instability in the joint.[25] Sitting for long periods may be painful, and there may be difficulty with activities involving hip flexion, such as putting on socks, walking uphill or climbing stairs. However, all of these symptoms can have other causes – hip flexor tendinitis, hernia or disc issues for example. An MRI is needed for a definitive diagnosis.

A common culprit for labral tear appears to be hyperextension of the hip joint together with external rotation, as in Warrior I (back leg) or a ballet *arabesque* (ballet dancers as well as yogis are believed to be more at risk for labral damage).[26] Subsequent pain may arise not in hyperextension but in hip flexion, as in *paschimottanasana* (Straight-Legged Forward Bend). Around

75 per cent of labral tears appear to be the result of repeated micro-trauma over a period of time.[27]

Ambitious practice may play a role in labral degeneration. *Yoga Journal* 'influencer', Laura Burkhart, explains how pushing for advanced postures was generative of her own labral tear:

> My body started telling me it was exhausted and didn't want to do long practices or extreme poses. Did I listen? No. I had big plans, work to do, classes to film, and bills to pay. One day, while demonstrating Compass Pose [*parivrtta surya yantrasana*], I pulled my left knee into my armpit and immediately felt a deep pain in my left groin. My initial reaction was frustration with my body for not keeping up with me. I pushed past the pain and continued doing everything I'd been doing. A week later, while teaching I demonstrated Side Plank [*vashistasana*] with my top (injured) leg in Tree Pose [*vrksasana*] and heard a 'pop'. That was the straw that broke the camel's back. I was in so much pain that I could barely sleep or walk for five months. During that time, to teach I either sat in a chair or hobbled around in pain.[28]

A further factor for Laura was giving up weight training, a decision she took, 'in order to increase my flexibility to get into *vishvamitrasana* [Friend of the Universe Pose], which would eventually be photographed for [a] Master Class article in *Yoga Journal*'.[29] The decision 'paid off'; advanced postures came within her reach – but at a cost. With a history of 14 years of dance followed by 16 years of yoga, specific work for strength was an aspect of movement practice that Laura couldn't afford to dispense with.[30]

While it seems pretty clear that labral tears *can* cause pain and limit mobility, there's an important caveat. Ariele Foster, physiotherapist and yoga teacher with a specialism in hypermobility, points out that some degeneration of the labrum is likely a natural part of the ageing process, and for the majority of people may be entirely asymptomatic.[31] (According to Ray Long, orthopaedic surgeon and founder of Bandha Yoga, up to 96 per cent of cadaver specimens have hip labral tears.)[32] Ariele cautions against ascribing all hip pain to labral degeneration, even where an MRI shows degeneration to be present, because, 'Correlation doesn't equal causation.' If you've been diagnosed with a labral tear, I recommend reading Ariele's article, 'Yoga and Your Hips: Deciphering Femeroacetabular Impingement and Hip Labral Tears'.[33] The same goes for all joint degeneration, by the way. Just because it's there, it doesn't mean it's causing your pain.

If you are teaching a student with a labral tear, guide them to do the following things:

- Avoid any movement that causes pinching, clunking or pain. Exactly what kind of movement that is will be individual to the student, so you will need to do some exploration together with them; however expect external rotation, extension and/or flexion of the hip to be a potential problem.

- Avoid extreme hip articulations.

- Stay actively engaged in postures.

- Work for hip stabilisation rather than 'opening'.

Amy, a CT-typical yoga teacher who has experienced a labral tear, says, 'I found hip extension quite irritating, as well as things like *baddhakonasana* [Bound Angle Pose], where the head of the femur potentially puts pressure on the labrum, and extreme flexion would pinch.' She suggests, 'using a bolster or similar to create space between thigh and torso' in Child's Pose (*balasana*), and in *baddhakonasana*, 'elevating the knee slightly with a block or bolster and placing a heavy sandbag close to the hip end and squeezing down the line of the femur'.[34] Joelle, who we heard from at the head of this section, says, 'External rotation, for example, in Warrior II or Half-Lotus [*ardha padmasana*], cause me some pain and irritation, but a block or support under my knee makes it possible to sit externally rotated.'[35]

However, what hurts and what helps depends on the precise location of the tear. Joelle was told by her consultant to avoid hip extension, but in practice hasn't found it an issue, whereas for Sasha, a CT-typical yoga teacher, *asana* was only problematic when she went too deeply into hip extension. She says:

> Engaging strongly with the glutes helped to put the brakes on, e.g. in lunges. Walking for any distance was the main aggravation. Relief came from working on stabilising the hip joint with lots of glute and hamstring strengthening, and, yes, it did take months of work.[36]

With conservative practice, rest and rehabilitation, it's often possible to reduce inflammation and manage labral tears without surgical intervention. Amy emphasises that labral tears can get better but that it takes time and that the key thing is to, 'identify irritating factors and avoid those things for a while before reintroducing them gradually'.[37]

Pelvic floor dysfunction

When we think about pelvic floor dysfunction, particularly in tandem with hypermobility, most minds immediately jump to weakness and laxity, with the general response being to throw some Kegels at it. While *hypo*tonicity does indeed tend to be a primary issue for hypermobile people, secondary *hyper*tonicity can become as much, or more, of a problem, and there may be a complex combination of hyper and hypo, with some parts of the pelvic floor being lax and unresponsive to movement cues, and other parts tight and unable to relax. Iyengar yoga teacher, Leslie Howard, who specialises in yoga for pelvic floor health, says that in her observation while *hypo*tonicity of the pelvic floor is the more common dysfunction in the population at large, among yoga practitioners *hyper*tonicity appears to be more prevalent, and she cautions against prescribing *mula bandha* and pelvic floor lifts to our students without proper information about their actual pelvic floor needs.[38] Care is particularly important when we are dealing with sensitive hypermobile systems, in which muscles are easily provoked into spasticity by over-zealous attempts at strengthening.

Pelvic floor structure

It's sometimes argued that as the pelvic floor muscles move in concert, learning about the individual muscles is not so valuable. However, as someone with a basically *hypo*tonic pelvic floor in which one specific area (the attachments to the region around the left sitbone) is *hyper*tonic and easily provoked into nerve-pinching contraction, I've found it immensely helpful to have specific language for different geographical parts.

As I mentioned in Chapter 3 (see 'Working with *bandha*'), the central body of the pelvic floor is configured like an eight, with one end at the tailbone, the other at the pubic bone and the eight crossing over at the mid-point (or perineum). The figure eight also has posterior 'wings' slung transversely (across) from sitbone to sitbone. The anterior (front) part of the figure eight is made up of a bilateral (one on each side) pair of muscles called levator ani. However, levator ani is also differentiated into three more distinct pairs of bilateral muscles. Starting from the front, these are: puborectalis, pubococcygeus and iliococcygeus.

Posterior to (behind) these muscles, and not part of levator ani, is a muscle called ischiococcygeus, or (confusingly) just coccygeus. Together with some of the fibres of iliococcygeus, ischiococcygeus forms the transverse (crosswise) sling part of the pelvic floor, with attachments on the sitbones. Piriformis lies very close to ischiococcygeus, and may become involved in any hypertonicity.

If you'd like to see these muscles on a simple diagram, I suggest Figure 2 (in 'The Pelvic Floor') at TeachMeAnatomy: https://teachmeanatomy.info/pelvis/muscles/pelvic-floor.

Exploring pelvic floor movement

Students often view the pelvic floor as a static structure, and are under the misapprehension that it's part of the task of yoga to make sure it stays that way – whereas in fact the pelvic floor is designed to move organically with the breath, in synergy with the thoracic diaphragm. Whether your student is hypo- or hypertonic in the pelvic floor, or a bit of both, the beginning of making positive change is becoming familiar with this natural, wave-like movement.

Depending on the knowledge and experience of your student, you may need to start by explaining the diaphragm and diaphragmatic breath. For example:

> The diaphragm is a large muscle that attaches to the underside of the lower ribcage. When you breathe diaphragmatically – a normal, relaxed breath – the diaphragm domes down on the in-breath (pushing the abdominal organs down and up so that the belly rises to accommodate them), and the pelvic floor pulses subtly down in tandem with it. On the out-breath, the diaphragm domes back up, and the pelvic floor also subtly lifts.

Students may arrive in your yoga room having internalised a paradigm of control with regard to their pelvic floor. To shift the emphasis here, I like to use sea creature imagery to convey a sense of rhythmic organic pulsation. Give your student some time to feel into these movements and get to know them.

If your student's pelvic floor is very tight or is shut down due to trauma, there may be little or no movement, or the movement of the pelvic floor may no longer be syncopated with the movement of the diaphragm. In this situation, I suggest that you invite your student to imagine the movement just naturally arising in their body, without effort. Sometimes, this is enough to re-initiate actual movement, but it doesn't matter whether that happens or not. Be mindful to frame not-feeling as one of the possible discoveries in this exploration, and as valid and useful. If you're teaching in a group situation, always articulate imagining as a possible approach, emphasising that the potential benefits are just as powerful as being able to feel a physical movement. This is an exercise it's not possible to get wrong.

If your student can feel rhythmic movement, invite them to slightly exaggerate it: on the inhale, allowing their pelvic floor to really relax and expand, so that the pubic bone, tailbone and two sitbones spread away...and on the exhale drawing the pelvic floor in and up, and pubic bone, tailbone and two sitbones towards each other. The intention is to develop pelvic floor articulacy, finding more and more places to soften and let go...and engage and contract. Invite your student to imagine any spots of tension releasing...and lax and unresponsive places waking up. Sensation can happen between the sitbones, between the tailbone and the vagina or penis, between the vagina and clitoris, up inside the vagina, up inside the anus... and so on. Being comfortable with using the proper words for the different parts in a straightforward way will help to dispel any feelings of shame or embarrassment your student may be experiencing. Avoid euphemisms, which will have the opposite effect, signalling that these are forbidden regions of the body, which may not be experienced or spoken of.

This exploration can be deep, not only from a physical point of view but also from an emotional one. Name for your student the possibility of experiencing sexual sensations, and of awakening memories of sexual and/or birth experiences. Some of these may be pleasant and some may not. Invite them simply to hold whatever happens in the container of their awareness, and if any experience feels overwhelming or too much, to stop, and refocus on where they are now and what they can see, feel and touch in the present moment. Emphasise the importance of going at a comfortable pace and not pushing through difficulty or distress. Recognise when a referral may be appropriate.

Cat or Cow – hyper or hypo?

In Chapter 3, we looked at Cat–Cow (*bitliasana–marjaryasana*) as a teaching tool for protraction and retraction of the shoulder blades (see 'Plank, *chaturanga* and shoulder stability'). These two postures can also help our students to get a handle on when and how the pelvic floor is contracted, and when and how it's stretched.

Have your student come to kneeling in the usual way and arc up into Cat (spinal flexion, posterior pelvic tilt), pressing strongly down into the floor through their hands and knees, and drawing their front body in towards their spine. In this position, invite them to notice how their tail bone moves towards their pubic bone – and their pelvic floor lifts in and up (engaged). Now have them shift into Cow (spinal extension, anterior pelvic tilt), still maintaining engagement. Hypermobile students may tend to hang in Cow, so emphasise staying a little engaged. Invite them to notice how their tailbone tips up and away, opening up (stretching) their pelvic floor. Students with hypotonicity will benefit from finding a sense of *mula bandha* as they move into pelvic floor opening (see 'Working with *Bandha*' in Chapter 3).

Once your student is familiar with these two orientations in Cat–Cow, they will begin to be able to feel how the movement of their pelvis affects their pelvic floor in similar ways in other postures. Remember the swan-diving forward benders in Chapter 3 (see 'Forward bends, "yoga bum" and hip versus lumbar flexion')? When swan divers fold forwards, their coccyx is angling back and away, and their pelvis is in a deep anterior tilt, which means that their pelvic floor is being strongly stretched. A forward bender working with more abdominal engagement (to lift their pelvis somewhat out of anterior tilt) will be actively drawing their coccyx towards their pubic bone, rather than sheering it away. In other words, their pelvic floor is engaged. You could say they have some Cat in their Cow or that their muscles are co-engaged. Is this a good thing? It depends. If they are weak and loose in the pelvic floor, yes, probably; if their pelvic floor is tight and needs release, the student is usually going to be better off finding more Cow in the movement.

Working with hypotonicity (too loose)

If you have established that your student is hypotonic in the pelvic floor, one of the primary tools for cultivating strength with awareness is going to be sensitive practice of *mula bandha*. Since I've already discussed *bandha* in detail in Chapter 3 (see 'Working with *bandha*'), I'm going to refer you back to that section for suggestions for introducing *mula bandha* to your students. And we'll be considering how too much *mula* can be harmful where the pelvic floor is *hyper*tonic in a moment. In this section, we're going to look at some further approaches to *asana* that can be helpful when the pelvic floor is loose and weak. Remember that there is a fine line between hypo- and hypertonic. Introduce strength work slowly and in small pieces, checking in with your student during the practice and at subsequent classes about any effects they have experienced and modifying your work accordingly.

There are many postures that facilitate pelvic floor engagement. What follows is a small selection to get you going. Once you have understood the principles, you will be able to come up with lots more yourself.

The elevator

It's not unusual for students with a weak pelvic floor to think they have been engaging – i.e. lifting – their pelvic floor muscles when in fact they have been bearing down, which is actually the opposite movement and is going to increase hypotonicity. Bearing down is what we do when we pee, poo or give birth vaginally. It's a push out rather than a lift up. If tilting their pelvis and exploring the movement of their pelvic floor on their breath hasn't helped your student to identify the sensation of lift, try this Kegel-type exercise, described by *Yoga Journal* editor, Meghan Rabbitt:

> Picture the pelvic floor muscles between your two sitting bones. Inhale, and as you exhale, draw the muscles together as if they were the two halves of an elevator door closing to meet in the middle. Once this door is closed, lift the elevator up and then release. Next, imagine the pelvic floor muscles between your pubic bone and tailbone. Inhale, and as you exhale, draw those muscles together in the same elevator-door fashion, lift the elevator, and then release. Now, draw all four elevator doors together at once, meeting at one point in the middle, then lift and release.[39]

The suggested repetition is five times. However, I'd probably start with three for a hypermobile student. Work up to practising two or three times a week.

Squeezing the inside thighs

Have your student lie on the floor with their legs bent and give them a yoga brick to place between their thighs. Ask them to squeeze the brick (engage their adductors), feeling the two sides of their transverse abdominis, just above their pubic bone at the front, draw in towards the midline. You want your student to work both slow- and fast-twitch muscles, so cue them to intersperse longer holds with short squeeze-and-release movements. Don't overtax them. Building up slowly is best.

Your student can also squeeze a brick in *samasthitihi* (Equal Standing)/ *tadasana* (Mountain Pose). Make sure you're using a light brick, not a wooden one – you don't want to break any toes! Again, intersperse longer holds with short squeeze-and-release movements. From standing, your student can lower into *utkatasana* (Chair Pose) and hold for a few breaths – or, if they are not yet strong enough to squeeze the brick for long, they can rest and then enter *utkatasana*.

Your student can also squeeze a brick in *dandasana* (Staff Pose) and *paschimottanasana* (Straight-Legged Forward Bend), in tandem with the forward-folding approach described for swan divers in Chapter 3 (see 'Working with too much hip flexion'). Ultimately, the idea is that your student can create the squeezing movement without the prop.

Half-Bridge (*ardha setubandhasana*)

This exercise is all about creating posterior pelvic tilt. Have your student set up for Bridge Pose (*setubandhasana*). Ask them to press their feet into the floor and tip their pelvis up off the floor, keeping their lower back long and flattish, so they are like a wedge, rather than a bridge. Hypermobile students may tend to lift too high, tipping themselves into an anterior tilt: cue them to lower down a bit and allow the lumbar curve to diminish. Invite your student to notice their pelvic floor doming in and up, and transverse abdomini engaging. Here, too, have them both lift and hold, and lift and lower as repetitions. Your student can also add a brick between their thighs if they find it helps them to create engagement.

Three-Legged Dog

Have your student enter Downdog in the usual way. Ask them to lift their right foot about 4 cm (2 inches) off the ground and hold it there for a few breaths. Their legs remain parallel. They should feel their pelvic floor lifting and engaging. Change to the left side.

Gomukhasana legs

Have your student come into *gomukhasana* (Cow Face Pose) in the usual way. Cue them to squeeze their inside thighs towards one another as they hold the posture for a few breaths. Then change sides. The squeeze may be easier to feel in the ashtanga vinyasa version of *gomukhasana*, a balance rather than a hip stretch, in which the legs are tight in together (more adducted) and the student sits on their heels.

Working with hypertonicity (too tight)

There are teachers who believe that pelvic floor hypertonicity is a silent epidemic in the yoga world, particularly in ashtanga vinyasa (in which *mula bandha* is used throughout *asana* practice) and in forms that focus on cultivating core strength. Heba Shaheed, physiotherapist and founder of The Pelvic Expert, explains that, 'People who spend a lot of time working out and holding onto their core muscles can develop tension in their pelvic floor because they keep these muscles switched "on" without giving the muscles times to relax and let go.'[40] Leslie Howard adds:

> It's…very important to remember that a tight muscle is not a strong muscle. A tight muscle is living in a state of contraction. It's not good at stretching or releasing or softening. If you cough and you need to contract your muscles, but your muscles are already contracted, there may not be very much more for that muscle to go.[41]

In this section, we're going to look at some postures for releasing and softening a hypertonic pelvic floor, restoring its normal capacity both to relax and to contract, and so to move synergistically with the thoracic diaphragm. As with hypotonic pelvic floor, there are many postures that are therapeutic for hypertonicity. These are just a few to introduce you to the principles and get you started.

Supta baddhakonasana

For *supta baddhakonasana* (Reclined Bound Angle Pose) invite your student to come to rest on their back, draw both feet in towards their groin and let their knees fall out to the sides. For maximum relaxation, offer your student a bolster to lie on (with the bolster tracking their spine, lower end against their sacrum). If necessary, support their head with a folded blanket or block. For hypermobile students, I suggest support under the knees (blocks or blankets) to prevent overstretching in the hip. You are looking to take the hips out of their maximum range of motion. Once your student is settled, invite them to imagine their pelvic floor relaxing and letting go, with the two sitbones, the tailbone and the pubic bone all releasing away from one another. As long as they are comfortable, your student can stay here for five minutes or so.

Ananda balasana

For *ananda balasana* (Happy Baby Pose) have your student come to rest on their back and, taking hold of their feet, bend both legs so that the soles of their feet are pointing to the ceiling and their knees are moving towards their armpits. If your student can't reach their feet, give them two belts to loop over. For pelvic floor stretch, it's important that your student remains in anterior pelvic tilt, so make sure that their tailbone is oriented towards the floor and their lumbar spine is slightly arched (extended). This is more important than having their knees close into their armpits or being able to catch their feet with their hands. Again, the invitation is to imagine softening and release in the pelvic floor. The hold time for a CT-typical student might be five minutes, but I suggest a minute or two for a hypermobile practitioner, less if they are unstable in the hips. Be guided by what feels comfortable for your student.

Malasana

Have your student come into *malasana* (Garland Pose/squatting), feet hip-width apart or a little wider. They can have their feet parallel to one another or turned out laterally – just make sure their knees are tracking their second two toes. Check that their knees are comfortable and not straining. If your student finds it hard to balance, have them lean their bottom against a wall. If their heels are floating, place a block or a rolled-up mat or towel under their heels. Invite them to imagine their pelvic floor relaxing and spreading. They can stay here for a minute or two.

Prasarita padottanasana

To enter *prasarita padottanasana* (Wide-Legged Forward Bend) have your student step out a little more than one of their own leg lengths. The stride can be adjusted a little in or out for individual needs. Their feet are parallel to one another. In order to create an anterior pelvic tilt that will stretch the pelvic floor, the forward bend needs to happen primarily from the hip (pelvic flexion) rather than the spine (spinal flexion). If your student can flex from the hip and bring their hands to the floor, ask them to do that. If they are tight in the posterior chain and tend to go into a lot of spinal (rather than pelvic) flexion, have them bend their knees (making sure that their knees don't medially rotate into a knock-kneed shape) and give them a chair or some blocks to place their hands on when they fold – or they can place their hands against a wall. If they are still in posterior tilt, choose a different posture. Have your student hold here for a few breaths, imagining their sitbones broadening away from one another and their pelvic floor spreading, from sitbone to sitbone and from tailbone to pubic bone.

Supported Bridge

Whereas the Half-Bridge variation in the previous section focused on posterior pelvic tilt and pelvic floor engagement, this Bridge offers a relaxed anterior tilt, designed to open and release the pelvic floor. Have your student lie on their back, arms by their sides, feet on the floor, hip-width apart and parallel, a little way from their sitbones. Ask them to press up into a bridge, lifting their hips and arching their lower back away from the floor. Place an upended brick under their sacrum and invite them to rest their back on it. If your brick has sharp edges, you may need to cover it with a folded towel for comfort. For a more restorative version of this posture, have your student lie over a bolster. (The bolster goes under the student's hips and horizontal to their spine.) If your student cannot lift up so high, lay the brick on its side or flat, but make sure that they are in anterior pelvic tilt. If your student cannot lift high enough to create the tilt, choose a different posture. Your student can rest here for up to five minutes, focusing on softening and releasing in the pelvic floor.

The role of mula bandha

It's my belief that by teaching *mula bandha* in an intelligent way we can offer students an opportunity to become familiar with the structure and movement of their pelvic floor and to feel into its tonicity, so that they can make informed choices about any pelvic floor practices they adopt and how they approach them. Unfortunately, not all the teaching on offer in this area is based on sound knowledge of pelvic floor physiology. It's not uncommon in the ashtanga world for *mula bandha* to be described as squeezing the anus. While there's nothing inherently harmful in this action (in fact it's very close to a yogic practice called *ashwini mudra*), if you do it consistently for 90 minutes, you're going to end up with a very tight arse and your pelvic floor out of kilter.

In any yoga class, it's likely that at least a few students already have hypertonicity of the pelvic floor, and that others are at risk of developing it, so if you're teaching *mula bandha* it's important to offer cueing that emphasises awareness, with some optional subtle engagement, rather than insisting on strong contraction, and to advise students explicitly against lengthy periods of gripping. Shelly Prosko, a physiotherapist and yoga therapist with a pelvic floor specialism, says:

> The way I teach *mula bandha* does not necessarily equate to a PFM [pelvic floor muscle] contraction. And many yoga teachers agree it is an 'awareness' and an energetic sensation of the pelvic diaphragm – not a squeeze or contraction. This is because we do know that more holding, tightness, and tension can potentially do you more harm than good. This overuse and holding can fatigue the PFM's, so that when it is time for them to perform their duties and actually contract to stop the flow of urine, they fail. Additionally, this holding can create or exacerbate a variety of pelvic pain disorders.[42]

If you are an ashtanga vinyasa teacher, be aware that where a student has active and uncomfortable pelvic floor hypertonicity, they may need to abandon *mula bandha* entirely for a time while they work on softening and re-establishing the relationship between pelvic floor and diaphragmatic breath. For some students, consciously engaging *mula bandha* only on the out-breath has helped to restore pelvic floor rhythm. Your student may or may not choose to return to using a full *mula bandha* in their practice, depending on how the *bandha* affects their pelvic floor tonicity once healthy function is restored.

For more information on *mula bandha* see Chapter 3: 'Working with *bandha*'.

Leslie Howard has a good course on hypo- and hypertonic pelvic floor, 'Yoga for the Pelvic Floor: Keys to Lifelong Health'. Find it online at: https://yogauonline.com/yogau-product/6661.

Postural orthostatic tachycardia syndrome (POTS)

As we saw in Chapter 1, POTS is a form of orthostatic intolerance that frequently (some would say always) co-occurs with genetic joint hypermobility. It can have a profound and disabling effect on the person's life or it can be a bit of a nuisance but pretty manageable. Like hypermobility, POTS often goes undiagnosed, especially at the less severe end of the spectrum. Many hypermobile students have no experience of life without POTS, and if the symptoms are relatively mild, may not be aware that there is anything out of the ordinary here ('Doesn't everybody get dizzy if they stand up too quickly?'). Where POTS is severe and debilitating, it may be quite obviously outside the normal range of experience.

In a yoga class, the most obvious signs of POTS are likely to be light-headedness, faintness, breathlessness and rapid increase in heart rate following positional changes such as:

- rising to sitting from a reclined position, for example *savasana*

- lifting to upright from a standing forward bend, for example *prasarita padottanasana* or *parsvottanasana* (Intense Side Stretch)

- lifting to upright from a head-back backbend, for example *ushtrasana* (Camel Pose), or *urdhva dhanurasana* (Upward-Facing Bow Pose) in ashtanga-style drop-backs.

Extreme heat usually makes orthostatic issues worse, so hot yoga classes are generally contraindicated for students with POTS.

POTS-friendly asana

While orthostatic intolerance doesn't go away, keeping generally fit and active is widely acknowledged by medical professionals – and POTS people ourselves – as being key to minimising its effects. Because yoga is a mindful, controlled activity, and practice can be done slowly, it often feels a little more accessible than most physical activities to those who generally experience palpitations, faintness and a racing heart as a consequence of exercise. The following are some simple strategies for enabling students with POTS to participate as fully as possible in *asana* work.

Head down

Have dizzy POTS students exit postures such as *prasarita padottanasana* slowly...slowly...slowly...and with the head down, so that the heart area unfurls first and the head last, keeping the chin slightly tucked for a few breaths before finally bringing the head fully upright. If the student's orthostatic issues are severe, have them step their feet in, with the head still down, and lower to Child's Pose before slowly uncurling to sitting as above, and from sitting slowly rising to standing. A chair can be a useful support for this transition – and the student can also move from sitting on the floor to sitting on the chair as an intermediate position, and from the chair to standing.

The skeletal-muscle pump

The movement of skeletal muscles in the extremities plays a role in the circulation of the blood (particularly the venous return to the heart) by squeezing the veins and so pushing the blood along them. Because veins are made of connective tissue, this muscular action is extra important for hypermobile people, in whom the vascular system may be slack and circulation therefore inefficient, with blood pooling in the feet, lower legs and hands. For people with POTS, long, static, standing holds, such as those often practised in the Iyengar system, can therefore be very challenging from an orthostatic point of view (as well as from the point of view of muscular hypotonia and lack of fascial and ligamentous support in a hypermobile body).

It took me decades to realise that the uncomfortable, numb, thick, tingly heaviness I sometimes feel in my lower legs and feet when I'm standing static is a sign of blood pooling. You can help your POTS students out by alerting them to the significance of sensations of this kind and cueing them into lower limb activity as follows.

ORTHOSTATIC MUSCLE SQUEEZES

Orthostatic squeezes – in which muscle contracts without creating movement – activate the muscle pump, stimulating circulation. They also, of course, create muscular engagement: win–win! You can help your POTS students in standing postures by offering hold times short enough for them feasibly to remain active throughout. Alternatively, have your student squeeze and release selective muscles repeatedly. If they are newer to yoga, less fit and more proprioceptively challenged, this approach can also help them to feel the difference between hanging in a posture and maintaining an active stance.

TREADING AND KNEADING

Having students with POTS keep supporting limbs in motion during longer 'static' postures can help them to maintain something closer to normal circulation. So, for example you could suggest:

- treading feet (and hands) in Downdog

- bending and straightening legs repeatedly in *utkatasana*, *parsvottanasana* and Warrior postures. This brings the added benefit of active muscle strengthening.

Arms down

When the arms are above the head, the vascular system has to work harder to circulate blood. While the majority of people with POTS will be fine with bringing their arms up briefly, for example as part of a sun salutation, holding the arms in a raised position for an extended period of time, as for example in Warrior I, may be more of a problem, making the person feel faint and dizzy. You can help POTS students by offering the following alternatives:

- Bringing their hands to their hips. This variation can be helpful where a student would also benefit from opening their collarbones. Cue the student to lift their thorax, spread their collarbones laterally and draw their elbows towards one another behind their back, imagining that each arm is an extension of its collarbone. Make sure they don't over-arch in the lumbar spine.

- Bringing their hands to prayer position. This variation can help to lift and stabilise the torso. Cue the student to press their thumb mounds into their breastbone...and lift their breastbone into their thumb mounds...while also pressing the palms together and opening their elbows to the side.

Note that both these modifications present alternative challenges. Rather than just giving your student a get-out, which can feel demoralising, offer them something to work on. They are more likely to engage with your suggestion if they feel they will be developing their *asana* work as a result.

Counterpose

Head-down counter-postures such as Child's Pose can be helpful for students with POTS, for example after a head-back backbend. Remind the student to come back upright from the counterpose slowly and bring the head up last. *Viparita karani* (Legs Up the Wall) assists venous return and is a useful counterpose after standing. Be aware, though, that for students with POTS, blood may quickly exit the feet and legs (because, when upside down, the walls of the veins provides less resistance in a hypermobile vascular system), so hold times here will also generally need to be shorter than for CT-typical students.

Limit static upright hold times

Remind everyone (not just your POTS students) that the stated hold time is just a suggestion and that the 'correct' duration for a posture is the one that works best for the individual. Highlight dizziness, faintness and sensations of blood pooling as indications that it's time to come to rest in Child's Pose, move through a vinyasa into the next posture or gently shake it out – as fits the style of yoga you're teaching.

∗ ∗ ∗

Some students with POTS will choose to accept a little light-headedness as just part of the deal, knowing that they are unlikely to actually pass out; others will not be comfortable with feeling dizzy at all. Personally, I've found that my orthostatic tolerance for dizzy-making postures has improved with sensible practice. I'm not aware of any research in this area, but it would be interesting to know if my experience is generalisable. Obviously, never pressurise a student to do a movement that makes them feel light-headed or otherwise unwell, and never put a student in a situation in which they're likely to pass out. It's common sense, isn't it?

Pranayama

I've had some quite critical responses from yoga teachers over the years for opting out of pranayama in yoga classes. Many teachers seem to believe that pranayama is a gentle practice and that it's safe and beneficial for everyone. If you skip it, they often assume that it's because you're resistant to quieting your mind and finding inner stillness.

Molly (yoga student with HSD)

As Molly notes, there is a general belief in the yoga world that *pranayama* is a benign practice that everyone can do safely without any modification. It isn't. There are several groups of people for whom most *pranayama* is contraindicated, and those with POTS (i.e. the majority of your hypermobile students) are one of them.

It's axiomatic in yoga that deepening the breath is a good thing. However, most people with POTS hyperventilate to some degree.[43] This isn't the kind of hyperventilation you can observe, for example as tight chest breathing or gasping for air; it's detectable only by medical testing. When we over-breathe, we eliminate too much carbon dioxide. While having too *much* carbon dioxide in the blood stream can harm the organs, having too *little* is also problematic and can cause tingling in the limbs, muscle cramps, dizziness, fainting, brain fog and anxiety.

It's perhaps not surprising, then, that hypermobile yoga practitioners I've talked to have described *pranayama* practice as uncomfortable, dizzy making, distressing, anxiety inducing and disruptive to nervous-system functioning. For me, too, *pranayama* has usually been unpleasant, the effect generally being to increase my tendency to breathlessness and make me feel light-headed. Julia, a trainee yoga teacher with hEDS, says, 'I have had negative effects from *pranayama* on my nervous system and my breath, which years later I'm still paying for.' She concludes:

I now approach pranayama with caution and respect, and wish others would be more circumspect. We really do need more research here.

In the course of my own POTS diagnosis, I was lucky enough to meet Dr Stephen James, consultant in cardiothoracic anaesthesia and exercise capacity, and director of the Breathlessness Clinic. Steve's interest is in the little-researched subject of how POTS affects breathing, and he is also a yoga practitioner, so I reckoned he would be the ideal person to ask why those with POTS might find *pranayama* practice unpleasant. He says:

I think the physiology of the dizziness from *pranayama* practice would be down to the following:

1. Baseline hyperventilation, usually secondary to increased rate and depth of the normal breath, lowers the carbon dioxide in the blood.

2. Lowered carbon dioxide leads to decreased blood flow to the brain, increased nerve excitability, and decreased oxygen release from haemoglobin around the body which contributes to fatigue. The level at which this happens varies between individuals and how long each individual has been at different carbon dioxide levels.

3. *Pranayama* practice tends to increase carbon dioxide clearance as the amount of breath going in or out is slightly increased. This further lowers the carbon dioxide levels and symptoms occur. The decreased blood flow to the brain causes all the head symptoms and is reproducible in most people with or without POTS.

4. The dizziness and other symptoms cause a physiological stress experience, which in most people sets off some degree of sympathetic drive, increasing their breathing rate and extending the problem. A concurrent increase in heart rate occurs but there are other factors commonly at play with this as well.[44]

So what should you advise a student with POTS to do during formal *pranayama* practice? For newer students and those with more serious POTS symptoms, I would suggest a comfortable, relaxed diaphragmatic (abdominal) breath. In other words, normal breathing. No special counts. No deepening. No lengthening of inhale or exhale. I would also suggest that they lie down for *pranayama* practice, because (a) it's more comfortable if you have POTS and (b) if everyone else is doing fancy breathwork, there's no guarantee that they won't join in, even if you have suggested this may not be a good idea. Should they make themselves faint, at least they won't have anywhere to fall.

For me, it's a rule never to teach any *pranayama* to any student (hypermobile or not) until I can see that they have a healthy, established diaphragmatic breath. If this is clearly present and your student wants to explore formal *pranayamas*, I suggest you introduce them with plenty of caveats about suitability, one at a time (so that if there are any ill effects, you will be clear which breath practice caused them) and ideally one to one. Check regularly whether the student feels dizzy or short of breath, and if they do, abandon the practice. You may have to be investigative here. For 30 years or so, I persevered through dizziness in *nadi shodhana* (Alternate Nostril Breathing) because I thought it was normal. I eventually worked things out for myself, but I wish a teacher had encouraged me to explore the appropriateness of this practice for my physiology at the outset.

What of ashtanga vinyasa and *ujayi* (Victorious) breath, which is practised throughout the posture work in the four ashtanga series? Since there is no scientific research on POTS and *ujayi* as far as I'm aware, I can only speak from personal experience here. I use *ujayi* as per normal in my own ashtanga practice and have not experienced any problems. However, *ujayi* as a stand-alone practice (when standing, sitting or lying static) is for me as horrible as all the other *pranayamas*. Perhaps this has something to do with adrenaline and appropriate use of the sympathetic nervous system (to stimulate energetic movement). I don't know. While hypermobile students I've taught have sometimes had difficulty maintaining the required core body engagement to establish and/or maintain an *ujayi* breath for *asana*, I haven't – yet – come across a student who has experienced exacerbation of POTS symptoms. That's not to say there isn't anyone who does.

The takeaway for teachers: expect that formal *pranayama* practices may be unpleasant for students with hypermobility and POTS, may make them feel faint and may even cause long-term nervous-system disruption. This is not because these students are doing the practices 'wrong'; it's because their cardiopulmonary system is functioning differently from that of their CT-typical, POTS-free counterparts. If a hypermobile student appears restless during *pranayama* practice, bear in mind that it may be that they feel as if they're going to pass out rather than that they have a 'busy' mind or are resistant to settling.

Sacroiliac joint problems

In Chapter 3 we looked at some ways to present potentially risky postures in such a way as to preserve SI joint health in the vulnerable hypermobile population (see 'Triangles, side angles, twists: preserving sacroiliac joint stability'). In this section, we're going to be considering the needs of hypermobile students who arrive in your class with existing SI joint pain and/or instability.

Like any other joint, the SI can subluxate. An added complication here is the bumpy edge-shape of the sacral segments – the five fused vertebrae that make up the sacrum. These fit into the ilia like jigsaw pieces, so once they have slipped out of place, it can be difficult for them to find their way back. (Think of a zip that has gone out of kilter.) SI joint subluxation can be chronic, and it can cause pain and inflammation, which further hampers the resetting of the joint.

SI joint problems usually manifest on one side (not necessarily the one with the dysfunction), occasionally on both, and may present as:

- a pain about the size of a penny piece on the SI joint

- dull, achy lower back pain, which may spread to the hip, buttock and/ or groin – sometimes with more acute episodes caused by muscles spasming in the lower back and hips

- sciatic-type pain (shooting/sharp/stabbing) in the buttock/back of thigh

- stiffness and reduced movement in the lower back/hip/pelvis/groin

- instability in the pelvis/lower back – as if it might collapse on standing/ walking/moving from standing to sitting.

Other back/hip conditions can produce very similar symptoms, so it's important that SI joint problems are diagnosed by an appropriate professional.

Subluxated sacrum

When we're working with SI joint issues we need to discriminate between those in which the sacrum is currently sitting out of true (subluxated) and needs to find its way back in, and those in which the sacrum is sitting correctly but is inflamed, poorly supported and in need of stabilisation. Let's look first at the subluxated sacrum.

Students with an SI joint that frequently subluxates may have their own special manoeuvre that helps it to 'relocate' – or may have a friendly professional (osteopath or physio) who knows how to manipulate it carefully back into place. The following is one conservative approach to realignment, versions of which are offered by some physios. You can try it yourself even if your SI joints are fine – do it on both sides, so you don't create an imbalance. If you do currently have an SI joint subluxation, just work with the side that experiences relief as a result. This exercise should feel good, especially if you are hypermobile and inherently somewhat lacking in myofascial support in the pelvis; if it feels uncomfortable, painful or just wrong: stop!

1. Lie on your back, feet hip-width apart and level with one another.

2. Lift your knees to 90 degrees (the position called 'table top' in some Pilates and body conditioning classes). Put your right hand on top of your right thigh and your left hand behind your left knee, keeping the knees and feet lined up in table top.

3. Press your right knee into your right hand, using the hand to create resistance, and at the same time push your left leg back into your left hand, again using the hand to create resistance, while maintaining table top – the feet and hips do not move. This is an isometric hold. Maintain it for 15 seconds.

4. Do the second side if appropriate.

5. Bring your feet back to the floor. Place a brick or block between your thighs and squeeze it for about 20 seconds.

If you're doing this exercise with a student, make sure they are clear that they should stop if they experience discomfort, and check in with them to make sure that any sensations they are feeling are along the lines of relief. Typically, one side will be uncomfortable (abandon that one) and the other side will offer the needed release. If both sides hurt, abort the experiment.

If the joint does go back in, hurray! However, your student is not all set to rock and roll. It takes time for the sacrum to 'settle' and the ligaments and fascia to reset. Even though the student may immediately be out of pain and able to move normally, they should be discouraged from launching straight back into their usual yoga practice. It's best to wait until the following day, when the focus needs to be on sacral stabilisation.

There are also a number of yoga postures that may help the sacrum back into joint. These work on the basis of opening the SI joint in order to allow space for the sacrum to drop back in, with the segments and the corresponding bony grooves on the ilia lined up. As such they are not necessarily good for long-term sacroiliac stability and should be seen more as first aid. Which posture works for which person is individual and requires some gentle exploration. There are a few things your student should know before they start:

- An effective SI joint release provides a sense of comfort and relief, not only during but also afterwards. If the posture is painful or just doesn't feel right, come out of it immediately. It may be doing more harm than good. If the posture has two sides, try it on the other one, because…

- As we saw in the exercise above, SI joint release most often needs to be done on one side only.

- Just because a particular posture helped someone else's SI joint back into true, that doesn't necessarily mean it will help yours. Pay attention to your own experience and proceed accordingly.

- Postures that reset the SI joints are sometimes the very same ones that may overstretch and destabilise them. Like any medicine, they should therefore be used in specific situations and in an appropriate way – followed up by ongoing stabilisation work.

The following are a few general suggestions to explore – carefully. A gung-ho approach is not going to be helpful. Sensitivity and mindfulness of sensation are required here. Your hypermobile student may want to hang out passively in the postures; however, they are more likely to find SI joint release if they practise with muscular engagement. Co-contraction (or balanced muscular force) helps to create even joint spaces and avoid further injury.

Backbends

As yoga anatomist and ashtanga vinyasa teacher, David Keil, notes, 'No one knows exactly what the SI joint is doing when you're in a backbend, including the researchers that have studied SI joint movement in as in-depth a way as possible with the technology that is currently available'.[45] Nevertheless, some hypermobile students with SI joint issues find relief in backbends. Senior Iyengar yoga teacher, Roger Cole suggests that, *supta virasana* (Reclining Hero Pose) can help to realign subluxated SI joints 'by directly pushing the top of the sacrum backward into place'.[46] Obviously, your hypermobile student should try this only if their lower back and knees are comfortable in this posture. If they are not, *supta virasana* supported by a bolster may be accessible. Some of my hypermobile students have found that *shalabhasana* (Locust Pose) can reset an errant SI joint. An advantage of this posture is that it involves only a little spinal flexion. Backbends that take the hips and spine to end range can in themselves be destabilising for the SI joints.

Twists

A gentle twist (in which one side of the sacrum rotates forwards and the other backwards) can also in some cases help to reset the SI joints. However, as Roger Cole warns, 'the wrong twist can easily make matters worse',[47] so if your student is going to experiment, it's best they do so cautiously, backing off if they experience any pain or discomfort.

Hip hikes

Hugging one knee into the chest tips one ilium up (the one with the knee towards the chest) while pitching the other down and away, therefore potentially opening up an asymmetrical space between the ilia and the sacrum. For most people with an SI joint 'out', one side of this posture will be painful and should be avoided, and the other will provide relief. This is the side to practise.

Abductions of the femurs

In postures such as *baddhakonasana* and *padmasana* (Lotus Pose), the thigh bones act as levers on the ilia, drawing the SI joint apart and potentially making space for it to find its way back into true. All the above precautions apply. If your student is in a lot of SI joint pain, this kind of manoeuvre may be very painful and contraindicated.

∗ ∗ ∗

Roger Cole notes that the key to putting the SI joints back in alignment may be in a posture that combines elements of all of the above:

> For example, practising *shalabhasana*…variations with just one leg lifted combines backward bending with one-sided pelvic tilting and works muscles against the resistance of gravity. Combining a *padmasana* action with a backbend (as in some forms of *matsyasana*, or Fish Pose) can often create both the space and the movement needed to put the sacrum back where it belongs.[48]

In-joint but painful sacrum

For some hypermobile students, SI joint pain is caused not by current subluxation but by general myofascial laxity allowing too much sacroiliac movement, with irritation and inflammation arising as a result.

Mild SI joint pain of this kind can often be managed and gradually reduced by the approaches to SI joint stability outlined in Chapter 3 (see 'Triangles, side angles, twists: preserving sacroiliac joint stability'). If the pain is more acute, your student may need to avoid some of these postures – *utthita trikonasana* (Triangle Pose), *janusirsasana* (Head to Knee Pose) and twists – entirely for a period of time, while they focus on rehabilitation and stabilisation, ideally with the help of an appropriate professional. Alternatively, Donna Farhi has an online programme, 'Yoga for Lower Back

Pain: Keys to Sacroiliac Stability and Ease of Movement', for working with more severe SI joint dysfunction. You can find it at: https://yogauonline.com/yogau-product/7746.

Other potentially troublesome and to-be-avoided postures are those involving abduction of the femurs (or spreading the legs wide), for example, *baddhakonasana*, *upavishta konasana* (Open Angle Pose), *samakonasana* (Equal Angle Pose/box splits) and Warrior II. Note that, as mentioned above, these are the very same postures that can, in some instances, reset the SI joints – because they draw the joints apart and make space for the bones to realign. They will not be helpful where the SI joints are in place but are sore and inflamed, perhaps with surrounding muscle spasm.

Some versions of Warrior I may also be problematic for those with SI joint pain. Usually, this posture will be more comfortable and less potentially destabilising if the back heel is off the floor and the foot and knee face forwards – as opposed to the heel on the floor and the back leg externally rotated. This latter is a perfectly good alignment in general, just often not appropriate in this situation. The heel-off Warrior enables the pelvis to face forwards all in one piece, and without the rear leg exerting rotational force backwards. If the student has mild SI joint discomfort and prefers to externally rotate their back leg and ground their back heel, try cueing them to orient their shoulders – not their hips – forwards, so that their pelvis can remain as one unit and the whole torso (not just the hips) rotates towards the front leg. If the second shoulder doesn't make it far forwards enough to line up with the first, that's fine.

Spondylolisthesis

Spondylolisthesis is a condition in which one of the vertebrae, usually in the lumbar spine, slips out of true with its neighbours. It can be completely asymptomatic, but if the displaced vertebra presses on a nerve it can cause lower back or buttock pain, pain radiating down one leg, numbness in one leg or (more rarely) weakness in one leg.[49] Eventually the transverse process may break off the body of the vertebra, creating major local instability. Spondylolisthesis can be congenital or a consequence of age-related joint degeneration. Among the hypermobile population, a history of practising extreme backbends may be a factor. Pilates teacher, Karen Ellis, who has spondylolisthesis, says:

> Doctors speculated my breakage happened by way of ballet dancing – where
> I forced my back into hyperextension, think *arabesque* and *grande jeté*, for

many years. Once my spondy was discovered, specialists told me never, never, never do [spinal] extension.[50]

The most common direction of slippage is forwards (anterolisthesis), in which case, as Karen says, deep backbending is the main contraindication, but vertebrae can also slip backwards (retrolisthesis), in which case it's forward bending that is not advised – so this is a situation in which you need detailed information from your student. That said, as with most conditions, any movement that makes pain worse and/or further limits movement possibilities is to be avoided. Baxter Bell, yoga teacher and medical doctor, says, 'Now, I don't think this implies that you cannot do any of those actions, but it would be wise to limit those movements to a more limited range (not moving to the full position you are able to take) and assess how that movement impacts your symptoms.'[51] Good practice also when working with hypermobility of course.

Students with anterolisthesis

While deep backbends are not advisable with anterolisthesis, postures such as *shalabhasana* and *setu bandha* (Bridge Pose) practised low, controlled and with repetitions, as described in Chapter 3, will be helpful for the strengthening and stabilising that is important for students with this condition (see 'Backbends for strength'). If your student is tight in the posterior chain, as those with anterolisthesis sometimes are, they will also benefit from hamstring and gluteal mobilisation. *Supta padangushtasana* (Supine Big Toe Pose), with a yoga belt, is a good place to start, as the spine is neutral and supported by the floor in this posture.

Retrolisthesis

Students with acute retrolisthesis may need to avoid forward bends entirely. If the student has less pain and more movement possibilities, guide them to approach any forward bend as if it is a backbend, bending their knees if necessary and tipping forwards in spinal extension, stopping just before the point where their spine needs to shift into flexion. In other words, they are aiming to 'swan dive' (see 'Forward bends, "yoga bum" and hip versus lumbar flexion' in Chapter 3). If you teach a vinyasa style, involving many forward bends practised at speed, I strongly suggest that you refer any potential students with retrolisthesis to a more appropriate style of practice, with a knowledgeable teacher. They are at risk in a vinyasa class. A practice designed for those with lumbar disk herniation will often be appropriate.

For more information on spondylolisthesis see the 'Spondylolisthesis' section in Chapter 1.

Thoracic Outlet Syndrome (TOS)

The thoracic outlet is the space below the collarbone where nerves and blood vessels pass through the lower neck/upper chest area into the arm. Thoracic Outlet Syndrome occurs when the nerves, and sometimes also blood vessels, in this area are compressed, usually by tightness in pectoralis minor and in the scalene muscles, the latter of which attach to the first rib and pull it up towards the collarbone, closing up the thoracic space. The symptoms are a vague hand/arm pain, difficult to pin down to a precise location, and tingling in the hands and fingers. TOS is sometimes mistaken for carpal tunnel syndrome or a repetitive strain injury.

TOS is particularly common among hypermobile people, a major cause in this population being inferior shoulder subluxation (when the humerus slips forward and down out of the socket) due to muscle hypotonicity and joint laxity.[52] The habitual posture of many people with this kind of subluxation will be shoulders rounded forwards and dropped down.

When a student has TOS, it's helpful to gently coax neck, shoulder and upper chest muscles to relax, so opening up the thoracic space. Once the muscles have let go a little, there will usually be a role for general shoulder strengthening to improve the integrity of the joint, but strong muscle building is not appropriate where muscles are hypertonic. Maintaining arms raised – as in Warrior I or *utkatasana* – will aggravate TOS for most people. Suggest to the student that they keep their hands on their hips or in prayer position, thumbs at the sternum.

Yanking on the arm or shoulder to try to stretch it is likely to cause muscles to go into even tighter spasm. The emphasis when working to release TOS is on *gentle* and *mobilisation*. Strong stretches are not going to be helpful here. Roger Cole, describes a key intention of practices for TOS relief as being, 'to lower the first rib away from the clavicle'.[53] This image may help your student to understand where release needs to happen and space needs to be made. Postures that will move them in this direction are those in which the chest opens and the shoulders roll back.

Restorative matsyasana

Have your student lie over a rolled blanket or bolster placed horizontal to their spine at the mid-point of the thoracic region. The student's head can be on the ground or supported by a block or two. For most people, the posture works best with the arms down, a little way from their sides, backs of the hands on the floor (as in *savasana*). The arms can be supported with blocks or folded blankets or towels if necessary. Make sure that your student is well supported in the joints but that there is room for expansion and opening to happen. Invite the student to notice:

- their front ribs lifting and separating

- the shoulder points – where the head of the humerus protrudes at the front of the shoulder – broadening away from each other and dropping back towards the floor

- their shoulder blades falling towards each other (into retraction)

- their chest lifting and broadening

- the manubrium (the top part of the sternum) lifting.

As long as they are comfortable, they can rest in this position for five minutes.

Mobilise the scalenes

Another key intention with TOS is to loosen and relax the scalenes. Roger Cole explains:

> Whenever the scalenes contract, they grow broader, potentially putting pressure on the nerves between them. This compression is amplified if the muscles and surrounding fascia are thickened by chronic tightness, or if they go into spasm.[54]

The scalenes are responsible for tilting the neck, so if your student habitually holds their head to one side, it's likely that one set of scalenes is hypertonic.

You will probably be familiar with the basic form of this exercise. This version is customised for hypermobile students, and the detail is important. It may make a difference between the movement being beneficial for your student and actually making their neck situation worse, so take time to read through and be sure to explain the subtleties to your student.

You may have done this exercise with a hand on your head. We are going to use a towel. This is because:

- a person with TOS will probably find the arm-up position uncomfortable or impossible

- arm-up is likely to make a person with POTS feel dizzy or faint

- using a hand tends to encourage the person to pull on their head, which is not the intention here.

If your student has POTS, they will usually be more comfortable doing this exercise sitting down.

1. Have your student lower their right ear towards their right shoulder until they feel a comfortable (not extreme) stretch on the left side of their neck. They flip the towel over the left side of their head and hold the ends with their right hand. Ask them to inhale and press their head up into the towel for a count of about five (less if they start to feel breathless), and then exhale slowly and naturally to release and relax their right ear down towards their right shoulder – not pulling it down with the towel, just letting it relax. Cue them to imagine their first rib falling away from their neck. Repeat three times.

2. Now have them let the towel go and drop their right ear towards their right collarbone, finding a gentle edge and holding there for a few breaths, imagining their first rib falling away from their neck.

3. Now have them drop their chin towards their right collar bone (so they are looking at the floor), again feeling their first rib dropping away and so opening up the thoracic space, and holding for a few breaths.

4. Have the student bring their head upright (slowly if they have POTS). Invite them to take a few moments to notice what they can feel and mark any changes for themselves. Then do the second side.

This exercise is about relaxing and mobilising. It's important not to strain or hold the positions too long, even if they feel good. If the neck is overstretched, muscles may respond by going into spasm.

As an added bonus, your student will also be releasing and mobilising the trapezius and sternocleidomastoid.

Vascular issues

As we saw in Chapter 1, there are particular considerations with regard to physical activity for people with the vascular type of Ehlers-Danlos (vEDS) and Marfan Syndrome – conditions in which the vascular (circulatory) system is particularly fragile. Inappropriate exercise can be potentially life-threatening for those in this group, so the contraindications here need to be taken very seriously.

Mild to moderate exercise is generally considered helpful for people with both vEDS and MFS, so if you're teaching a gentle yoga class, there shouldn't be any particular problem here. Just make sure that vEDS students are well padded in any lying-down practices to avoid bruising. If your class is somewhat more challenging, you need to be aware of the following risk factors:

- Long (isometric) holds in strong postures: isometric contraction causes blood pressure to rise and increases the risk of blood vessel rupture.

- Fast-paced sequences that take the person beyond aerobic range (about 50 per cent of capacity).

- Demanding inversions, such as shoulderstands and headstands.

- Heavy lifting, for example, basing in an acroyoga practice (as opposed to lifting light weights for strength and tone, which is beneficial).

- Straining: for newer students with vEDS/MFS, this may mean that sun salutations are out – whereas for those who are fitter, a slow-paced sun salutation could be OK.

- Classes in which the person feels they have to keep up and in which they are not encouraged to rest whenever they feel tired. Be aware that even if you repeatedly give your student permission to rest, they may not feel able to take it when others in the class are moving fast and the group energy is rising.

- Hot yoga: heat causes the heart to beat faster, creating greater vascular demand.

- Classes designed to push limits, encouraging more, longer, stronger.

- Strong *kriyas* (cleansing practices) and *pranayamas* (breath practices), for example *kapalabhati* (Shining Skull Breath), *dhauti* (Purification

Breath) and *bhastrika* (Bellows Breath), which may place stress on the vascular system.

What constitutes 'moderate' shifts a little in line with the person's general fitness levels, and it's entirely possible that a somewhat more physically demanding class may be suitable for a very active student with vEDS/MFS, but you need to be sure that they are aware of the potential risks and that they have talked to a cardiologist about what's appropriate for them as an individual. Bear in mind, too, that different people have different attitudes towards risk, and while some students with vascular issues will prefer a conservative approach, others may lean more into challenge. As long as the person is fully informed, in my view it's their call. As a teacher, it's our responsibility to make sure the student understands whether a posture involves strong isometrics or a *kriya* is likely to raise their blood pressure and so on – and with less experienced students we may need to be very proactive here.

Yin and Restorative Yoga

Five years ago, I was constantly hyper. I never relaxed. My nervous system was a mess. I would say now that I had low-level trauma derived from being a black autistic guy in a white neurotypical world. I tried meditation but couldn't sit still. Then I found restorative yoga, and everything changed. I wouldn't say I'm totally chilled now, but I know when I'm off centre and need to get on my mat for a stillness and quiet break.

Eddie (yoga practitioner with hEDS)

There's a lot of confusion out there about yin yoga and restorative yoga, with many people (including some yoga teachers) believing them to be the same thing, while others assume that 'yin yoga' is a generic term for a gentle form of *hatha* yoga. As you'll see from this chapter, knowing exactly which yoga is what is important when we're considering what might be an appropriate practice for someone with hypermobility. So let's start by defining some terms.

What is yin yoga?

The origins of yin yoga lie in the Taoist yoga taught and practised by martial artist, Paulie Zink,[1] a style that includes both long, slow holds typical of what we now think of as yin, and dynamic postures. Back in the 1980s, Paul Grilley[2] spent a year studying with Paulie. He subsequently tweaked, twisted and developed what he had learnt, dropped the dynamic work and taught his new, slow, passive approach to teachers such as Sarah Powers.[3] It was Sarah who coined the new name, yin yoga.[4]

Bernie Clark, yin yoga teacher and author of *The Complete Guide to Yin Yoga* explains that:

Most forms of yoga today are dynamic, active practices designed to work only half of our body, the muscular half, the 'yang' tissues. Yin yoga allows us to work the other half, the deeper 'yin' tissues of our ligaments, joints, deep fascial networks, and even our bones.[5]

In other words, yin yoga is concerned with those tissues prominently affected by the genetic hypermobility syndromes. So what does it mean to 'work' these tissues in the context of yin yoga? According to senior yin teachers such as Paul and Bernie, a key intention of yin yoga is to 'stress' the fascial tissues. Whereas muscles can be stressed in a healthy way by fast repetitions, the appropriate stressor for fascial tissue is slow, passive loading maintained for a period of time – yin holds are generally five minutes and upwards. Bernie says, '*Stress* is the force we apply to our tissues and *stretch* is the resulting elongation, if any, that results from the force.'[6] However, stretching is not the only possible outcome of stress; according to Bernie, stressing the joints can also create strength and stability, because, 'During the long-held, static stress on our connective tissue, biomechanical changes occur at a cellular level: the fibroblasts, chondrocytes and osteoblasts that rebuild our fascia, ligaments, cartilage and bones respond to the mechanical strains that they experience.'[7] Strengthening ligaments and fascia? That sounds like a good thing for hypermobile people, doesn't it? We'll be talking more about if, when and how later in this chapter (see 'Is yin yoga appropriate for hypermobile people?').

While Bernie is clear that yin yoga is a practice for stressing rather than stretching the fascia, if you ask students, and indeed teachers, what yin is all about, most will talk about deep stretch in passive postures held for a long time. In what I think of as the classic style of yin (the one I learnt back in the day from Paul Grilley and have encountered since then in many generic yin yoga classes), any propping tends to be introduced to enable a student to access a posture, rather than to support joints or reduce range of motion. However, as yin yoga has gained in popularity, it has evolved into rather a broad church. At the other end of the spectrum from 'classic' is an iteration much closer to restorative in feel and intention. In his book *Brightening Our Inner Skies*, my colleague, yin yoga teacher Norman Blair, describes a version of yin practice as concerned with comfort as with challenge.[8] If you want to see a posture fully propped for relaxation and ease, check out the first image in the '*Savasana*' section, on page 182 of *Brightening Our Inner Skies*.

The metaphysics of fascia

Yin yoga's preoccupation with fascia is more than just physical, though. At the heart of yin lies meridian theory. Paul Grilley explains:

> Spiritual adepts from the earliest times have described an energy system of the body that is vital to its health. In India they called this energy *prana* and in China they called it *chi*. The Chinese Taoists founded the science of acupuncture, which described in detail the flow of *chi* through pathways they called 'meridians'. It is *chi*, in all its forms, that keeps us alive.[9]

Central to Paul's approach to yin is the work of Dr Hiroshi Motoyama, a yoga-practising Shinto priest who is also a double PhD scientist with a long track record in researching the science of bodymind. His work suggests that the locus of the meridian system is within the fascial tissues. Another well-known researcher in the field, Dr James Oschman, expands upon this theory:

> All movements, of the body as a whole, or of its smallest parts, are created by tensions carried through the connective tissue fabric. Each tension, each compression, each movement causes the crystalline lattices of the connective tissues to generate bio-electric signals that are precisely characteristic of those tensions, compressions and movements. The fabric is a semiconducting communication network that can convey the bioelectric signals between every part of the body and every other part.[10]

If this is indeed the case, the implications for hypermobile people – those of us whose fascial tissues have a different tensile quality – are immense, complex and wide-ranging. As far as I'm aware, these possibilities have been discussed little, if at all, within the medical and scientific establishment, and are generally considered a bit woo-woo. The possibilities for future research are fascinating though. If you're interested in developments, organisations to follow are the Fascia Research Society (https://fasciaresearchsociety.org) and the Fascia Research Congress (https://fasciacongress.org).

Another prominent thread of yin yoga practice lies not in the Tao but in Buddhist mindfulness meditation practice. Teachers such as Sarah Powers and Norman Blair (who is a student of Sarah's) have focused on yin as a practice of presence. Sarah says:

> Yin takes you deeper into where you are, not out to where you think you should be. This approach challenges us to rethink what *asana* is about. It marries meditation and *asana* into a very deep practice... Yin yoga challenges you to sit in the pure presence of awareness. It's hard in a different way than

active *asana* practice, but in a way that's more profound and satisfying as well as more beneficial to the deeper tissues.[11]

As such, a gentle well-propped yin practice may offer potential as a mindfulness practice to those hypermobile students for whom sitting meditation is inaccessible (see 'Sitting meditation' in Chapter 2).

What is restorative yoga?

Restorative yoga doesn't want to stress your fascia, or any other part of you, although it, too, involves long, slow, passive holds. Its remit is to relax, renew and restore, using plenty of props to make sure that your body is fully supported. A typical restorative hold time is between five and 20 minutes, and a key intention is to create conditions for practitioners to drop into the parasympathetic nervous system, where rest, integration and profound physical and emotional healing may occur. Because intense, hard-edge stretching can trigger a sympathetic nervous-system response (not least if you're hypermobile and worried you're about to dislocate!), end range of motion is off the menu here.

Restorative yoga was originated by B.K.S. Iyengar – hence the incorporation of many props. While some current approaches have cut loose from their anchorage in the Iyengar system, becoming more free-form in their orientation, others remain heavily Iyengar influenced. The downside of the latter may be an unhelpfully didactic approach to propping – which can present difficulties for neurodivergent hypermobile people with particular sensory needs – and a formulaic relation of posture to ailment. Whereas, when taught by a teacher with trauma training and awareness, restorative has the potential to be a powerful trauma-healing practice, the ethos of the more traditional kind of restorative work can sometimes be the opposite of trauma-appropriate. That said, as always in yoga, the 'what' of the style is often less significant than the 'who' of the teacher – their understanding, experience and particular orientation to yoga practice.

What is gentle *hatha* yoga?

Gentle *hatha* yoga doesn't really belong in this chapter. It gets a mention because it's often confused with yin and restorative approaches. A general descriptor really, rather than the name of a style, gentle *hatha* is a slow and not too physically demanding yoga practice, often geared to those with limited physical capacity. While this type of practice may include some yin and/or restorative sections, it's not necessarily passive (it may include basic standing and active sitting postures) and does not necessarily involve long holds.

Is yin yoga appropriate for hypermobile people?

After years of practising yin yoga and not having a clue what I was supposed to do or feel with my body, I've come to the conclusion that we hypermobile people should do restorative yoga rather than yin. I am convinced that the only way to do it safely and really let go is with the use of props.

Luis (yoga practitioner with HSD)

Well, now, this is a question and a half. As I mentioned in the Introduction, it isn't my intention for this book to be a dogmatic set of prescriptions and prohibitions. Hypermobile people are a diverse group of individuals, with differing capacities, needs and intentions for practice. That said, there are some general considerations to take into account when deciding whether yin yoga is a helpful practice for someone with genetic hypermobility – and if it is, what kind of yin and what might be some provisos.

Yin yoga as fascial stressor

Let's assume, first of all, that we're talking about yin yoga, as described by Bernie Clark, as a fascial stressor. For most living organisms, the right amount of stress provides the necessary stimulation for strengthening and repair. Proportion is key here. Too much stress tips the balance into injury and attrition. We know that hypermobile connective tissue is by definition more fragile and less capable of withstanding stress than the genetically typical version (although many factors, such as age, strength training and possibly the particular genetic variation the person has, may offer protection against damage in the short and sometimes in the longer term). Given that hypermobile connective tissue is generally already experiencing more stress than it can cope with just in the course of the activities of daily life, one question that arises is whether it actually needs any more. If more stress is appropriate, it seems sensible to assume that the amount that is going to be beneficial will be far smaller than that which benefits genetically typical fascia. Indeed, hypermobile people know this from our everyday experience of being in a body. We generally cannot do as much, for as long, as a CT-typical person can.

Yin yoga as stretching practice

I love yin yoga, but I am getting to the opinion that yin doesn't like me very much. The stretching feels soooo good, but I'm pretty sure I overstretch all the time. Moving out of a posture can be really painful. I'm not sure that I should actually be doing passive stretches.

Deborah (yoga practitioner with HSD)

While for teachers such as Bernie Clark the intention of yin yoga is to strengthen and stabilise the fascial structures, in a significant proportion of the yin yoga classes that happen every day in yoga studios and community centres across the land, stretching is a key objective. Consider the following, fairly typical, class descriptions:

Yin yoga is a calm class, where you will hold seated postures for long periods of time in order to increase flexibility and encourage a feeling of release and letting go. (Frame Studio, London)[12]

Here's a beginner yin yoga class for full body flexibility that doesn't require props. (Yoga with Kassandra, YouTube)[13]

Yin yoga is a stilling practice that cultivates space within both body and mind, whilst increasing flexibility, range of motion in your joints, and body awareness. (Yoga Soul, Manchester)[14]

As we saw in Chapter 2 (see 'Passive stretching'), hypermobile people tend to love a good old passive stretch – and a little targeted and carefully calibrated stretching, when practised in tandem with strengthening and stabilising work, can be helpful for releasing contracted muscle and restoring joint balance. 'Targeted' and 'calibrated' are key words here, though. Although yin is a slow, passive form, it's not necessarily gentle. Most yin postures have fearsome potential as stretches, and if practised to an extreme in terms of range of motion and duration can be highly aggressive for ligaments, tendons and fascia. A skilful teacher can help their hypermobile student to work preferentially into particular areas of tightness and constriction rather than flopping into familiar and already overstretched places.

While just enough yin can help a spasming muscle to let go, paradoxically too much yin can actually contribute to muscle spasm, with the nervous system responding to attempts to create more extensibility in a system that is already excessively lax by causing particular muscles or groups of muscles to clamp down hard (or harder) – a scenario many hypermobile practitioners will be only too familiar with. In this situation. a combination of Pilates-style conditioning, together with gentle mobilisation and myofascial release, is likely to be most helpful. (For information on myofascial release, see 'Myofascial release (MFR)' in Chapter 7.)

Yin yoga and edge

Yin yoga offers a fertile ground for the cultivation of edge: the art of finding the sweet spot that holds the potential for expansion into our experience in all dimensions. When we push too hard, the result is constriction and shutting down, our nervous system becomes hyperactive and we may feel pain and cause injury. When we fight shy of any kind of challenge, we may feel bored, zoned out or disengaged, and fail to experience growth within our practice. I will be discussing edge in a lot more detail in Chapter 7 (see 'Edge'), and I certainly do feel that working with it is an essential part of practice as a hypermobile person. Here I want to add a caveat or two. When yoga teachers advocate for yin as a practice for hypermobile students, they sometimes seem to be making an assumption that being aware of our own edge is (a) always possible and (b) a preventative against all harm. It isn't either of those things, especially if you are working with limited proprioception and vulnerable connective tissue. If you get injured practising yin yoga, it does *not* necessarily mean that you were paying insufficient attention to your edge or pushing it. And there are definitely times when, as hypermobile yoga practitioners, we are not adequately resourced in terms of proprioception, nervous-system stability and fascial integrity to engage with a practice that may potentially challenge us in all of these areas.

Yin yoga as letting go

In yin classes I was always told to let go, yield, etc. If I let go in paschimottanasana [Straight-Legged Forward Bend] or a split, I go to the maximum of my flexibility and it will either increase my hypermobility or will give me an injury.

Eva (yoga teacher with hEDS)

Slowing the adrenal response and cultivating parasympathetic mode is generally helpful for hypermobility – I'll be talking more about this in the section on restorative yoga below (see 'Restorative yoga for the hypermobile nervous system'). However, getting with the project of release and letting go can be a challenge for a hypermobile person in a yin yoga class. While the language of surrender may be intended to point to nervous-system relaxation, and ultimately to a kind of metaphysical ease, for a student with hypermobility, it may primarily connote pain and dislocation. This is not to say that those of us who are teachers should not be using words like 'release' and 'let go', but we do need to think carefully about what they might mean to particular groups of people in our class. (Hypermobile students are not the only ones who may experience difficulty here; those with unresolved trauma may also struggle with 'letting go' as a remit of practice when offered without qualification and adequate support.) Suggesting multiple approaches to being on the mat rather than facilitating one-track processes is generally going to be helpful and inclusive. One possibility for teachers might be to invite exploration of the continuum between holding on and letting go, noticing where more and where less holding is helpful (on physical, emotional and mental levels) and feeling into what is optimal in each moment (the edge) without needing to make anything change.

Practising yin yoga in a beneficial way

I think it's important that we each find our own safest practice. For me, a mindful modified yin practice is very nourishing. But I do not dislocate and most of my [other] practice focuses on building strength.

Sara (yoga practitioner with HSD)

There are those who would say that yin yoga is inappropriate for hypermobile students. The yin yoga class description for Yogahome (London), for example, includes the rider:

[Yin yoga] is recommended to all wishing to actively and deeply stretch their body, and therefore not recommended to those with hypermobility, hyperflexibility, spinal disc issues or unstable joints.[15]

But, as we have seen, yin yoga does not necessarily connote deep stretch, and there are easy ways to modify a yin practice in order to make it safe and beneficial for the majority of hypermobile people. In this section we're going to consider some of them.

Propping

I've been practising yin yoga regularly for about six years. I always use props, especially to support my hips and make sure I don't compromise my dodgy SI joints. This works well for me.

Femi (yoga teacher with hEDS)

For the average CT-typical practitioner, yin yoga is most likely to centre on freeing up joint movement and accessing versions of postures requiring more flexibility. Indeed, the first section of Bernie Clarke's book, *Your Body Your Yoga*, is entitled 'What Stops Me?'.[16] For hypermobile yinsters, on the other hand, the question is more likely to be along the lines of, 'Where are the brakes?'. On the whole, practising yin yoga safely as a hypermobile person means taking care to ensure that joints stay well out of end range of motion. Because those with joint hypermobility have reduced proprioceptive capacity, and therefore cannot necessarily tell whether our joints are at end range or not, modification frequently entails using props in such a way as to make reaching end range impossible. This might mean, for example:

- placing folded blankets under the knees in Reclined Butterfly

- folding forwards onto a bolster rather than the legs or the floor in Folding Butterfly, Dragonfly or Caterpillar

- placing a bolster under the up-side leg in Reclined Twist

- placing a bolster under the back in Reclined Saddle

- placing a folded blanket between the bottom foot and the knee that rests on it in Square (open Shoe Lace)

- sitting on blocks in Seated Saddle.

Creative exploration is the essence of propping for yin. The possibilities here are endless, and the application will be unique to each individual. Expect your needs – and if you are a teacher the needs of your students – not always to be the same. What worked yesterday, is not necessarily going to be what best serves today...next week...or next year. Neither will it be the same first thing in the morning as just before lunch or late at night.

Limiting hold times

While a typical hold time on offer in a yin yoga class might be five minutes, for me personally an appropriate hold tends to be a minute or so. As a restorative yin yoga teacher, a key principle that I want to impart to my students, especially the hypermobile ones, is: when you're cooked, get out of the oven. The optimal hold time is not the one that the teacher sets, but the one that works for the individual. It's always OK to come out of a posture at any point. If you're a teacher, make sure you communicate this permission to your hypermobile students – in such a way that they really believe it – and repeat it at regular intervals. I usually introduce the hold time something like this:

> You have five minutes to explore this posture. You can stay in it for the full five minutes, or you can stay in it for a minute or so and then come out. It's entirely up to you. Longer is not necessarily better.

Engaging muscles

> *I love yin, but I keep my muscles fully engaged instead of letting go. This feels a lot safer. I used to do yin more as a passive stretch, but I got injured.*
>
> Ty (yoga practitioner with vEDS)

I'm with Ty on this one. Rather than completely relaxing into yin yoga postures, I prefer to squeeze and release, activating certain muscles and softening others, so that I stay selectively engaged. While it's not unusual for hypermobile students to start out their yoga life happily hanging out at end range in their joints, with the process of time and experience, for many of us this kind of noodling comes to feel – and be – fairly precarious. Where the bones allow for extreme joint opening, active muscular support helps to preserve the integrity of the joint and to protect against subluxation and dislocation.

Muscular engagement also offers greater proprioceptive feedback, which may be why some yin practitioners – me included – find it more satisfying. In the worst-case scenario, passivity in the joints can lend itself to feelings of disembodiment and lack of containment.

Stimming, shifting and fidgeting

I love practising yin on my own, but if I go to a class I have difficulty with the emphasis on staying still. I feel physically uncomfortable and get more and more anxious. I sometimes have the impression that teachers think I'm not willing to stay with my thoughts and feelings, but this isn't so.

Nella (yoga practitioner with hEDS)

Whereas in a vinyasa-based practice we might be looking to experience stillness through the eye of movement, in yin yoga we are typically looking to experience stillness through being physically still. For some hypermobile people, the physical part of this can be challenging in unintended ways. Hypermobile tissues offer less than usual resistance to pressure, so hypermobile practitioners will often experience discomfort from floors and the weight of one body part on another more quickly than a CT-typical person might. Padding can help, but under 20 feather beds, some of us will still feel the pea. For this reason hypermobile students may need to change position frequently. We may also need to move because we sense tissues overstretching or joints losing integrity and about to subluxate or dislocate.

Hypermobile students who are also autistic may need to stim in order to stay present to their experience (see 'Stillness and stimming' in Chapter 4). Stims are sometimes interpreted as fidgeting by allistic teachers, and as symptomatic of resistance to the project. In reality, as we have seen, repetitive movement – thumb twiddling, hair twirling, face stroking and so on – is conducive to inner stillness for autistic people, and is to be welcomed in a neurodiversity-aware yoga space.

If you're teaching yin and aiming for inclusivity, my suggestion is that you give your students plenty of permission to move gently. While a yin yoga practice is not a walking meditation or a dance movement class, on the other hand we don't want our students to feel they have to be like mausoleum statuary. Teachers often worry about one student's movement distracting others in the room. In my experience, this only happens when movement of any kind has been outlawed. When subtle movement is articulated as a possibility, other students shifting and turning becomes like the creaking of the ship: just another texture of the voyage.

To set the context for movement-friendly yin practice, I might say something like:

Internal stillness has a quality of aliveness. It devolves out of being in a living body and having the capacity to tune in to that body moment by moment and honour its needs. Some people are drawn into physical stillness by a yin yoga practice. For others, mindful presence requires some movement. The yin yoga postures are not intended to be fixed and rigid, because bodies are not fixed and rigid but are cycles of blood and breath, atoms in flux. Notice if and when your body needs to move, and feel free to allow it to shift organically.

Is it still yin?

I've tried different approaches to yin, such as strengthening some muscles or not letting go completely, but I don't think this is really yin yoga – is it?

Kara (yoga teacher with HSD)

The only yin that works for me is supported positions that don't involve a stretch. Probably technically more restorative yoga than yin.

Asma (yoga teacher with hEDS)

Propping, engaging, moving…this does beg the question of whether we are still in the realms of yin yoga. If yin is defined as a passive form in which we follow the line of least resistance and let go into the joints, I guess not. Nor are highly propped approaches such as Asma's likely to be stressing the fascia very much. Does any of this matter? Perhaps only if you're a purist. For me, it's important to know the original purpose and intention of a yoga practice, and to understand how we are changing the purpose and intention when we colour outside the lines. If the adapted version accommodates those for whom the original is not accessible, I'm all for that.

But it feels fine

In Chapter 1, we discussed the relationship between hypermobility and hypermobility syndrome: hypermobility as a benign, perhaps even in some situations advantageous genetic difference and hypermobility that causes some degree of pain and pathology (see 'Hypermobility compared with hypermobility syndrome'). A question that frequently arises is whether those with hypermobility which is currently not problematic should be taking the same precautions against over-mobilisation as those for whom hypermobility is already generating difficulties.

While we know that factors such as strength and fitness, stress levels and perhaps the type of genetic variation are probably involved, a complexity of working with hypermobility is that there is no reliable way of predicting for whom hypermobility will become a syndrome. On the yoga mat, this means that some hypermobile practitioners will have no problem with strong passive stretching and may enjoy this kind of practice, and we can only make a guess at whether or not they will experience negative consequences in the longer term. What we do know for sure is that those with genetic hypermobility are at risk of going on to develop morbidities and co-morbidities, some of which may be relatively mild, others of which may be life-altering. Consider Jana's story:

As a young person, I was very fit and active. I did ballet and was a competitive ice skater. I never had a problem with the flexibility side of things – whereas I could see that some of my friends did – but I thought that was a good thing! It all started to go wrong when I was at university. I was unhappy away from home and under pressure academically. I wasn't able to skate much and started doing a Flex class regularly – so less strength and more stretching, which I now know destabilised me. It began with a dislocated hip, and one thing led to another. I had a string of injuries and started to experience intense fatigue. I had to leave my uni and go back to live at home. I was eventually diagnosed with hEDS and POTS. In my early thirties, I am studying again and am also doing a lot of Pilates to gain stability, but I still need to use a mobility scooter sometimes to get around, and I think that will be the case for the foreseeable future.

I take the view that it is important for yoga teachers (and other movement professionals) to be able to recognise hypermobility in their students and to have enough knowledge to educate them in a basic way about:

- what hypermobility is

- what the potential risks are

- which ways of working are most likely to be safe and beneficial.

With this knowledge, hypermobile students can make informed choices about how they choose to practise and what degree of risk is acceptable to them. When we're dealing with practice habits that support health and biomechanical function versus those that can potentially disable long term, the stakes are very high, and in my view it's appropriate for teachers to err on the side of careful and conservative. If you're a hypermobile student, remember that CT-typical teachers do not always appreciate the fragility of hypermobile tissues and the sensitivity of our systems. If you feel that a practice or approach is wrong for you, trust your instinct.

For more information on working with students whose hypermobility is currently experienced as benign, see, '"Resistant" students' in Chapter 2.

Restorative yoga for the hypermobile nervous system

As we saw in Chapter 1 ('Adrenaline levels, hypermobility and PTSD'), raised adrenaline levels, together with a nervous system that is chronically sympathetically dominant, are a feature of hypermobility. Hypermobile people who are also autistic are likely to be dealing in addition with chronically elevated levels of the stress hormone cortisol (also produced in the adrenal glands). The consequences for mental health may be far-reaching, and at the extreme end may result in self-harm, eating disorders and panic attacks, as well as playing into chronic fatigue and pain. In this section, we're going to be considering how restorative yoga offers a way of regulating the nervous system and pacifying the adrenal response.

A quick primer on the autonomic nervous system

The autonomic nervous system (ANS) is the part of the nervous system responsible for regulating unconscious body processes, such as heart rate, breathing and digestion. The ANS is subdivided into two branches which function reciprocally: the sympathetic nervous system (SNS) and the parasympathetic nervous system (PNS). When the SNS is more active, the PNS is more dormant, and vice versa.

The SNS is designed for situations of high alert, activity or crisis and is associated with the fight/flight/freeze response. In an SNS state, hormones such as adrenaline and cortisol cause blood pressure and blood glucose levels to rise, the heart rate to accelerate, muscles to contract and pupils to dilate. Blood flow is diverted away from the digestive and reproductive systems. The PNS, on the contrary, is associated with 'rest and digest'. It lowers the heart rate, relaxes muscles, slows breathing and directs blood flow into the in-testines and reproductive organs to facilitate relaxation, recovery, repair and – on an emotional level – integration.

Broadly speaking, physically challenging practices, such as sun salu-tations and backbends, and energetic *pranayama*, such as *kapalbhati*

(Shining Skull) and breath retentions, activate the SNS. Practices such as slow breathing, meditation, restful *asana* and guided imagery (as in yoga nidra) allow us to drop into the PNS. It could be said that restorative yoga is a specific for the parasympathetic nervous system.

What restorative yoga can offer

There are multiple elements in a good, well-rounded restorative practice that can help to regulate an overstimulated hypermobile nervous system.

Deep rest

As we discovered in Chapter 1, living in a hypermobile body can be fatiguing in multiple ways (see 'Fatigue'), the sum total of which may feel, and be, overwhelming. Restorative practice offers space for the body simply to *be* for a while in a space of total rest, without anywhere to go or anything to do. From an adrenal point of view, senior Iyengar yoga teacher Roger Cole explains that:

> The adrenal hormones are catabolic, which means they foster biological processes that burn energy and break down cellular structures. If you activate the adrenal glands over and over again without sufficient recovery in between, your body becomes depleted and exhausted, and you are susceptible to a variety of illnesses.[17]

Deep relaxation turns off production of adrenal hormones and promotes production of anabolic ones – those concerned with building, production and growth.

Secure(r) embodiment

A well-held and well-supported restorative practice can help to anchor a hypermobile practitioner into a body that may feel vague, erratic, permeable or unstably constituted. Emphasis on feeling into the body (rather than pursuing out-of-body states) is helpful here. The aim is to create a ground of embodiment which is secure and reliable enough to provide a safe basis for exploration of internal experience.

Support

Support through propping helps to maintain hypermobile joints – as far as possible – in a neutral position during complete relaxation. (How far this is possible is a moot point, which we'll be addressing later in this chapter – see 'Does restorative yoga present any risks for hypermobile practitioners?'.)

The intention here, however, is not only to ensure physical safety, but also to enable a sense of emotional security. For this reason, soft props (bolsters, blankets and so on) are preferable on the whole. According to restorative yoga teacher, Jill Pransky, we are looking to, 'support passive postures with props in such a way that the body and mind feel grounded, safe and integrated'.[18]

An opportunity for internal focus

It can be no news to anyone that we live in a society that has commodified attention. Restorative, yin and *hatha* yoga teacher, Melissa West, says:

> In the attention economy, there are many external factors from smartphones, computers, marketing, to social media that direct our attention, mostly up and out of our body. It is said that we check our phones 150 times a day and touch them 2,600 times a day. This not only causes a deficit of attention, but also overwhelm of our nervous system.[19]

Restorative practice offers us a dedicated space for following the skein of our attention deep into the centre of ourselves. By taking time to witness what we meet there with kindness and curiosity, we create opportunities for held emotions to be felt and discharged, for old hurts to be integrated and for intuitive wisdom to arise. Through this process, over time, we may become gradually more able to respond to our experiences – the good, the bad and the ugly – in a more reflective rather than reflexive way. For highly sensitive hypermobile people, who may often feel at the mercy of a storm of feelings, release from this kind of reactivity can be particularly needful.

Restorative yoga for pain management

We have already seen (in Chapter 1) how chronic pain of a variety of kinds is a factor for many people with hypermobility. For some, pain may be a dominant feature, and relief from it an urgent desire. For others, pain may be more intermittent, low-level and manageable, and here the main need is for good nervous-system regulation to mitigate against any escalation.

If you cut your finger or break a bone, pain is an indicator of physical trauma – and a preventative against using the injured body part in ways that will interfere with healing. We tend to assume therefore that when pain is present, so is physical trauma (together with the need for restricted movement), but this is not always the case. Chronic pain is the result of hyperactivation of the nervous system, often triggered by multiple small and larger traumas. Yoga therapist, physiotherapist and pain specialist, Neil Pearson, explains:

Many changes occur in the nervous system when pain persists, and these changes can increase the experience of pain independent of new injury. For example, research shows that the nociceptors become more easily stimulated and are able to send more signals when pain persists. At the spinal cord, similar changes occur, with the production of more receptors, the engagement of previously inactive receptors, and increasing resting excitement of the spinal cord neurons. All of these changes allow more danger signals to travel up to the brain. In the brain, changes can occur that distort perception of the painful body part, impair motor control and proprioception, interfere with perception of normal sensations, and sensitise the emotional and attention areas of the brain during pain perception.[20]

Luckily, as Neil points out, 'Science shows that there are techniques that can alter the nervous system and thus alter pain in a positive and lasting way.'[21] According to his review of the research, effective, evidence-based approaches include:

- education – knowledge does actually change physiology

- physical activity

- imagery (for example, imagining a body part as without pain and able to move freely)

- mindfulness practices

- meditation

- breathing practices.[22]

Conversely, it has been demonstrated that attempts to ignore or suppress pain do not lessen it, whereas, Neil says, 'Acceptance and observation do.'[23]

Hypermobile people with severe chronic pain have often become afraid of any kind of uncomfortable sensation. Because body parts are supported and movement is minimal, a restorative practice can feel like a safe-enough place to begin to re-encounter their body and offer attention to sensations. Rachana, a yoga practitioner with hEDS, says:

Going to a restorative class was incredibly scary for me. At that point, there was nothing I could do that didn't hurt. But I found the bolsters and blankets very comforting, and I began to realise that, if I was careful and didn't go to extremes, I could put my limbs in different positions without anything going wrong.

Mindfulness and meditation, with a focus on noticing and accepting our embodied experience, lie at the heart of restorative practice, and classes can include gentle education about pain processes, as well as appropriate guided imagery, where there is a focus on hypermobility and/or chronic pain. Whereas the kind of *pranayama* that might be offered in more active and upright classes is contraindicated for many hypermobile people (see 'Pranayama' in Chapter 4), observing naturally occurring breath while supine, as in restorative practice, is going to be appropriate and helpful for most. Not active as such, restorative yoga can provide a gentle impetus towards expanding possibilities for movement and initiate reconditioning.

Guidance for restorative teachers

As the teacher of a hypermobile student in chronic pain, you will need to offer a lot of context and holding, and it's important that you yourself understand something about the dynamics that prolong pain beyond the point where it indicates acute injury. While your student's pain is not a result of present-time organic harm or pathology, it is 100 per cent organically real, and before you can begin to help them to dissolve it, you first need to validate it – otherwise your student is likely to think you don't believe they are really in pain. Remember, people with hypermobility have often been dismissed and discredited repeatedly by 'helping' professionals, and may be sensitive to any suggestion that this is happening again. Conversely, being taken seriously can be very validating. Dan, a yoga practitioner with hEDS, says:

> It was very important to me that my teacher understood that I really was in a lot of pain most of the time, and that she believed that I actually would dislocate if I lay down unsupported. Previous teachers seemed to think I was being dramatic. Being believed was very healing emotionally.

It's important to begin gently. If your student feels that they are under threat, their nervous system will start to go into overdrive, and this is the opposite of what we're looking for. The objective is to enable them to feel safe and supported. Asking your student what they might need in terms of propping, and following their lead, will generally help them to feel that they can trust you. Remember that for some students the initiating injury or injuries may have been the result of overly pushy or inattentive yoga teaching, or teaching without awareness of the ramifications of hypermobility. A conversation on entering a posture might go something like this:

Teacher: I see you're choosing to miss this posture out. Is it painful for your hip?

Student: Yes, I can't put my leg in that position.

Teacher: If you need to leave this posture out, that's completely fine, but we may be able to find a way for you to be in a safe modified version where your leg is comfortable and supported. Would you like to explore that?

Student: Yes...maybe... As long as I don't have to do it if it hurts.

Teacher: No, I don't want you to be in pain, so I would suggest that you don't do any posture that hurts.

Student: OK, I can give it a try.

Teacher: I'm going to place a bolster here, with a folded towel on top. Would you like me to support your knee with my hands as you lower it down?

Student: Yes, that would be good.

Teacher: Now lower your knee down slowly and carefully... I'm going to move my hands out now... Let me know how that feels.

Student: It feels fine. I don't think I need the towel.

Teacher: OK, lift your leg a little bit and I'll take the towel away. Make sure you come out of the posture if you start to feel that you've been there long enough, even if it isn't the end of the set hold time.

While a remit of working with chronic pain in general is to re-establish a sense of robustness, when we are teaching a hypermobile student, we need to remember that their connective tissue is actually not robust, and that there is a basis to their fear and anxiety – even if it has escalated to an unhelpful point. Rebuilding confidence in their capacity to move has to be balanced with a sensible, hypermobility-informed approach to how much of what, how fast and how far.

Chronic pain that does not resolve may have its origins in emotional trauma, particularly if the person:

- appears disconnected from their body

- is disturbed by their internal imagery

- is afraid of focusing inside

- is unable to breathe in a regular, relaxed, diaphragmatic way

- has a pronounced startle reflex.

In this case, invite the person to practise with eyes open, and give plenty of permission for them to focus their attention elsewhere than inwards or on their body. An appropriate referral would be to a Somatic Experiencing therapist, a trauma-informed Phoenix Rising yoga therapist or a body-based psychotherapist.

Neil Pearson's article 'Yoga Therapy in Practice: Yoga for People in Pain' is full of great advice and suggestions for teaching people in chronic pain. You can find it at: https://paincareu.com/wp-content/uploads/2019/02/IJYT-Yoga_Chronic_2008.pdf.

There is more information on practising yoga when in pain in Chapter 7 (see 'Working with pain').

Does restorative yoga present any risks for hypermobile practitioners?

As we have already seen, the emphasis in restorative yoga is on complete physical support for absolute comfort and ease. In general, this is a pretty safe situation for a hypermobile person, but even a restorative practice can go pear-shaped. Bear in mind that for many hypermobile people, sleeping is a high-risk activity. Most of us with hypermobility are accustomed to waking up with joint pain and minor subluxations; those more severely affected may need to wear splints and braces at night to keep joints in a neutral position, and for a minority of hypermobile students, bracing may be necessary in a restorative practice too. Kim, a yoga practitioner with hEDS, says:

> I always loved restorative yoga but initially I had a lot of problems with relaxing in the long savasana because my knees would spontaneously dislocate. Then my teacher suggested I try using the braces I wear at night. That totally fixed the problem. I now use my wrist braces too.

Postures need to be not only supported but also supported in such a way that joints cannot splay and subluxate when the person relaxes. Joint integrity is more likely to be compromised where there are dysfunctional muscle patterns (which in hypermobile bodies there usually are), in which some muscles are very tight and unable to release, and others are switched off and fire inadequately, so that the joint is pulled askew. In this situation, in addition to a well-propped restorative practice, structural repatterning work with a suitably skilled physiotherapist, yoga therapist or other bodyworker will also be of benefit.

The bottom line is that no activity is completely safe and appropriate for every person all of the time, and as teachers we always need to be paying attention to the individual, modifying appropriately for their needs and referring where necessary. On the whole, though, restorative yoga with a hypermobility-aware teacher is going to be a good bet for most hypermobile students, whether they are currently very deconditioned and afraid of moving or physically fit and active.

6

Hypermobile Children and Yoga

My mum makes me come to yoga, but I do really like it. It makes my body not hurt so much, we move around a lot, and I have fun with Megan, my friend.

Poppy (eight-year-old yoga practitioner with hEDS)

This chapter is written, first, with parents and teachers of hypermobile children in mind, and includes some great advice on how to approach yoga with this student group from my colleagues Iris Waller and Melissa Palmer, who between them have many years of experience of teaching yoga to hypermobile children. Second, this chapter is aimed at adult hypermobile yoga practitioners and teachers of adult hypermobile students who are curious about how early developmental differences may continue to affect movement patterns in later life – an area I find fascinating.

The overview

For some children, hypermobility is life-impacting from early years, whereas for others it may present few if any issues and may go unremarked. Ehlers-Danlos Support UK notes that, 'It is not uncommon for a genetic condition to first become apparent during puberty, alternatively symptoms can be triggered by a trauma, such as a virus, many years down the line.'[1] As in adults, hypermobility in children is often dismissed, and it can be very difficult to obtain an accurate diagnosis. Ehlers-Danlos Support UK says:

> EDS/HSD is poorly recognised in children, with a long delay in the time to

diagnosis. This results in poor control of pain and disruption of home life, schooling and physical activities.[2]

Beth Smith, mother of Emily, who was diagnosed with hEDS at the age of 12, says:

> In retrospect, we know Emily had shown symptoms since she was two years old, but because EDS is not well known to doctors, she went undiagnosed for far too long… We know from our own experience that seemingly trivial complaints the doctors ignored when Emily was young – 'growing pains' at night, difficulty walking, difficulty writing, frequent sprains and strains, easy bruising, headaches, fatigue, poor sleep – were really early signs of EDS. Those signs were completely missed by every doctor who saw her, even as they became more and more obvious as she got older.[3]

While failure to recognise joint hypermobility traits and refer on the part of doctors is usually down to ignorance and the belief that joint hypermobility is extremely rare, there are those who insist that hEDS and HSD are fabricated syndromes. Even post-diagnosis, carers and children are not out of the woods in this regard. In January 2020, The Ehlers-Danlos Society reported on Facebook that it had:

> …been hearing from a growing number of families and individuals sharing their experiences of being diagnosed with a factitious disorder, either imposing ill-health on self, or, more typically a parent on a child. We note that Ehlers-Danlos syndromes are being listed as a condition to be concerned about when looking for a factitious diagnosis.[4]

It's common, too, in paediatric settings for parents/carers to be told – misleadingly – that there's no point in seeking diagnosis for their hypermobile child, because there's nothing that can be done for them. In fact, knowledge brings power and the capacity for skilful management, which can make an enormous difference. Before her diagnosis, Emily was a semi-bedridden wheelchair user. Four years post-diagnosis, Beth says:

> [She] has improved greatly… She is learning to drive and rarely needs her wheelchair now. She still struggles with dislocations, pain and fatigue, but she is better and we are deeply thankful for the care she has received that has allowed her to gain function back.[5]

For Emily, the effects of hypermobility were severe and receiving a diagnosis was life-altering. Even where hypermobility is not problematic for the child, in my view it's very helpful for it to be identified, so that parents, together with the child, can take simple steps to ensure that, as far as possible, not problematic is the way that it stays.[6]

Managing physical activity

The general recommendation for hypermobile children is that they keep fit and active, going for low-impact exercise (such as walking, swimming and gentle cycling) and avoiding high-impact and aerobic sports.[7] Where a child is passionate about an activity that isn't considered ideal for their joint health, personally I would always suggest finding a way to make it work for them. Having them stay strong and mobile is the most important thing, and they are much more likely to do that if they love their chosen physical activity. Clay, for example, was diagnosed with hEDS at the age of six:

> As a keen martial artist, he was told by his physio that [martial arts training] was helping to keep his muscles strong, supporting those wobbly joints, and to try and continue training... Clay trains up to three times a week at X Martial Arts school in Wakefield and is currently working towards his brown belt. He has recently competed in his second competition this year, winning himself a bronze medal in points sparring.[8]

The needs of a hypermobile child in a sports training programme, or a ballet, gymnastics or martial arts class, are going to be slightly different from those of their CT-typical peers. For example, dance physiotherapist, Lisa Howell, explains that a hypermobile child in a ballet class:

> ...must take care to keep very strong and stable around her [sic] joints to avoid injury. As there is less protection to sideways movements through the ankles and knees, girls with hypermobile legs often get injured in these areas more easily. She should do lots of balance work on a wobble board or similar to increase her stability around these joints. This is also true in the spinal joints.[9]

Whatever the activity, care needs to be taken that the hypermobile child is focusing on strengthening above stretching and that they are being given time to develop stamina slowly. Knowledgeable teaching can be preventative not only of present injury but also of serious problems at adolescence and beyond. Chris Cook, a former coach of young gymnasts, says:

> Gymnastics can be an excellent sport for children with hypermobility as long

as the coach knows what they're doing. Often, children who start gymnastics don't have the strength required to hold them in the correct positions with muscle alone, so they 'lock out' their joints such as elbows and knees to make things easier. This can be dangerous for children (or adults) with underdeveloped muscles and hypermobility. If the equipment and techniques are not correctly adjusted, certain exercises can put unnecessary strain and stress on joints, ligaments and muscles.[10]

Sounds familiar, doesn't it?! A good teacher will ask questions about the child's hypermobility and how it affects them. They may ask if they can liaise with the child's physiotherapist or any other professional involved in their care. They will proactively modify activities on an individual basis where necessary, and will be clearly interested in teaching the child in the most appropriate way possible. Beware of teachers who:

- push their students for more, bigger, faster (even in a pre-professional programme – slow and steady wins the race)

- manually stretch their students or have them manually stretch one another

- don't listen when you try to explain about your child's hypermobility and the particular needs that go with it

- focus purely on performance goals rather than attending to long-term student development and welfare

- lack the skills to adapt training to individual needs, imposing a one-size-fits-all approach on all students.

How early is hypermobility evident?

Hypermobility runs in families, so if you have it, it's likely that at least one of your parents did too and that so will some of any children you have. When I work with hypermobile parents and carers, I'm often asked how early it's possible to recognise hypermobility in a child. The answer is, from birth. Physiotherapist, Pam Versfeld, who specialises in movement acquisition in children, describes characteristic postural differences between genetically hypermobile and CT-typical newborns:

At birth, typically developing full-term infants lie with their arms and legs flexed. In fact, the muscles of the hips and knees are tight and cannot be completely stretched out. The slight tightness (stiffness) in the muscles of the hips and knees helps the newborn infant to lift the arms and legs up when kicking and reaching. Newborn hypermobile (and pre-term) infants lie with their legs and arms more extended and flat on the cot mattress. The usual tightness of the hip and knee muscles is absent, and the hips and knees can be fully extended. The laxity in the muscles means that it requires more effort to lift up the arms to reach for toys and kick the legs.[11]

Plus ça change, eh, hypermobile people?! On Pam's website, you can see juxtaposed images of a CT-typical baby girl and a hypermobile baby boy. Whereas the girl appears taut, with arms and legs drawn into her torso, the boy is splayed, with femurs very laterally rotated and arms flopping on the floor.[12]

Early movement acquisition

Within a few weeks of birth, CT-typical babies are able to control their trunk as they kick, move their arms, reach out for toys and so on. This activity strengthens their muscles for the developmental milestones of rolling and sitting. Hypermobile babies, on the other hand, have difficulty in stabilising from the centre, and therefore are less able to move their limbs, and so less able to gain strength.[13] I'm probably not the only hypermobile person who feels as if I'm still dealing with the repercussions of this vicious circle. As a result, hypermobile babies are often late to sit – and may sit with a rounded, collapsed-looking back,[14] like a tortoise's shell. Laxity of tissues tends to generate a state of being in which we are not sure we can rely on our body to do the thing we intend. Because this sense of uncertainty originates in the physical body, not in the cognitive mind, it may be present even in the earliest weeks of life, so it's not surprising that, according to Pam Versfeld, hypermobile babies appear more tentative in their movements and more cautious as they explore the world.[15]

Making it onto the knees requires a degree of tensility in the hips that many hypermobile babies don't have. Arm strength may be another issue. When lifting up from a prone position, hypermobile babies may lock their elbows and hyperextend their spine, while their shoulders ride up to their ears[16] – a familiar pattern to any yoga teacher who has taught Updog (*urdhvamukhasvanasana*) to adult hypermobile students, and one that limits the acquisition of arm strength. As a result, hypermobile babies may get around by bottom-shuffling rather than crawling: a creative solution to a problem, and one that enables them to become independent movers and explorers of their environment but which misses out some important developmental skills that generally are acquired on hands and knees. Crawling is important for stabilising the shoulders sufficiently for good arm control, which will enable the infant eventually to carry out tasks like feeding themselves and putting on clothes. It also assists in the development of the vestibular (balance) system, and of co-ordination, as the left and right sides have to work together rhythmically to create the crawling movement.[17] Hypermobile yoga students who have long-term and thorough-going difficulty with quadruped postures, such as *chaturanga dandasana* (Four-Legged Staff Pose) may turn out to be those who have missed out on the important shoulder and core-body stabilisation of the crawling phase. Rosie, a yoga practitioner with hEDS, says:

> I've always found *chaturanga* impossible. I've tried so hard, but I just can't seem to control my shoulders and middle section. When I found out from my dad that I got around by shuffling on my bum as a baby and never crawled, it started to make sense. Of course I don't have that control and muscle patterning.

A few months later, weak hips and hyperextending knees, together with feet splayed wide and laterally rotated, can make it difficult for a hypermobile baby to balance in standing and to shift their weight in order to take a step.[18] Whereas once upright a CT-typical baby will bend their legs to sit down again, hypermobile babies tend to collapse backwards with straight legs,[19] like a jointed wooden doll. All in all, it's no surprise, that as a rule it takes hypermobile babies a few months longer than their CT-typical counterparts to start walking. While the average CT-typical baby takes their first steps around their first birthday, according to Pam Versfeld, most hypermobile babies don't reach the same milestone until they are between 18 and 20 months old.[20]

Because organisation of the brain is tied up with movement, missing stages may lead not only to holes in muscular and proprioceptive development, but also to longer-term neurological deficits. Ann Green Gilbert, elementary school teacher, dance academic and creator of BrainDance, explains that:

> The developmental movement patterns help to wire the central nervous system, laying the foundation for sensory-motor development and life long learning. When patterns are missed or disrupted there may be missing gaps in a person's neurological development. These gaps may cause neurological

dysfunction that may later appear as learning disabilities, behaviour disorders, memory problems, sleep disorders, speech, balance or filtering problems, and other difficulties that may disrupt the flow of normal development.[21]

For more information on early movement acquisition, I highly recommend Pam Versfeld's Skills for Action website – www.skillsforaction.com – where you can see images of hypermobile infants at all the different stages of development discussed above.

The W-sit

While I was going through a box of old family photos, I came across this picture of me W-sitting, aged about eight. I remember very clearly as a child finding crossed legs an uncomfortable – sometimes tortuous – position to sit in, as my back muscles spasmed, and after a few minutes stabbing pain set in. It seemed like another incomprehensible perversity of school that crossed legs were insisted on there.

As you can see from the image, the W-sit looks like *virasana* (Hero Pose), except that the ankles are bent and the feet turned out. An anteverted (pointing forward) hip socket and femoral neck will naturally predispose some children (and adults) to be more comfortable sitting between their thighs. Femoral anteversion – an internal spiralling of the thigh bones which many children are born with – will further tend to make the W an easy, natural sitting position. (In most children, femoral anteversion starts to decrease naturally at around eight years of age.)[22] The W offers a wider base of support than crossed legs, and locks the hip joints 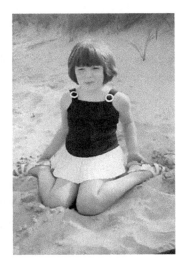 at end range, with the passive joint structures pulled taut to provide extra stability.[23] It therefore requires less core activation than crossed legs, so it's not surprising that the W is a go-to sitting position for many hypermobile children.

The W-sitting controversy

A Google search for 'W-sitting' will bring up a plethora of articles, half of them vehemently denouncing the W as deleterious to healthy child development in multiple ways, the other half pooh-poohing the W's allegedly disastrous effects. 'Why the "W" Sitting Position IS Bad for Kids' declares the headline of a 2017 article in the *Mirror*.[24] 'Why It's Totally Fine to Let Your Kid Sit in the "W" Position' counters Cassie Shortsleeve for Parents.com.[25] So what actually are the pros and cons of the 'W'?

Building muscle

It's pretty clear that if a child is regularly sitting in a position that requires little muscle activation, they aren't going to be building much muscle strength in it. This can be a bit of a Catch 22 for hypermobile children, who may not have the stability to sustain floor sitting for longish periods in any other way. One of the issues here is the amount of time that primary-school-aged children are often expected to be able to sit on the floor in one position. While a hypermobile child might be able to try on a repertoire of different positions for short periods of time during play, they may actually need the inherent stability of the W to remain comfortably seated long enough, for example, to listen to a story. I know that was the case for me.

Tightening of the hips

As in any situation where we adopt one position excessively, W-sitting can create patterns of extreme flexibility in one range of motion and tightness in another. Pam Versfeld says that W-sitters can have as much as 90 degrees of internal rotation, whereas the normal range is 45 degrees.[26] (I can vouch for that in my own body.) This is a problem where external rotation becomes correspondingly limited. In this case, when asked to sit cross-legged the child may sit with their pelvis in posterior tilt and their spine in flexion to accommodate the limitation in hip movement. These children may not be identified as hypermobile, because their muscular flexibility has become limited, but nonetheless the underlying issue is one of connective tissue laxity.

Lateral tibial torsion

When a child sits between their legs, their tibias laterally rotate. (This is one of the actions that is limited when an adult yoga practitioner can only sit on top of their calves in *virasana*.) Because children's ligaments are still very adaptable, if they habitually W-sit, the result may be permanent lengthening of those that permit lateral tibial rotation, and shortening of those that permit medial tibial rotation, together with lengthening of the ligaments on the medial side of the ankle and tightening of those on the lateral side. This may lead to a stance in which when the knees line up with the hips, the feet are turned out laterally, often also with pronation. This is not optimal for the biomechanics of walking and running, and can strain the knees, causing knee pain.[27]

Rotation of the upper body

It is argued that in W-sitting it's not possible to rotate the upper body. Physiotherapist Kelly Askins says this, 'makes it difficult for the child to reach across the body and perform tasks that involve using both hands together or crossing their arm over from one side to the other'.[28] I carried out a little exploration in my own body and discovered that, as I suspected, I can do all these things just fine while in a W-sit, so, personally, I'm not sure there's any validity to this objection. What is different is the fixity of the hips when these tasks are performed in a W-sit – whereas in a cross-legged position the hips shift around as the upper body moves. If the child spends a lot of time in the W-sit, this may have implications for the acquisition of balancing, running and jumping skills.[29]

Hand preference

A further potential downside to W-sitting, according to Kelly Askins, is that it may hinder the development of hand preference.[30] I suspect that the cart is being confused with the horse here. W-sitting overlaps with hypermobility, overlaps with neurodifference. There are known to be higher rates of ambidexterity among autistic children in particular (between 17 and 47 per cent, as opposed to 3–4 per cent in the allistic population).[31] Ambidexterity correlates with differences in brain processing, particularly in the areas of language and motor skills.[32] While W-sitting is an ingredient in the mix here, I personally doubt whether it can be said to have a unique causal relationship with ambidexterity, although I guess it might play into an existing predisposition for flexible brain processing over clear cerebral lateralisation (the specialisation of particular functions or cognitive processes to one side of the brain or the other).

I am slightly ambidextrous myself, and I've always viewed this as an advantage. In fact, as an adult, I've actively trained my ambidexterity at times. I am dyspraxic and I also process language differently from the norm. I'm hyperphantasic (a high visualiser) and 'see' all linguistic communication, kind of like a movie, before translating it into words. This means that my verbal processing is slightly slow, but on the upside my capacity for lateral thinking is far greater than that of someone whose cognition is predominantly linguistic. My world is exceptionally vivid, highly coloured, art-house beautiful, and I'm skilled at writing poetry, dreaming and internal travelling. Would I swap all of this for better cerebral lateralisation? Not on your life. Could it be, then, that neurotypical bias is at play in the preference of child developmentalists for lateralisation?

So is W-sitting a problem?

In my view, it depends. In and of itself, there's nothing intrinsically wrong with the W, and many CT-typical children naturally adopt it during play, along with sitting cross-legged, kneeling, squatting and so on. If a child is only and always sitting in the W, though, it would probably be a good idea to encourage them gently to diversify. Pam Versfeld suggests:

> When you see your infant sitting between his/her legs, gently move her [sic] legs to a better position and say something such as, 'Feet in front'. Once the infant gets the idea, you will find that he/she will move the legs when you say, 'Feet in front'.[33]

Just as it takes time and practice to create new kinetic patterns as a hypermobile adult, so too for a hypermobile infant. Initially, sitting with feet in front may feel strange and uncomfortable to the child, so it's important to go slowly and not insist on lots of time sitting that way. Pam says, 'You will need to spend time playing with [the child] in the new position, with lots of encouragement to get her to reach for toys and move from the new sitting position onto her knees and up into standing.'[34]

For older children who are interested, ballet – with a sensitive, hypermobility-aware teacher – can offer a useful antidote to W-sitting because the technique is based on external rotation at the hip and lining the knee up with the foot. The right kind of yoga, too, can be helpful.

But all children are flexible

It's true that children's bodies are inherently more pliable than those of adults. However, the kind of loose-jointedness that characterises hypermobile children is of a different order and is easy to spot once you are familiar with it. When I was assessed for hypermobility, one of the questions on the diagnostic questionnaire was: 'When you were a child, did you ever show off gymnastic positions to your friends?'[35] As an autistic child, I was far too intimidated by the complexities of social relationships for exhibitionism (though other autistic people have told me that displaying their Gumby skills was a way they related with others); I was also too floppy to do most party-piece contortions, but, nevertheless, my limbs did collapse into some weird and wonderful arrangements. These were not positions that CT-typical children were regularly assuming in the course of normal daily activities.

In hypermobile children, this kind of flexibility may also be symptomatic. As a child, I took ongoing joint pain (together with massive sensory overload, processing difficulties and huge levels of anxiety) as a given, and trooped stoically on without mentioning any of it to anyone. This is not an unusual picture. Ehlers-Danlos Support UK notes that children with EDS/HSD may experience:

> ...abdominal symptoms or growing pains. They may also present with neurodevelopmental disorders such as hyperactivity, dyspraxia, sleep and food issues, emotional problems and anxiety.[36]

And...as in adults, childhood hypermobility can be totally asymptomatic. A significant proportion of the children succeeding in pre-professional sports and dance programmes are hypermobile. For some, this is a period of grace before the onset of problems; for the lucky ones hypermobility never becomes an issue.

Is yoga good for hypermobile children?

According to physiotherapist, Leslie Russek, who specialises in hEDS, the answer is yes.[37] Deconditioning is a major concern with hypermobile children, and any physical activity that they enjoy and that they can participate in without stress about their ability to keep up or risk to their joints is one to be encouraged. Of course, it has to be the right kind of yoga. Like hypermobile adults, hypermobile children in a yoga class need to be working first and foremost for stability and strength, at a measured pace and in an environment where the well-being of the child is more important than achieving technical tricks. A good yoga class with a hypermobility-aware teacher can offer opportunities to:

- develop stamina. Some hypermobile children are habitually fatigued, and as a result may have withdrawn from physical activities geared to their CT-typical peers. As Leslie Russek explains to her young readers:

  > If you don't get regular exercise (for example, if you have pain or your joints are injured), your body becomes less able to exercise and you feel tired. It may seem backwards, but the solution is to get more exercise even though you are tired.[38]

  Yoga can offer gentle, well-paced conditioning ('Start low; go slow!' Leslie advises),[39] adaptable to natural fluctuations in the child's energy levels from day to day

- mobilise any areas that are overly tight. For example, simple external rotations of the femur (sitting like a frog or grasshopper legs) can help with hip tightness in habitual W-sitters – and mobilisation here may help to modify non-optimal gait patterns

- repattern. Crawling activities, for example, such as mimicking the movement of different animals, may help children who have missed out on this developmental phase to acquire some of the associated neurological patterning

- regulate the nervous system. Hypermobile children are often anxious and/or highly stressed by the difficult sensory environment of school, its social demands and the requirement to complete tasks designed for peers with more normal processing styles. Time spent in a quiet environment, where there is a friendly and open attitude to difference, and some time to rest, can make a significant difference in the child's ability to cope.

Hypermobile children in a yoga class

Joint hypermobility is very common, and it's an unusual children's yoga class that doesn't include at least a child or two affected by it. In settings where yoga is offered for children with Specific Learning Difficulties (SpLDs), such as dyslexia, dyspraxia, ADHD, dyscalculia and dysgraphia, the proportion of hypermobile participants will be much higher. However, there is little if any information out there about how to meet the particular needs of hypermobile children in a yoga class, and working with hypermobility is seldom covered in training for children's yoga teachers.[40] So what are some strategies for teaching hypermobile children in helpful and effective ways? I asked Iris Waller, children's yoga teacher with a specialism in autism and SpLDs,[41] and Melissa Palmer, a children's yoga teacher who has hEDS and is the parent of four hypermobile children.[42] These are some of their suggestions.

Getting students interested

Iris notes that most children are not in a yoga class because they have chosen to be there. Children's yoga teacher, Jodi Smith, adds:

> In some cases, yoga is a mandatory part of a school program. Other times, it's the parent's choice for their child to attend class. Either way, a child's interest in yoga may not be high if they feel forced to do it.[43]

In this situation, the first priority is to engage the child by making activities interesting and fun. Jodi says:

> As a yoga teacher, my job is to gauge the feelings and interests of the class and adjust to meet the children. My job isn't to force them into something but to introduce elements that will make their time in yoga class meaningful.[44]

In some instances, however, a child may be more interested in yoga, and it may be possible to do more detailed hypermobility work, implementing more of the adult strategies detailed in this book – particularly if the child is older and if you are working with them one to one.

Keep joints in motion

- As we have seen (in 'Fatigue' in the 'Muscular system' section in Chapter 1), being static can cause pain in hypermobile joints, and hypermobile children may therefore present as inattentive or unable to settle. Iris says that when working one to one with a hypermobile child, she often gives them a gym ball to sit on, enabling them be in motion while listening. Balancing on a gym ball requires the child to turn on stabilising muscles, which in hypermobile children may be underdeveloped, so this strategy is a win–win.

- Like hypermobile adults, hypermobile children will struggle with long, standing, static holds. Iris suggests keeping postures flowing to avoid joint pain and fatigue.

- We saw in Chapter 4 that for hypermobile people who are also autistic, 'fidgeting', or stimming, helps with nervous-system regulation and aids concentration (see 'Stillness and stimming'). Rather than trying to enforce physical stillness, Iris suggests that you support the child's native strategy for staying present. She says: 'I often give them props to have while they practise – fidget spinners and so on – so that they can listen better.'

Time to rest

CT-typical adults tend to think of children as balls of boundless energy, but hypermobile children often experience fatigue. Melissa notes that moving practices can be exhausting for hypermobile children, and it's important to include rest periods between active sections of the class.

Buttons and shoelaces

As we have seen (in 'Early movement acquisition' above), differences in early movement acquisition can have an effect on development of manual skills among hypermobile children. Iris warns teachers to allow extra time at the beginning and end of sessions for helping hypermobile children with tasks such as doing up buttons and shoelaces.

Feel the floor

Melissa emphasises the importance of grounding for hypermobile children. Contact with the floor through hands and feet offers a wealth of sensations and consequently many opportunities to increase proprioceptive feedback.

Offer weight

Melissa uses sandbags or weighted beanbags in many of her classes. These offer feedback on body boundaries and can be calming for a hypermobile system.

Go slowly

Like hypermobile adults, children with hypermobility may have difficulty with reproducing shapes and picking up simple choreographies. Melissa advises slowing everything right down. A gentle pace will also tend to calm hyperactive nervous systems and reassure everyone that there is plenty of time to learn.

Balancing

Melissa and Iris both point up issues with balance among hypermobile children. Iris says:

> In classes, I only do very modified standing balances with hypermobile kids, as they tend to over-compensate immediately, and in a group it's very hard to adjust that. I might do a Tree [vrksasana] with one foot on top of the other with some clapping.

If, on the other hand, you have the opportunity to work one to one, graduated work with balance, in increments the child can manage while maintaining good biomechanics, could be very helpful.

Sitting cross-legged

As we have seen above (in 'The W-sit'), hypermobile W-sitters may have difficulty with sitting cross-legged. If you're teaching one to one, work to strengthen and selectively mobilise can help to make a biomechanically functional cross-legged sitting position comfortable at least for a short period. If you have only a limited time with a big group, in which this kind of detailed work is not possible, Iris suggests having all the children sit on a bench for any seated postures – rather than in a biomechanically distorted cross-legged position that reinforces unhelpful postural habits.

Standing postures

In a large group, in which there is little time to work individually, Iris suggests sticking mostly to seated and supine postures, perhaps together with Mountain Pose (tadasana) and Warrior (virabhadrasana) I or a modified Triangle (utthita trikonasana).

Weight-bearing on the arms

Arm movements that strengthen and stabilise the shoulders can be helpful, but in a class setting, Iris avoids weight-bearing on the arms – 'no Downdog (*adhomukhasvanasana*) and no Cat (*marjaryasana*)'. It's too risky for hypermobile children, who may have significant shoulder laxity.

Hyperextensions

- As we saw above (in 'But all children are flexible'), showing off extreme postures as a child is actually a criterion for hypermobility diagnosis. You can expect some hypermobile children to be very proud of the weird things they can do with their joints – and, of course, winning an audience response (impressed, appalled or grossed out) only encourages them to do it more. Needless to say, these kinds of activities can actually be harmful, reinforcing laxity in developing fascial structures and potentially leading to chronic dislocations and joint degeneration later in life. But consequences that may ensue in the different universe of adulthood are unlikely to have much reality for a child. You are most likely to dissuade children from performing their hypermobility in harmful ways by responding neutrally, eschewing amazement and disgust, and reorienting everyone towards the movement approaches we are looking to cultivate in a yoga class.

- Hypermobile children are unlikely to be aware that they are hyper-extending their knees or their elbows, and – like hypermobile adults – may need a lot of teacher input to feel neutral alignment and be able to reproduce it. Iris says, 'I may ask them to straighten their arm, for example, and tell them exactly when to stop, then do the same in the posture.'

- For children with posterior knee hyperextensions, Iris suggests placing rolled-up blankets or folded towels under the knees in seated forward bends.

Overstretching

Children's joints are not fully developed. Bones, ligaments and tendons are still highly malleable and vulnerable to any forces that might distort them. For example, dance physiotherapist, Lisa Howell, explains that:

A developing pelvis – anything under the age of 18 to 22 – will still have a Y-shaped cartilage in the hip socket. This is designed so that the acetabulum (the hip socket) can grow as the head of the femur grows. It's not a solid hip socket. So if we're putting a lot of strain through the pelvis while that is still cartilaginous, we can change the shape of the hip socket. This is not necessarily a good thing. I've seen some radiographic evidence where we've actually done damage to [ballet] students' hips by having them in programmes that are encouraging over-stretching over a period of time.[45]

For this reason, good pre-professional dance and sports programmes err on the side of training for strength and are relatively conservative about introducing new or more extreme articulations. There is no place in a children's yoga class for postures requiring preternatural flexibility, even if some of your hypermobile students can easily produce these positions. Hypermobile children, like hypermobile adults, need graduated work for strength and stability.

Work with feet

To help with over-pronating feet, Iris suggests exercises such as:

- pretending to walk super-silently around a room full of sleeping chicks

- rising onto tiptoes

- pulling an imaginary towel towards you with your toes

- imagining Cinderella shoes that are too small – crunch the toes up, then press the ball of the foot down (show children what the ball of the foot is) and release the toes.

Body awareness

CT-typical teachers may assume that all children are aware of what they are feeling physically, but for hypermobile children sensate experience may be largely vague and unconscious. Melissa suggests including lots of time for guided exploration of physical sensations. For example, the teacher might ask:

- Where are your feet?

- Can you feel your feet?

- Are there any sensations in your feet?

- What words might go with the sensations, for example: hot/cold/sharp/soft/prickly/tingly.

Family involvement

Iris points out that hypermobile children often do better in family classes, which enable parents/carers to understand their child's biomechanical challenges and also give the adults some strategies to help. Bear in mind that hypermobile children usually have at least one hypermobile parent, sometimes aware of their own hypermobility and sometimes not. Hypermobility-aware family yoga can be a revelation and a tremendous help to all the hypermobile members of the family.

7

Practising Yoga with Hypermobility

Yoga Serenity Prayer
Universe, grant me the serenity to accept there are poses I cannot do,
courage to try the ones I can
and wisdom to know the difference.

Michelle Marchildon (the Yogi Muse)

This chapter is about practising yoga in a safe and beneficial way with a genetic joint hypermobility syndrome. It's based on my own experience of being in movement practice as a hypermobile person and on the experiences of my hypermobile students and clients. We will be considering questions such as: how can you engage with yoga in a way that will be positive and helpful for you? Should you be doing yoga at all – and if so, what kind of yoga and with what kind of teacher? How can you best collaborate with yoga teachers who may have varying degrees of hypermobility awareness? How can you turn around physical incapacity and work with pain? You'll also find some experiential work here.

You may be encountering this chapter injured, fatigued or in general perplexity about if or how you 'should' be practising yoga. Know that your body isn't a problem to be solved, a wild beast to be pacified or an enemy to be slain; and practice is not a destination to get to, but a holistic learning process uniquely calibrated to your own needs. The capacity to practise well as a hypermobile person involves a meeting of good information with the willingness to offer attention, curiously and with an open mind, to the teacher that is your body.

Hypermobility often appears to be the gift given by the bad fairy, until you actually start to play with what you've got in the box. There are huge challenges of course, but there are also many opportunities to learn, not just about biomechanics, but also about who you are as a human being, and how you can feel, live and be that person in the kindest and most skilful way possible. This is the stuff of practice.

'I've been advised not to do yoga'

I've just been diagnosed with hypermobility and have been told I should stop doing yoga. I'm absolutely devastated. I rely on yoga to keep me sane and ease out some of the pain of hypermobility. Do I really have to stop?

Fumi (yoga practitioner with hEDS)

It's unfortunately quite common for diagnosing professionals to advise hypermobile people to avoid yoga. This is not totally without reason; there are definitely types of yoga and particular approaches to yoga practice that I would suggest you give a wide berth to – I'll be talking more about which these are and why later in this chapter (see 'Which type of yoga?'). However, when a medic tells a hypermobile person that yoga is contraindicated, I think we have to unpick what they're really recommending. Long-time yoga practitioners know that 'yoga' encompasses a huge and diverse range of practices and intentions. Most hypermobility doctors, on the other hand, have no substantive experience of yoga, and tend to conceive of it as a passive stretching programme – something that people with HSD, hEDS and MFS definitely do need to steer clear of. What hypermobility doctors do universally advocate for their patients is careful, measured strengthening and stabilisation. This is something that the right kind of yoga is very well placed to provide, alongside a range of other physical activities.

Yoga practice offers other benefits that hypermobility-informed medical professionals acknowledge to be immensely helpful for their patients. As we saw in Chapter 1, muscles in a hypermobile body may be tight and spasmy. A sensible, balanced yoga practice that focuses on mobilisation rather than stretching (more on the difference between these later – see 'Mobilisation versus stretching') can be very helpful in release of myofascial tension and the general neuromuscular repatterning that can follow. As we saw in Chapter 5, gentle restorative practices can facilitate regulation of the over-adrenalised nervous system typical of hypermobility, reducing anxiety, promoting healing and pacifying excessive pain responses.

Something needs to change

While yoga can potentially offer substantial benefits, for many hypermobile practitioners being formally diagnosed with a hypermobility syndrome prompts the recognition that their current practice needs to shift in some significant ways. This might mean:

- slowing down

- focusing more on structure and stability and less on stretching

- orienting towards offering attention to sensations, feelings, emotions and thoughts

- learning how to use yoga practice to regulate internal states

- moving away from goals and achievements, and towards intentions and experiences.

For some yogis, a shift in style of practice is necessary. Itziar, a yoga practitioner with HSD, says:

I was doing very fast vinyasa flow classes where the teachers didn't explain the postures or give many corrections. I was getting injured because I mostly didn't know what I should be doing, and even when I did, I didn't have time to actually implement what I knew would make the posture safe for me. I now go regularly to a much slower class with a very experienced Iyengar teacher, who explains everything in detail. Every once in a while, I do a vinyasa flow class just for fun.

Adding in other movement forms (Pilates, the Feldenkrais Method®, Alexander Technique, swimming, etc.) is also important in making an existing yoga practice viable and beneficial. We'll be talking more about this later (see 'Yoga addiction versus cross training and supportive practices').

Deconditioning...and reconditioning

Two years ago, I was running marathons. Now I can barely walk to the corner shop.

Tom (yoga practitioner with hEDS)

As I mentioned in Chapter 1, some of my most debilitated hypermobile clients have progressively reduced both:

- their range of physical activity and

- the amount of physical activity they do…

…to the point where their window for possible movement is tiny and their capacity for physical endurance severely restricted. This is a fairly common scenario, and it's easy to see how it can come about. In a study on the exercise beliefs and behaviours of those with joint hypermobility, physiotherapist Jane Simmonds and colleagues conclude that, not surprisingly, 'Pain, fatigue and fear are common barriers to exercise.'[1] Researchers Scheper *et al.* explain that in hypermobility:

> Overuse injuries occur with minimal provocation and may lead to activity impairment to preserve joints. This results in 'pay later' behaviour for participating in certain activities, characterised by overactivity, followed by underactivity to recover. Consequently, there is a downward spiral of less activity due to fear and more pain with less provocation, leading to deconditioning.

In addition:

> Fear of pain will trigger avoidance of painful muscle contractions, leading to submaximal muscle performance. For persons with joint hypermobility, submaximal muscle performance will, however, have the immediate negative consequence that their compensation mechanism, essential for joint stability, will fail. Functional consequences, [such] as impaired balance and lower balance confidence, will further fuel fear of movement and catastrophising thoughts about pain and vice versa.[2]

How this may look in reality is illustrated by the experience of Keely, a yoga practitioner with HSD:

> *I had dealt with frequent injuries and joint pain related to hypermobility since I was a kid, but was pretty capable and active into my early twenties – I just owned a lot of ice packs and ankle and knee braces. In high school I was on the swim team, and in college and grad school I regularly rock-climbed and did yoga. I commuted 12 miles round trip daily by bike in my first year of grad school.*
>
> *In my second year of grad school, though, I spent a lot of hours at a computer daily, was running for exercise, and was in a very minor accident (got knocked over on my bike by a car going less than 10 mph) which resulted in a minor shoulder injury that further destabilised an already loose joint.*

Over the course of the next two years, as a result of that combination of stressors, my existing pain issues increased, and muscle tension and spasms in my neck/shoulder/upper back began to interfere with my ability to work. I quit running at a doctor's recommendation, then climbing and yoga due to pain. After I decreased my activity levels I lost strength, and as I lost strength I started to have problems with joints I'd never had problems with before.

Anoushé Husain describes a similar downward trajectory with EDS:

At 16, I stopped karate. A sport that I was in love with, but also the thing that was keeping my joints way more stable without realising… The reduction in activity and my subsequent ill-health are no coincidence. By the age of 23, I had had operations every couple of years for my joints and then was going through cancer treatment, which meant I was even less active (and frankly my body was wrecked).[3]

Reversing the spiral

Luckily for us, bodies are to a large extent plastic and – outside of end-of-life situations – can pretty much always be coaxed back into greater capacity and function. Anoushé Husain took up climbing to regain fitness and physical stability. It is possible to turn things around, as Corinne's experience demonstrates:

I used to do a huge amount of sport until an injury put an end to it at age 21. I became a comfort eater and put on weight. About 3 years ago, I started going to a dance fitness class but couldn't do anything above my head as my shoulder hurt, but I kept going. I then decided to start ice skating. I adored it and skated for up to 3–5 hours at a time even though it could hurt.

My love of fitness grew and I decided to become a personal trainer. Whilst doing the course, my pain got worse but sports massage helped. Still undiagnosed and not knowing why I had so much pain, I started to do rehab exercises and strengthening exercises and started to see an improvement.

Over time, I have lost loads of weight and strengthened. I still have flare-ups, but am learning more about listening to my body and what works for me. Getting the EDS diagnosis explained so much. Now I work with what I can do. I take part in the fitness classes I teach, plus go to the gym about three times a week. I started off deadlifting 8 kg last year and am now at 40 kg. Last year I couldn't do anything overhead, and now I can do assisted chin-ups and I also do lat pull-downs of up to 14.5 kg. For me these are massive achievements. I have times when I have set-backs but it's about working through them and coming out the other side.[4]

Laura, a 26-year-old student with hEDS, has a similar story of exercise success through adversity:

Already having years of ballet training under my belt really gave me the determination to get back on my feet; however, making improvements to your quality of life is just as much a mental battle as it is a physical one. I started slow with core exercises, focusing on simple Pilates movements and stretches that I could do laid down in my bed. Similarly, I spoke to physiotherapists who provided small repetitive exercises to do that would work my muscles hard without stressing the joints to any extent. I returned to ballet, and whilst it was not as easy as it had previously been, my ballet teacher allowed me to drop in and out of exercises as it suited me to allow me to work myself back to where I was before, and to continue to improve. Eventually I worked myself back to a place that was similar to the condition that I had been previously: still dislocating hips and experiencing leg pain, but my body had adjusted to the chronic pain and learned to block out a substantial amount of it. Equally, my fatigue improved as I was encouraging my body to want to rest through working my muscles.[5]

The following are a few guidelines for reorienting yourself to activity if you have become deconditioned and unfit:

- Just because you can't do an activity perfectly doesn't mean you can't do it at all. Do as much as you *can* do – even if that's only five minutes or just using your arms. Start somewhere. There's no objective standard you have to meet, and you don't have to be as good as (or better than) everybody else. It's about showing up and getting what you need from the activity.

- Go slowly and steadily: this is definitely a tortoise-over-hare situation. Give your body plenty of time to adapt and be aware that it takes longer for a hypermobile body to create muscle and build stamina.

- Expect some set-backs. These are normal and part of the bigger process. Yoga practice is less about achieving goals and more about meeting our experiences and allowing them to shape and inform us.

- As Corinne's story illustrates, while listening to your body is an essential skill, reconditioning also entails continuing – with care and consideration – through some pain. It's impossible to gain muscle strength without experiencing a little fatigue and soreness. This is normal and to be expected. If pain is excessive, row back, do fewer repetitions and shorter holds, and give yourself longer to rest in between. If possible, check with a teacher or physio that you are doing your chosen exercise in a biomechanically helpful way. There's a lot more discussion of different types of pain and how to work with them below (see 'Working with pain').

- Mark for yourself where you have gained capacity – can do one more repetition, lift one more pound, continue for five more minutes. Give yourself an opportunity to celebrate small positive steps – rather than surreptitiously moving the goal posts.

One-to-one professional support

Starting to move again after a period of inactivity can feel terrifying. Knowing what's safe enough to do, where to find an appropriate edge in terms of duration and intensity, and which signs and symptoms are normal, tolerable parts of beginning to improve fitness and which sound a warning note…can all feel overwhelming. This is where one-to-one support from a knowledgeable, hypermobility-aware movement professional can be gold. There are a whole host of different kinds of specialist who can be helpful here, but they may include:

- one-to-one yoga teacher

- yoga therapist

- physiotherapist

- Feldenkrais Method® teacher

- Alexander Technique teacher

- Pilates teacher

- somatic movement educator or therapist

- personal trainer.

It's not necessarily the case that just because a movement professional is fully qualified they will know all about hEDS/HSD/MFS. Things are getting better, and generally there is more awareness of joint hypermobility syndromes across the board, but it is still by no means a given that a professional selected at random will be able to offer you appropriate guidance. Hypermobility is complex to work with; you will need to do your research in order to find someone with the relevant knowledge and experience to help you in an effective way.

If you can't locate a hypermobility specialist (the situation is improving but, let's face it, we're not exactly popping out of the woodwork), an experienced movement professional who is good at listening, curious and gentle in their approach can still be a good fit. While a strong foundation in their own sphere of expertise is essential, the capacity of your movement professional to relate to you with empathy, to create a climate of positivity and possibility, and generally to be a healing presence is also crucial. You need to feel heard, reassured, encouraged and held within the space of the studio or consultation room.

It can take time to turn around pain, debility and biomechanical dysfunction, especially when you are hypermobile and need to proceed in very small increments, but you should feel a clear benefit from the work you are doing. As I have already mentioned, reconditioning sometimes involves encountering certain kinds of pain, but you should not be experiencing an overall increase in general pain levels or greater limitation in your movement possibilities. For a professional, working with hypermobility needs to be collaborative and somewhat exploratory. Not everything will be immediately helpful, and a good teacher/therapist will want you to feed back to them so that they can modify their approach in an ongoing way. If, however, you have discussed any increases in pain and debility with the professional and still nothing has changed – or it's getting worse – look elsewhere for help. If the professional is dogmatic and unwilling to work in partnership with you – run for the hills (or limp slowly)!

Chronic overactivity

I have a traditional six-day-a-week, third-series ashtanga practice. I'm hypermobile and my back is starting to really hurt.

Ivana (yoga practitioner with HSD)

I discovered ballet when I was 19, and it wasn't long before I was doing class every day. Yes, that's literally every day, seven of them a week. It was obsessive. I kept this up into my mid-thirties and rarely experienced any joint pain – when I did, it got better in response to rest and treatment, in the normal way. I took my miraculous body for granted. It was a seamless transition into the relatively rather relaxed five- or six-day-a-week practice tradition of ashtanga vinyasa. (You get Saturdays off, plus the days of the new and full moon.) The transition to ashtanga represented a desire to move in more meaningful and holistic ways. It was a shift away from the production of aesthetic surfaces and towards movement as a practice for embodied knowledge. It was also a response to the early effects of age on my body, and was meant to be a general deceleration and scaling down in terms of the difficulty and intensity of the movement I did daily. However, I was conditioned to ramp things up, and the structure of ashtanga, with its progressive series of postures presenting escalating degrees of physical challenge, gave me plenty of scope. (I think ashtanga also offers opportunities to see through the glittering allure of attainment, but I hadn't made that leap of understanding at the time.) I bought into the dogma, and for two years I did the five-/six-day-a-week thing. And it started to hurt and it started to exhaust me.

This is not a diatribe against ashtanga. In fact, for me, because of its capacity to be adaptive (when taught by an experienced and creative teacher in the Mysore style), ashtanga vinyasa is one of the more promising forms of yoga for some hypermobile people (more on this later – see 'Which type of yoga?'). Rather, this is a reflection on my attitude towards my yoga practice, my physical needs and my hypermobility at the time. I was caught in the turbulence of a sea change between miracle body and fragile body, and it took some time to understand and accept the transition, to feel into the alterations I needed to make in my approach and to embody them. Perhaps you yourself are in this situation now. In a sense, of course, we are all always in this kind of process, always adapting, understanding, accepting, embodying, and the capacity to be in the flow like this is potentially one of the priceless bad-fairy gifts of having a joint hypermobility syndrome.

Yoga therapist, physiotherapist and pain specialist, Neil Pearson, says:

> In the face of ongoing pain, we typically decide that there are two ways to approach movement and activity. In some situations, we believe the movement will be dangerous to our body, and so we avoid the movement. However, this avoidance leads to increased sensitisation of the nervous system and to more avoidance of movement. Alternatively, we grit our teeth and push through the pain, ultimately stopping when the pain is too bad to carry on. This strategy gets the job done, but causes our protective systems to act as if they have to scream at us before we will stop. The first strategy is 'flight', the second is either 'flight' or 'fight'. Neither is an effective approach to calming down a wound-up, hyper-sensitive nervous system.[6]

While it's crucial to remain active with hypermobility – to retain (or regain) as much of your movement capacity as possible – it's also important not to aim too high, push too hard or do too much. Many people with hypermobility are initially chronic overdoers and need to learn moderation. Less is often more in terms of maximising physical capacity, and this is especially so with hEDS, HSD and MFS. Increments of progression that might be fine for a non-hypermobile person are often too much for our more delicate tissues and our more limited energy levels. Any time I'm given an exercise by a physio, for example, I generally reduce the number of starting repetitions by two-thirds. I know from experience that this will usually be about right for me, whereas if I start with the 'normal' person's target, within a couple of days I'm likely to be in too much pain to do the exercise at all.

It's important to recognise that with a hypermobility syndrome, capacity will fluctuate from day to day. This is not a problem because you are just an ordinary human, and life is not a never-ending Olympics for which you have to be at constant peak fitness. There is room for natural undulations in what you are able to do, and it's more than OK – it's healthy and positive – to listen and respond to them. On days when you feel more tired and more in pain, for example, you could generate energy and quiet your nervous system by relaxing into a restorative practice rather than bashing out a challenging ashtanga vinyasa series. If you try to route march yourself through your planned activities come what may, you will probably crash and burn. Amy, who has EDS, refers to this capacity to flow with what's possible in real time as 'living in the grey'. She describes a conversation with a counsellor soon after her diagnosis:

> I explained that…even the simplest of things, like my inability to go to the gym that morning, sent me on a downward spiral. I looked at him, as a mixture of snot and tears ran down my face and said, 'I can't live like this. I mean, I can't even go to the (hiccup) gym because of my elbows.' He looked at me, with great kindness, and said something that I will never forget. He said, 'Why can't you go to the gym? Did you talk to your instructors and see if you could modify? You see things as black-and-white, but they don't have to be that way.'

Amy concludes:

> Living in the grey takes a great deal of effort… I still sometimes have to remind myself that the world will be OK if I don't make black-and-white choices. In the end though, this new thought process has been a beautiful gift.[7]

What yoga has to offer

Yoga is a reflective practice that invites the presence of the whole person, rather than just a body reduced to a set of biomechanical relationships. It therefore offers many benefits that movement based purely on physical rehabilitation does not. You are invited to bring your sensations, thoughts and feelings onto your mat – to a degree that feels helpful and right for you – and to notice the thread of your breath. By listening and discriminating between different kinds of internal messages that may be available, you open the gate to a more conscious relationship with your body. It's all about slowing down, paying attention and feeling your way into the landscape of sensation in an open and curious way. Much of what our body knows is not yet available to our conscious mind, so this is a way of cultivating new fields of awareness, of making more of what you know as an embodied being available for your use.

The experience of practising yoga is very individual, but some of the things that commonly happen over time include the following:

- By engaging with 'all of it' we start to join up the dots, to become more interconnected between parts and to feel more contained by our physical body.

- Through observing sensation and witnessing how it interplays with emotional responses and patterns of thinking, we become more responsive and less reactive to challenging sensations, such as pain, and to difficult experiences, such as loss of capacity to work or socialise.

- We become more engaged with process and less concerned with end result. Practice is a journey rather than a destination, and this attitude tends to spill over from the mat into the rest of our life.

- We become able to pay attention with all of ourselves, and to respond as a whole, embodied individual. As a result, we have a sense of secure internal guidance. We are able to follow our own internal compass and to make more appropriate decisions for ourselves.

From a physical point of view, yoga can be a helpful and unthreatening point of entry into movement after a period of inactivity because it has the potential to be so very gentle and easy. If you're experiencing fatigue, a yoga nidra or restorative practice can generate energy rather than requiring it of you. As your capacity for movement increases, so the degree of physical challenge can be very gradually stepped up within your practice – and decreased again in periods when you are in more need of rest and calm.

Which type of yoga?

One of the questions I'm often asked by yoga practitioners newly diagnosed with hypermobility is which kind of yoga they 'should' be doing. Unfortunately, there's no simple, one-size-fits-all answer. Each hypermobile person is an individual. We each have unique biomechanical patterns, a unique combination of co-existing conditions, a unique capacity for proprioception, a unique degree of musculoskeletal stability, a unique level of fitness, unique preferences, a unique history, unique intentions for our engagement with yoga… Consequently, there is no one style of yoga that is absolutely contraindicated for all hypermobile people all the time, and no one style that will always work for everybody. Having said that, there are forms of yoga that will probably work better for the majority of hypermobile people, and which are less likely to cause pain and injury for most – and others which on the whole you are best advised to avoid.

As much as the style of the practice, what makes the difference between an unhelpful experience of yoga and a beneficial one is often the setting the class takes place in, and the knowledge and experience of the teacher. A very experienced teacher who has an awareness of hypermobility and keeps class numbers low could outweigh a style that seems less than promising for a hypermobile student. We'll be looking more at choosing an appropriate setting and teacher in the following sections.

What was, when I did my first class in 1981, just 'yoga' has mushroomed into a plethora of brand names, spin-offs and personalised styles – way more of them than I can possibly cover here. What follows are some of the more mainstream forms that you will come across often in community centres, studios, gyms and anywhere else yoga takes place. In this chapter, I'm covering active practices; yin and restorative yoga have a chapter all of their own (see Chapter 5).

So…in no particular order…

Vinyasa flow/flow yoga

Back in the day, when I started practising, the image of 'yoga' in the public mind was generally one of church halls and middle-aged ladies in leotards and footless tights. Yoga was assumed to be gentle and static. With the absorption of yoga into the health and fitness industry, public perceptions have radically changed – as have the practices. What most people think of as 'yoga' now is likely to be some version of vinyasa flow: a fast-paced, dance-like practice, in which practitioners segue their way through sequences of interlinked postures without pausing. While some teachers offer a more careful and considered form, at the more geared-to-fitness end of the spectrum, vinyasa flow may be rather like a stretch-oriented version of aerobics, with a mainly young and female demographic, a playlist and the teacher cheerleading at the front.

If you're thinking this doesn't sound ideal for hypermobility, on the whole it isn't. For most hypermobile people, the stream of constantly changing movements are difficult to reproduce in biomechanically helpful ways. In a typical vinyasa flow class, a large part of the role of the teacher is to keep the class moving through the choreography at an even pace. Classes are generally follow-along – participants are not taught the sequences first but copy the teacher, who stands at the front and does the 'flows' with the class. This means that the teacher has limited ability to see what students are doing, and few opportunities to guide them out of less optimal positions and into what may better serve them from a biomechanical point of view. This is problematic for many students, and especially so for hypermobile ones, who tend to have poorer than average proprioception and biomechanical control, and are therefore likely to end up in unfeasible and potentially injurious physical situations.

If you're coming to yoga for the first time, vinyasa flow is not a place I would suggest you start. If you already practise this form and really, really love it, my suggestion is that you experiment with doing just one class a week. Back this up with two more classes in a slower style, where there is an emphasis on structure and placement, in which you are taught (rather than led) and offered personalised guidance. Your vinyasa flow practice is most likely to be safe and beneficial if you approach it with a strong physical foundation.

Ashtanga vinyasa

Ashtanga vinyasa is the parent form from which the vinyasa styles descend. It consists of set (but adaptable) series of linked postures. (Vinyasa styles use the basic vinyasa, or linking, structure of ashtanga vinyasa and riff on it.) There are two formats in which ashtanga vinyasa is taught, and which of these you encounter it in will make a big difference to how safe and helpful your experience of ashtanga is likely to be.

Mysore practice

*I've benefited so, so much from doing Mysore classes. My teacher is
very knowledgeable. She's taken me right back to basics and made me
work to get strong and stabilise my hyperextending joints. In normal
yoga classes, I was throwing myself into shapes without knowing what
I was meant to be doing. Now I have to properly understand each
posture before I'm given a new one. I really love working this way. It's
empowering.*

Anna (yoga practitioner with HSD)

Mysore style is the way that ashtanga vinyasa is traditionally taught. (Mysore
refers to the location of the *shala*, in India, that the ashtanga practice
originates from.) In a Mysore class, students are gradually introduced to a
set series of interlinked postures, which they are then able to practise without
being led by a teacher. The teacher (or teachers – many *shalas* have a lead
teacher plus assistants) works individually with students in the class to help
them understand the structure and dynamics of each movement, to feel its
relationship with breath, to create appropriate modifications and so on. In
a good Mysore room there is a high ratio of teachers to students, so there is
always someone to help when a student is stuck, wants some technical input
or needs some other kind of support in working with a particular *asana*.

I am myself a Mysore teacher, and am probably very biased, but my
experience is that Mysore practice can be a great situation for a hypermobile
student. There's no one and no-thing to keep up with, and ideally you get to
build a long-term relationship with a skilled and experienced teacher who
knows you and your practice well, and can help you to adapt as appropriate
to you in terms of physical challenge and duration on a day-to-day basis.
What's not to like?

Well, there is an important note of caution to be sounded here. In the
Mysore rooms I run, the ethos is collaborative: we want to be in partnership
with our students. We also work adaptively, using lots of props to help
make the practice accessible to everyone. This is not the case everywhere.
Some Mysore *shalas* adhere much more closely to the traditional sequence
of postures, outlaw props and operate a top-down teaching system. Strong
adjustments (definitely not advisable for hypermobile practitioners) may be
the norm, and you may be pushed to try for flexibility that is not appropriate
for your body – even if you can achieve it.

If you're interested in trying Mysore-style ashtanga, look for a *shala* in which the practice is in service to the student, rather than the other way around. Avoid teachers who insist on making strong adjustments or who want to manipulate you into pretzel positions, who are goal oriented or focused on moving you rapidly through the series. Seek out teachers who ask you about your experience in postures, who listen without judgement and who are more interested in helping you to find structure and stability in the postures than pushing you into gymnastic *asana*. *Shalas* like this are not always easy to find, but they do exist and are hypermobility gold.

Led ashtanga classes

Led ashtanga is much more what most people would expect a yoga class to look like. The teacher stands at the front and directs, and everybody does the same postures at the same time. When practised to speed and without the kind of customisation for individual needs that can happen in a Mysore class, ashtanga vinyasa is fast and physically challenging, and I don't recommend it for the majority of hypermobile people. If you're new to yoga, this is definitely not a place to start. Look for a solid, sensible, student-centred Mysore room, where you can be taught the basics slowly and build up postures one at a time.

Iyengar yoga

> *Iyengar isn't the most flashy form of yoga, but I've found it very helpful for working out where I should be engaging in postures and getting better alignment. Another benefit for me is that it's slow. With Marfan Syndrome, I need to avoid anything too fast paced or aerobic.*

> Zoe (yoga practitioner with MFS)

In Iyengar yoga, close – some might say forensic – attention is paid to anatomical details and to alignment in postures. Props are used extensively to ensure that postures are practised with the required muscular engagement, and teacher training is rigorous – way beyond the 200-hour minimum recommended standard for generic yoga. For all these reasons, Iyengar can be a very helpful practice for a hypermobile person.

There are challenges, though. One is that the lengthy stream of precise verbal instructions that characterises Iyengar teaching can be hard to translate into movement and sensation if you lack proprioception. Another is that the precision of the teaching does not always allow for individual anatomical differences, for personal needs and preferences. Then there is the length of time that active postures are held for. Dora, a yoga practitioner with HSD, says:

> While I get a lot from doing Iyengar, you do have to be a bit careful about the strength aspects. I have got injured from holding a Warrior (virabhadrasana) posture for a couple of minutes. My muscles just gave out and I sank into my joints. I couldn't support myself that long.

Iyengar was my first yoga practice, and I remember those very long Warriors! At that point, I didn't have much capacity for switching on muscles, and I didn't realise that the pain I felt in my feet, hips and shoulders in standing postures was due to sagging myofascial structures that were not equal to keeping me upright. A hypermobile person in an Iyengar class will probably need to reduce hold times, and will do best with a teacher who is sympathetic to this and understands the reasons why.

Hatha yoga

> I find hatha classes a bit more accessible than some of the flow ones. They take less energy, and include some resting time, so I find I don't get too fatigued, which is important for me, as I'm still not quite over a period of chronic fatigue.
>
> Tariq (yoga practitioner with hEDS)

Properly speaking, 'hatha' refers to any physical form of yoga practice (including all those described here); in popular usage, however, the name 'hatha' has come to designate a slower and more static type of class, in which the teacher teaches a posture and then the students practise it while the teacher offers help and guidance. There are no linking movements; instead, there are pauses between postures, during which students may be invited into a resting position for a short while. If you're coming to yoga for the first time as a hypermobile person, a hatha class is a good bet. The format makes it not too physically demanding (so it's good for those with vascular-type EDS or MFS), and you're likely to have a good idea of exactly what you're meant to be doing and how.

One downside of hatha classes for those who are less debilitated by their hypermobility may be that they don't offer enough scope to build strength and stamina. It all really depends where you're starting from.

Scaravelli-inspired yoga

Vanda Scaravelli, who created this approach to yoga, didn't want to be the progenitor of a style; hence, classes are usually referred to as 'Scaravelli inspired'. Whereas other forms of yoga (for example Iyengar yoga and all the vinyasa types) require muscular effort, in a Scaravelli-inspired practice the intention is freedom of body and ease of movement. Yoga teacher, Lucy Greaves, explains: 'Scaravelli's key innovation was her focus on working with gravity: surrendering the weight of the body and dropping the bones towards the earth, and using that grounding sensation to help extend the spine up to the heavens.'[8] Classes are slow explorations of a small number of postures, and teachers generally offer imagery and metaphor to convey the feeling of different movements.

If what you really need is substantial muscular strength to bolster your resting muscle tone and give more active support, a Scaravelli class is probably not the place you're going to get it. If, on the other hand, you already have another strength and fitness oriented practice, Scaravelli can be a gentle, creative way to explore yoga postures from a more intuitive point of view. Scaravelli-inspired teachers tend to invite awareness and suggest movement pathways rather than telling you what to do. As Lucy Greaves explains, 'It's up to you to decide if you're doing a posture "right", rather than relying on a teacher to "correct" your shape.'[9] While for some hypermobile people, this may be a friendly way of easing into movement, for others it can be important initially to receive clear and directive movement cues, and a more instructed type of class may be more suitable.

Bikram and hot yoga

Bikram yoga consists of a set series of 26 postures, practised in a room heated to 105 degrees Fahrenheit – a temperature in itself a potential problem for some with POTS and cardiovascular issues. Some hypermobile people have told me they enjoy hot forms because the extreme heat releases spasming muscles. Patra, a yoga practitioner with HSD, says, 'I love the way that muscle knots release in a very hot studio, and I find I can get much further into positions.' And therein lies the problem. The releasing effect of heat on tight and painful muscles may initially feel great, but performing challenging yoga postures while in this state is likely to further destabilise the musculoskeletal system in the long run. As a hypermobile person, the last thing you want is to be moving further into your end range of motion.

Another issue for hypermobile students is that Bikram teachers work from a set script which includes cues that no hypermobility-informed teacher would offer their hypermobile students (locking back your knees in standing postures, for example), and which may make joint issues and general biomechanics more problematic. According to an article on Healthline website:

> The script calls for [teachers] to encourage students to stretch further into their poses and to not leave the room if they feel overwhelmed by the heat. Instructors sometimes follow students out of the room to persuade them to come back in. Some liken the instructional style to boot camp.[10]

It has been known for a Bikram teacher to stand by while students enter postures with dangerously poor alignment and without adequate preparation. I have witnessed this myself, as have other teachers I have spoken to. In any style of yoga there are more and less skilful teachers, but the format and ethos of a Bikram class mitigates against teachers acting for students' biomechanical security. It's a high-risk situation, and I would suggest you avoid it.

Hot yoga rooms are generally also heated to at least 100 degrees Fahrenheit, but what is practised in them may vary hugely from class to class. A quick Google search yields hot vinyasa, hot yin yoga, hot Dharma Wheel, hot aerial yoga, hot yogasana, hot Jivamukti and hot Rocket Yoga, to name a few. If a style is not appropriate for the majority of hypermobile students at normal room temperature, it's going to be even less so at temperatures that tend to increase joint mobility. On the whole, stick to warm but not hot practice spaces – they're less dangerous for most of us.

Rocket Yoga (a.k.a. 'The Rocket')

Rocket Yoga is a fast and furious adaptation of ashtanga vinyasa, with the gradual progression and strong foundation building that you will find in a good Mysore class removed. According to itsyoga.com, the website of Rocket founder, Larry Schultz, 'These advanced routines are appropriate for all levels of students.'[11] Spot the problem here? If you have hypermobility and you have never done yoga before, I suggest you avoid immediate immersion in fast-paced sequences of challenging postures like the proverbial plague. Find a style of yoga in which you will be introduced to postures in a slow, thorough and methodical way. One of the bywords of Rocket is, 'it gets you there faster'; in reality there are no shortcuts, and trying to pre-empt the process of yoga in this way is likely to fast track you only to the physiotherapist's consulting room – especially if you are hypermobile.

Sivananda yoga

Sivananda was one of the first styles of yoga (along with Iyengar) to become popular in the West. Aligned with the way yoga is practised in Indian ashrams, it's a holistic approach, encompassing breathing practices (*pranayama*), relaxation, vegetarian diet and meditation as well as *asana*. If you're allergic to playlists, designer leggings and feeling the yoga burn, Sivananda could be the way to go.

Sivananda classes start with a sun salutation (focused more on mobility and less on strength than the version practised in ashtanga and in most vinyasa classes) followed by a set of 12 basic postures, practised slowly, usually with pauses. Sivananda postures aren't crazy, so you're less likely to hurt yourself here than in, say, a Rocket class, but you may not build a lot of strength if that's what you're looking for. On the whole, although Sivananda teachers do talk about 'toning', in my experience there's actually more emphasis on mobilising in this practice. That said, if you love Sivananda, you can go outside yoga to fitness practices for your strength and stability work.

Viniyoga

The American Viniyoga Institute describes viniyoga as, 'an approach to yoga that adapts the various means and methods of practice to the unique condition, needs and interests of each individual'.[12] Viniyoga teachers create individual sequences of postures for each student, and emphasise function over form (producing movements in a beneficial way rather than creating beautiful shapes), so this can be an ideal practice situation for a hypermobile student. Viniyoga can be taught in a small group class – with lots of different modifications and adaptations for individual students – but is often taught one to one.

Chair yoga

If you are very debilitated or have POTS symptoms that make it hard to stand, chair yoga can be a helpful way to begin to regain strength and mobility. Most chair yoga is aimed at older and frailer people, but it's also possible to create a physically challenging practice on a chair. This is something that a one-to-one teacher with relevant experience might be able to help you with if you'd like to explore.

In summary

Yoga can be helpful for hypermobility, but it can also be harmful. If you come across a form of yoga you're not familiar with, don't just cross your fingers, rock up and put yourself at risk; do some homework. If there's an online description of the class and the style, read it – and if it doesn't answer your questions, talk to the gym, studio or ideally the teacher about what the class and the style are like. If they don't seem to know really, or are unwilling to talk to you, this is great information – look for a class elsewhere!

In general, avoid any style in which:

- the pace is very fast

- the room is very hot

- teachers stand at the front and do the class with the group

- teachers don't offer much in the way of personalised feedback

- there isn't much leeway for adapting (with the help of the teacher)

- there's more focus on entertainment than offering attention to internal experience

- the marketing is full of gimmicky rah-rah, focused on selling you a lifestyle or preoccupied with physical appearance

- beginners are encouraged to try very physically challenging, gymnastic-type postures.

Give the style a try if:

- it goes at a steady pace

- there is an emphasis on feeling into effective biomechanical patterns

- there are opportunities for the teacher to offer individualised feedback

- there are opportunities for the teacher to listen to students and adapt appropriately

- you are encouraged to offer attention to embodied experience

- there is an emphasis on building a foundation slowly and securely.

Playlists

While there's nothing intrinsically wrong with music in a yoga class, bear in mind that the less external distraction there is while you practise, the more easily you will be able to attend to internal experience. A little ambient sound may help you to make the shift inwards, but a 'kickass playlist' is there to entertain you. Save it for dancing round the kitchen, or go to a conscious dance class. When you are practising yoga, you need to be able to concentrate on what you are moving and how.

Which setting

Just as styles of yoga have proliferated, so have the settings in which yoga can be found. Yoga now takes place in dedicated yoga studios (some small and independent, others part of large commercial chains), boutique fitness studios, gyms, complementary health centres, leisure centres, church halls, community centres, parks, workplaces, rooms above pubs… While no one setting is absolutely guaranteed to be appropriate for a hypermobile yoga practitioner, some are going to be more (and others less) likely to serve a person with hypermobility well. The following are a few general guidelines.

Large chains and commercial enterprises

All businesses, including yoga studios, have to be financially viable in order to survive. That understood, there are some ventures for which the primary motivations are to offer intelligent yoga grounded in embodied awareness, to promote inclusive community, to uphold high ethical standards…and there are others for which the main objective is to achieve market dominance and make as much money as possible. In general, the quality of what is on offer to you in terms of excellent teaching and practices grounded in integrity will be conditioned by the intention and ethos of the organisation providing the classes. While a primarily commercial goal does not preclude knowledgeable and experienced teachers, the likelihood is that in this kind of setting most teachers will be poorly paid and therefore relatively newly qualified, and even where a teacher has a considerable body of experience, they may be hampered from using it because the management requires them to teach in such a way as to bring in large numbers of students (rather than with depth and authenticity).

Big chains can make huge economies of scale and tend to market aggressively to bring new members in. It can be tempting to go for a chain yoga studio membership when it's offered at a huge discount, especially if your earning capacity is limited by hypermobility-related disability. Bear in mind, though, that one class with a carefully chosen, experienced and hypermobility-informed teacher is worth a dozen with random teachers who may have no awareness of hypermobility and may be unable to help you to work in biomechanically beneficial ways – or, potentially, to help you individually at all, because they are spinning plates to keep a large and variously able group of strangers on track.

Gym classes

Much of the above also goes for yoga classes in gyms. While there are some honourable exceptions, those who bring a wealth of experience to their teaching and offer classes of integrity, in general gym-class yoga teachers tend to be relatively young and newly qualified. Of course, there's nothing wrong with that *per se*; we all have to start somewhere, and new teachers can bring a refreshing blast of excitement and enthusiasm. The problem for hypermobile people is that hEDS, HSD and MFS are complex to work with and require a teacher with a degree of hypermobility awareness and considerable experience of facilitating functional movement patterns.

While there are always exceptions, gym classes tend to be large – 30 or 40 is not uncommon – and it's easy to get lost in the crowd. This is a particular issue for those hypermobile people who appear on the surface to move well and are able to shoehorn themselves into postures requiring flexibility – but are in fact experiencing pain, muscular hypotonicity and hypertonicity, proprioceptive difficulties…and so on. Even if the teacher has the knowledge and experience to notice, in a huge group they are unlikely to have the time to offer you any substantial help.

For many of those who are also autistic or highly sensitive, the noise, fluorescent lighting, omnipresent screens and general busyness of the gym environment is going to be prohibitive, no matter how great (or not) the classes.

Large and long-established yoga studios

These large commercial studios with multiple locations and recognisable branding exist for the most part only in big cities. The yoga fame and kudos of working at a 'top' studio is attractive to many teachers. As a result, these studios are able to be selective about who they employ, most requiring five to ten years' of pre-existing teaching experience, so you can be fairly sure that a teacher at an established high-profile studio will be well grounded in teaching practice and will have something of substance to offer students.

The main downside here is in the kind of relationship you are likely to be able to forge with your teacher in this setting. Class sizes in big, well-known studios are frequently large. It may all be a bit anonymous and can feel like practising in a high-end supermarket, with your teacher unlikely to get to know you well or to be able to offer you much individual help and guidance. This is, of course, particularly problematic when you are hypermobile and may have complex patterns of pain, proprioceptive challenge and biomechanical difficulty – which may also change from day to day.

Then there's also the issue of cost. You need a good income to be able to afford classes at the big, established studios. If hypermobility and co-existing conditions limit your ability to work, class costs and membership fees may be out of reach.

While the studios themselves are usually very quiet, changing rooms, shops and cafes at some (not all) of the very large studios can be surprisingly busy and noisy and may be off-putting to hypermobile people who are also autistic. Some of the big studios use incense throughout the building – potentially difficult if you have sensory sensitivities or MCAS.

Small independent studios

As you might expect, a diverse range of intentions and approaches come under the 'independent' umbrella. Many small independents are the beloved baby of a long-time, dedicated yoga teacher and are founded in a desire to offer yoga classes of real worth, substance and integrity. In terms of suitability for a hypermobile practitioner, check out the ethos of the studio – look at promotional materials, ask about the studio in local social media groups, talk to the studio owner. Do the classes seem sensible, well-paced, informed by good movement principles and concerned with the welfare of students? Avoid studios offering gimmicky classes (Harry Potter yoga, karaoke yoga, beer yoga – yes, these do all really exist) and those specialising in hot yoga, Rocket Yoga or anything else that goes at a lick or encourages students to 'have a go' at gymnastic postures that really require years of foundation building and then may still be inappropriate for the majority of people.

Small studios usually can't be as fussy as the big ones in terms of minimum standards they require of the teachers they employ, and it's advisable to ask about the background, training and experience of any teacher whose class you are considering attending; nevertheless, a good studio will freight its teaching team with one or two teachers with a track record of teaching, extensive personal practice and solid training. They are the ones to seek out if you are practising with hypermobility.

Independent studios tend to be small, so a plus is that class numbers will usually be low and teachers are more likely to be able to get to know you and your needs. If you are also autistic and have sensory issues, this is likely to be a quiet environment, and it will be easier here than in the big studios to talk to the management about any issues you encounter with incense and other potential sensory triggers.

Independently run classes

Independently run classes (organised by the teacher themselves) can be found in community centres, church halls, home studios, hired studios – and just about anywhere there is available space. Some classes in small yoga studios are independently run: rather than being paid by the studio owner to teach a specific type of class, the teacher rents the studio and runs their own class in the space.

Don't assume that because a class is taking place in your local church hall or community centre, it won't be as good as one in a yoga centre. Very experienced teachers often choose to run their own classes so that they can teach, market and organise in a way that works for them. You may find a greater diversity of offerings and more individual styles and approaches in independent classes – some of which would not be given the time of day in more homogenised commercial settings but which may have very valuable perspectives to offer. Of course, independent classes are run by relatively inexperienced teachers too, so you need to evaluate the appropriateness of the class and the teacher for someone with hypermobility in the usual way.

A big advantage of independent classes is that the teacher will generally have much more of a relationship with their students: they are likely to be able to greet everyone by name, be familiar with their practice, and know about and remember any conditions the person may have – very helpful for those with hypermobility.

Community centres can be quiet or noisy, depending on the time of day and what else is running at the same time as yoga, but they are generally not as hyper-stimulating as gyms. They are usually also embedded in the community, so may not require you to travel far, which can be helpful if you are experiencing fatigue.

Independent teachers often offer concessionary rates, and many will never turn away a student who genuinely wants to make a commitment to yoga but can't afford to pay. As hypermobility and co-existing conditions may make it impossible to work full time, or at all, some flexibility over fees can be very helpful.

Which teacher?

While the type of yoga you practise and the setting in which you practise it are important, probably the most crucial factor in having a helpful experience of yoga as a hypermobile practitioner, is working with an appropriate teacher. With so many yoga teachers around these days, you might think it would be relatively easy to locate the right one for you, but in fact many of the hypermobile people who contact me have spent years searching unsuccessfully for a teacher able to help them to practise in a positive and relatively injury-free way. In order to understand what's going on here, it may be useful to know something about the current culture of yoga and the way yoga teacher training fits into it.

Some things it's helpful to know about yoga teacher training

Back in the day, yoga was a niche activity, considered by most people to be comical or odd. How things have changed! According to *The Guardian*, 'yoga' was one of the most googled words in the UK in 2016; the US yoga market was worth $16bn in 2017, and the global yoga market $80bn and growing.[13] Yoga teacher training is an important element in this financial sector. 'Double Revenue at Your Yoga Studio with a Teacher Training Program' proclaims the title of an article on Causely,[14] and, indeed, in a competitive market, offering a teacher training makes the difference between financial viability and going under for many yoga studios.

While the reality of teaching yoga is prosaic, and for many teachers involves hard work for low pay, the engine of advertorial and social media puffs out a steady obscuring smoke. #YogaTeacher features exotic locations, lithe young bodies, radiant health and designer clothing. It's a glamour-spangled lifestyle that is very attractive, particularly to young (and mostly white) women. Huge numbers of people are seeking yoga teacher training, and there is no shortage of opportunities for them to train. In terms of the supply of yoga teachers, this situation has created a funnel-shaped demographic, with a small number of experienced (and often sought-after) teachers at the narrow end and an oversupply of newly trained teachers making up the greater part of the yoga teacher population at the wide end. While it's easy to find a yoga teacher, it's much more challenging to locate a teacher likely to have the experience to work with the many complexities that generally characterise hypermobile students.

It should be pretty obvious, I think, that in order for a yoga teacher to have anything of substance to teach, they first have to have a significant body of personal practice to teach from. This is a period of time (in my view a decade is about the minimum necessary) in which they have engaged regularly in exploration of their own somatic experience on their own mat. Few students entering teacher training have anything like this. Most teacher trainings require a minimum of two years of yoga practice – and attending a weekly yoga class in a setting where there are many participants and little individual teaching can satisfy this condition. There are also plenty of teacher trainings that require *no* prior experience of practising yoga – yes, that's right, *no* experience. According to one respondee on Quora, who had recently qualified as a yoga teacher:

> It's not really necessary to have any experience before joining a yoga teacher training course, and I've seen many yoga students who enrolled in a yoga teacher training programme without having any experience. In fact, most people who pursue yoga teacher training courses are beginners.[15]

A quick Google search will bring up a plethora of accredited yoga teacher trainings that will take your money and book you onto a course right away, no questions asked and no evidence of practice experience required.

As a mentor of yoga teachers, I have met some new teacher training graduates who have practised yoga for many years and who have received thorough training over a lengthy period...and I have met some others who have no personal practice and a very sketchy grasp of the concepts and techniques of yoga. These teachers have scant understanding of the biomechanics of yoga postures in their own body, never mind anyone else's; little understanding of the dynamics of the student–teacher relationship; and are unable to hold a safe and secure class space. These are not the teachers you need as a hypermobile practitioner.

The older generation of teachers

I am part of a generation for whom the path to teaching yoga quite often was: you practise yoga for a very long time and then someone asks you to teach. I had been practising yoga for 22 years when I taught my first class. I had a recent yoga therapy training and a short adjustment one, but the 200-hour standard had not been invented, and I had nothing equivalent to what constitutes a yoga teacher training today. I mention this to make you aware that having a teacher training certificate is not the be-all and end-all, and not necessarily the best recommendation of a teacher. Some of the most experienced and knowledgeable teachers around learnt in the crucible of their personal practice and then through doing – and in some cases apprenticing. Of course, an older person hasn't necessarily been practising yoga for decades, and you need to check this out with your potential teacher. But be aware that practice and experience may in some instances trump training.

Some things it's helpful to know about yoga-teacher accreditation

There is no legal regulation of yoga teaching (or yoga therapy) in the UK or in the US: anyone can teach yoga (and anyone can practise as a yoga therapist); no training or experience are necessary.[16] However, there are several voluntary accrediting bodies and there is a generally agreed 200-hour minimum standard of teacher training in both the UK and the US. The accrediting bodies you will mainly come across when looking for a teacher are:

- Yoga Alliance (US)
- Yoga Alliance Professionals (UK)
- The British Wheel of Yoga (UK)
- Independent Yoga Network (UK).

You need to be aware that what can be covered even in a very good 200-hour yoga teacher training is quite limited (and not all 200-hour yoga teacher trainings are good). Being registered with a professional body does not mean that a teacher will be equipped to work with a student with hypermobility. You will still need to ask the teacher about their training, experience and general suitability to work with you.

The main accrediting bodies for yoga therapists are:

- International Association of Yoga Therapists (IAYT) (US based but registers yoga therapists internationally) – yoga therapists who satisfy IAYT criteria are C-IAYT registered

- British Council for Yoga Therapy (UK) – whose members can apply for registration with the Complementary and Natural Healthcare Council (CNHC).

While standards for yoga therapy registration are more rigorous than those for yoga teaching, yoga therapy is a broad category, including a very wide range of different approaches. You will need to check that any yoga therapist you are considering working with has the skills and experience you're looking for and is aware of the particular issues of hypermobile people.

What to look for in a teacher

Teachers who have helped me have all listened, believed what I said and been willing to help me work with what my body can/cannot do on any given day. When I've been frustrated (I often have), they have encouraged me to stay present to my own frustration – and to focus on the things I can do rather than the things I can't.

Kitty (yoga practitioner with HSD)

For me, a good teacher is someone with kindness and creativity, who is willing to research and think laterally and laugh with me when I present myself in class in my spinal collar and with my elbows, knees, ankles and wrists all braced – and still make the class inclusive for me.

Tiane (yoga practitioner with hEDS)

Teacher–student is a relationship, and like any other relationship it's highly personal. A teacher who is perfect for one student might be anathema to another – and vice versa. That said, there are some key skills, attitudes and capacities that on the whole fit a teacher to work well with hypermobility. Search out teachers who:

- actually teach: who take time to explain the what, the how and the why of postures – some teachers will do this through anatomical explanation, some by suggesting images, some by demonstrating particular actions that need to happen – and many teachers will use a combination of all these methods

- leave their own mat frequently to give personalised help and guidance

- ask permission before physically adjusting you, who adjust sensitively and for whom the purpose of an adjustment is to:

  - help you understand the dynamics of the posture

  - hold the structure of a posture for you so that you can feel it (even if you can't yet create it for yourself)

  - help you to identify where you need to engage more and where to let go

  - help you to identify where you are hyperextending

  - offer emotional support

  - help you to integrate or metabolise a movement.

  There's lots more about adjusting in Chapters 2 (see 'Adjustment') and 3 (see 'Adjustment: speaking in hands'). Although this information is aimed at teachers, it will also help you to work out what to consent to – and what to decline – if a teacher offers you an adjustment.

- listen to you and are able to respond sensitively and empathetically

- can offer appropriate modifications and suggest alternative ways of accessing a posture

- hold strong, clear, kind boundaries, with whom you feel safe, secure and contained, and with whom you feel empowered to speak, suggest, explore, experiment and create

- recognise the proprioceptive challenges involved in hypermobility and are able to work with them patiently – even when this entails repeating the same verbal cue or the same physical adjustment again and again

- understand that endurance is compromised in hypermobility and that hold times and numbers of repetitions need to be modified in order for practice to be strengthening for a hypermobile person

- understand that for many people fatigue is an aspect of hypermobility and respect the need of hypermobile students for rest – between postures, between practice days, within sequences and so on

- understand that the patterns of hyperextension and hypotonicity that typify hypermobility are usually very slow to change and that making these shifts has to be seen as a long-term project

- are willing to be creative and work adaptively

- encourage you to find an edge that is appropriate for you (see 'Edge' below)

- ask for medical details on their first encounter with you, ask clarifying questions and listen to your answers

- are in an ongoing conversation with you about your practice and its effects on your body, and are responsive to any needs you may have for adaptations and modifications.

What to avoid in a teacher

I've frequently been encouraged to do postures that are way too hard for me because I am very flexible, whereas really I know I should be working at a much more basic level and focusing on activating the right muscles.

Isie (yoga practitioner with HSD)

On the whole, steer clear of teachers who:

- stand up front and do the class with you. Some hypermobile students like to copy because, with poor proprioception, monkey see, monkey do can feel a lot easier than learning and embodying movements independently. However, practising this way is problematic for a number of reasons. For one thing, a teacher who is doing the class themselves is not focused on what's happening in it and is unlikely to notice if some participants are flailing around and have not understood the dynamics of the movements they are being asked to produce; nor does this teacher have opportunities to offer individualised help to students. Another important consideration is that all bodies are different, so the way a posture looks on the teacher's body may not be the way it needs to manifest through yours. When you copy postures, you are working with surfaces; when you embody the principles of postures, on the other hand, you are creating opportunities for postures to emerge in a unique way through the structures and processes of your own body. Shortcuts here lead only to unhelpful biomechanics and injury. You will develop proprioception, range, strength and skill as a mover by taking the long route: slowly, and with the help of your teacher, feeling your way into each *asana*

- encourage you to try physically challenging or 'advanced' postures before you have done the groundwork to practise them safely

- project their own responses to, or beliefs about, hypermobility onto you – for example:

  - they're impressed by your hypermobility and push you to go further than is appropriate for you in postures requiring a lot of flexibility

  - they blame you for your hypermobility, criticising you for not building enough strength, hyperextending or appearing floppy

  - they assume that you're not paying attention/lazy/not interested... when you take longer than CT-typical students to learn a posture

  - they assume that you are a 'pushy' or aggressive practitioner when you get injured more frequently than CT-typical students

- use physical adjustment to stretch you or to pretzel you 'deeper' into postures

- are dogmatic, imposing cookie-cutter rules of alignment, received sequences of postures or non-negotiable ways of doing things

- seem clueless about how to work with your hypermobility and just leave you to get on with it.

It's fine – and actually a good idea – to contact a potential teacher before coming to a class to let them know that you are hypermobile and ask about their approach and background. While most teachers are very busy and won't be able to enter into an extended email conversation with you, a sound and responsible teacher will be happy to share some information and give you an idea about the suitability of their style and training.

Don't necessarily rule a teacher out just because they have no pre-existing experience of working with hypermobility – especially if they have a good reputation and a long track record. Skills at working with movement patterns are transferrable across a wide range of different bodies, as is the capacity to work adaptively. Your teacher may be willing to do some research or training in the specific area of hypermobility. I sometimes offer one-to-two sessions to a teacher and their hypermobile student to help them find strategies, explanations, alternatives and general ways of working together more effectively.

Don't assume that just because a teacher is very experienced they will automatically know all about hypermobility – notice a theme here? While awareness is growing, hypermobility continues to be poorly understood and frequently unrecognised in the yoga world, and senior teachers may have distorted or limited ideas about what it means to be hypermobile. Make the usual enquiries about the appropriateness of this teacher to work with you.

Out on a limb: reorienting towards structure

I loved stretching – oh, how I loved stretching! It took me the longest time to get that by constantly pulling on my joints I was actually creating more pain and instability – and I wasn't even getting more flexible anyway! What really turned things around was understanding that what I actually needed was a bit more stability. Then I started to realise that there were other things I could feel apart from my joints more or less popping out of their sockets.

Annie (yoga teacher with MFS)

As hypermobile practitioners, we often begin our yoga journey strung out in our limbs and hanging in our joints. We hold ourselves up by opening the joints to their maximum (hyperextending) and stacking bone ends together to create a precarious kind of stability. It's a house-of-cards situation: it only stands up because each card is leaning on another. Supporting (or not supporting) ourselves in this way is a problem for a number of reasons:

- Joints are meant to be held firmly together, and repeatedly wrenching them apart destabilises the joint structure, potentially leading to injury. Iyengar yoga teacher and physiotherapist, Julie Gudmestad, explains:

    Many yoga students are quite surprised to learn that joints can become too flexible. But in many joints, ligaments and tendons play a major role in preventing excessive motion; if those tissues become too loose, the joint can move in ways that cause damage or set the stage for injury.[17]

- Over time, pressing bone into bone can create degeneration of bone surfaces and contribute to early-onset osteoarthritis.

- When we don't have good, active physical support, we are, in my experience, more likely to feel anxious, ungrounded, uncontained and overwhelmed. Our nervous system may be chronically activated and more likely to become stuck in sympathetic states – in some cases even giving rise to low-level trauma.

- As we saw in Chapter 1, hypermobile bodies are slack because collagenous structures (ligaments, fascia) are lax, and because muscle tone is low. While you can't change the genetic coding of your collagen, you can improve muscle tone by strengthening muscles in active postures and through cross training (see 'Yoga addiction versus cross training and supportive practices' below). This improved tensility carries over to baseline resting muscle states – and may help to give you a more comfortable night's sleep, with fewer subluxations and muscle spasms.

Working preferentially for strength in a yoga practice may initially present something of a challenge to hypermobile practitioners, who often prefer passive stretching and tend to flop into position. But with attentive practice, it is possible to reorient towards strength and stability as intentions. It's important to understand that (barring specialised passive approaches – see Chapter 5) yoga postures are intended to engage muscles in contraction as much as stretching, and that by giving equal weight to the contractive components we can find structure and containment, and the capacity to relate our outlying body parts back to the centre. Once you have made this shift, the new exploration will generally be so much more subtle, intricate and absorbing – and will offer so many more rewards in terms of decreased pain levels, musculoskeletal integrity and general physical capacity – that the old ways will no longer appeal.

A word of caution: creating strength and stability is not about gripping muscles or doing many repetitions of demanding endurance exercises. Most personal trainers agree that if your intention is to build strength, a small number of repetitions combined with substantial rest times is necessary – and that's for CT-typical people. Go slowly, be conservative. If you overshoot your actual capacity, you will injure yourself.

Edge

If we were to reduce yoga down to the bones, it's breath, movement and attention that would be left at the bottom of my saucepan. And whenever we breathe, move and attend to experience, we generate an encounter with a fourth thing, usually referred to in yoga as 'edge'. Beginning yoga practitioners often equate 'being on the edge' with 'going to the limit' – which for a hypermobile person tends to mean hanging out at end range of motion. Going to the limit is one particular experience of edge – but only one.

Many hypermobile people – and I have been one of them – love to dance on the brink of the precipice. This preference is often driven at least in part by a deficit in proprioception: for a lot of us extremity is that rare situation in which we receive fairly constant proprioceptive feedback. It's often only when injury or exhaustion forces us to re-evaluate how we are engaging with our practice that we begin to question the wisdom of habitually hanging on by our fingernails. In other words, we are compelled to renegotiate our relationship with edge.

For me, edge can best be described as the way we choose to place ourselves in relation to a particular sensation, emotion, thought or memory arising from our embodied experience. Rather than a singular position it's actually more like a spectrum of possibilities. Senior yoga teacher, Erich Schiffmann, describes edge like this:

> Each pose has a 'minimum edge' and a 'maximum edge', as well as a series of intermediary edges between these... [The maximum edge] is the point where the stretch begins to hurt. It is the furthest point of tightness beyond which you should not go. If you were to force yourself beyond this point, you would definitely be in pain and might hurt yourself or pull a muscle. The minimum edge is where you sense the very first sensation of stretch, the very first hint of resistance coming from your muscles.[18]

Erich's description implies that the edge is actually the middle: the centre point (or multiplicity of centre points) between too little and too much... too weak and too strong...too slack and too tight...too comfortable and too strenuous...a location that can be difficult for a person with impaired proprioception to divine. By setting an intention to feel our way out of end points, however, we can start to explore this middle ground, and as we slowly familiarise ourselves with the territory, we become more able to inhabit it.

What constitutes appropriate edge varies from person to person, posture to posture, day to day, moment to moment. There will be times in your practice when it feels helpful to press a little harder into your edge and times when it feels more useful to draw back. In other words, edge is not one location or a final arrival; it's never discovered, mapped, done and dusted. Edge is an ongoing process, an endless dance of shifting experience. Nor is edge really separate from us. There's no thin black line out there against which we in here pit ourselves. Edge is intrinsic, a unique product of the interplay between our individual body and psyche with a particular posture in a particular moment in time.

Being in conscious relationship with edge doesn't guarantee that we will be safe and injury free as a hypermobile yoga practitioner, but it does offer us some checks and gauges. Edge is a tool of enquiry that can help us to cultivate our sense of dwelling in our own movement and of being contained within our own body. As we experience these things with greater consistency and increasing subtlety, we become more able to tune into our actual embodied needs. Things become more real and more substantial. We may also start to feel a little more at home in the world, less anxious, less overwhelmed and less dependent on any unhealthy coping mechanisms we habitually resort to – cutting, starving, bingeing, headbanging and so on.

Experiential work: exploring the edge

You can take 20 minutes for this exploration or you can take an hour or longer. Its power is in repetition – do it as often as you are able to, and integrate it into your regular yoga practice.

You will need a quiet space where you are not likely to be interrupted, a yoga mat (or whichever kind of surface you choose to practise standing postures on) and any props you require to rest comfortably. If you are not able to stand or to lie on the floor, you can do this exploration in a chair.

1. Start lying down on your mat or chosen surface (or sitting in your chair) in a comfortable position, using props if you find them helpful. Begin to tune into your internal experience. Notice physical sensations... Notice any emotions you are aware of... Notice thoughts coming and going... Notice breath coming in...and going out... Whenever you become aware that your attention has drifted, gently bring it back to noticing your experience in the moment: what's happening now? Take at least a couple of minutes to enter the terrain of your body in this way.

2. You are going to practise Downdog. If Downdog is not possible for you, choose another standing posture that involves structure and offers opportunities to stretch. If you're in a chair, you will now come

into your active posture. This could be as simple as sitting upright, with your legs and feet parallel and your muscles engaged, spine away from the back of the chair if possible. Bring yourself into the posture in whichever way is familiar to you. Start to notice your physical experience. When you identify a sensation, ask yourself these questions:

- Where in my body do I feel this sensation?

- What kind of sensation is it – hot or cold, moving or still, pulsating, shooting, achy, deep or superficial…?

- Do any colours or images go with this sensation?

- Do any emotions go with this sensation?

- Do I feel called to stay with this sensation…move more deeply into it…or back off?

- And when I stay/move more deeply in/back off, what happens?

Hold the posture for as long as you are comfortable in it, and then drop back into any resting position that works for you – lying down on your back, Child's Pose (*balasana*), resting back in the chair, for example.

3. As you rest, reflect on what you noticed in the posture. Did anything feel familiar? Did anything feel new? Do you tend to press on in, or do you tend to draw back from sensation, or do you do something different? Were there moments when you felt as if you were on your edge: in just the 'right' place? Did the edge change as you followed it? Did you lose it or could you stay with it?

4. Move back into Downdog or your active posture. This time, notice how much effort you are making to sustain the posture. Notice what happens if:

- you work more energetically – engage more strongly to hold the shape

- you let go a little bit, allow yourself to relax, become softer.

Know that this is an open exploration. There is no 'correct' approach, no better/best. When you feel ready, drop back into your resting posture.

5. As you rest, be aware of anything you noticed in the posture. Did you find any sweet spots on the spectrum between maximum and minimum effort? Did anything feel familiar? Did anything feel unfamiliar? Did you learn anything?

6. Move back into Downdog or your active posture. This time, notice in particular any thoughts or feelings that arise. Be aware that you can choose to move towards any thought or feeling...and you can choose to move away from it. When you feel ready, drop back into your resting position.

7. As you rest, be aware of anything you noticed in the active posture. Were there internal positions or perspectives that enabled you to include more of your experience without feeling triggered or overwhelmed by it? Were these positions or perspectives constant or did they change? Did you find your internal edge at any point? Were you able to stay with it or did it come and go?

8. Let go of the enquiry and take some time to rest quietly, allowing thoughts, feelings, sensations and awarenesses to come and go. Give yourself at least five minutes to rest like this. If your practice has been longer, take ten minutes or more.

Mobilisation versus stretching

It often seems incomprehensible to those with normal collagen that a hypermobile person would want or need to stretch. Nevertheless, the *experience* of being hypermobile is often one of tightness and restriction, and the desire for some form of physical release is very real. Rosemary Keer (senior physiotherapist and hypermobility specialist) and Jane Butler (hand therapist and hypermobility specialist) note:

> Many hypermobiles like to stretch, but have been advised not to by health professionals for fear of damaging their tissues or joints through over-stretching. An unpublished audit at Guy's Hospital in 1986...revealed that patients with joint hypermobility found stretching helpful. This came as a surprise to the audit's authors, but has been borne out repeatedly in clinical experience. Stiffness is a common complaint, with many hypermobiles saying they 'feel like a 90-year-old'.[19]

According to Keer and Butler, this felt stiffness could be due to disuse of muscles in response to pain, or it could be that, 'hypermobile individuals are more likely to use their global muscles for stability and are therefore subject to more increased [sic] muscle tension and spasm'.[20]

While lots of passive stretching is not recommended for hypermobile people, it is not true to say that we should never stretch. Keer and Butler note that, 'Stretching can be a helpful antidote' to stiffness, tension and spasm, but with the important caveat that, 'it is important that the hypermobile individual does not overstretch, which is potentially easy to do'. They explain that:

> It becomes necessary to differentiate between stretching performed in order to regain and maintain muscle length, relieve muscle tension, or restore and maintain joint range, and stretching to increase an already hypermobile range of motion. It is good to stretch, but care is required. Educating an individual about how they can stretch safely without overstretching into their hypermobile or more vulnerable areas will help develop better body awareness, a skill which can be used in the future to ensure safe exercising.[21]

The following are some of the things you can do to make stretching low risk and likely to contribute to healthy biomechanics:

- Avoid hanging in (or hyperextending) your joints.

- Stretch actively, staying out of end range and engaging muscles to offer support and resistance.

- Stick to short hold times – usually shorter than those suggested for CT-typical people.

- Stretch selectively, where there is contraction or excessive tension, and not globally.

- Balance stretching with even more strengthening – tightness is often due to a lack of muscular support: while stretching can offer temporary relief here, it does not provide a longer-term solution.

- Learn to discriminate between the sensations of tension (conservative stretching may help) and inflammation (do not stretch).

- Swap out some stretches for myofascial release.

Myofascial release (MFR)

Originally a technique offered by specialised massage therapists and some physiotherapists and osteopaths, myofascial release is increasingly being taught and practised as a self-massage technique. If you're hypermobile, you may already have a collection of tennis balls, lacrosse balls, golf balls, prickly balls, squishy balls, foot rollers, foam rollers and Thumbbys™[22] that you like to lie on. The practice of applying tools like this to release body knots and kinks is myofascial release.

As we saw in Chapter 1 (see 'Fascia'), 'myofascia' refers to the interwoven fabric of muscles, tendons and fascia. Painful, contracted spots within this fabric are known as 'trigger points'. The defining sensation of a trigger point is of deep, aching tightness – and slow relief if you press into it. An MFR therapist will locate trigger points by the feeling of the tissue: whereas myofascia should be pliable and elastic to the touch, trigger points are tight, stiff and resistant when lightly pressed. According to the website of John Barnes, the originator of the Myofascial Release Approach and the granddaddy of hands-on myofascial work:

> Trauma, inflammatory responses, and/or surgical procedures create myofascial restrictions that can produce tensile pressures of approximately 2,000 pounds per square inch on pain-sensitive structures that do not show up in many of the standard tests (x-rays, myelograms, CAT scans, electromyography, etc.).[23]

No wonder your tight shoulder really hurts, eh?!

Why is it good for hypermobility?

While myofascial release can have a positive effect on overall flexibility, its primary intention is not (or doesn't have to be) increasing end range of motion; rather, the main purpose is to break up adhesions, creating greater fluidity and function in the whole myofascial fabric, as well as increasing blood flow and therefore improving oxygenation of tissues. Because it focuses on the fascial network as a whole, MFR is unlikely to create instability and dislocation – as tugging on the joint may do. In my experience, too, offering close, mindful attention to your body in this way can also increase proprioception quite markedly, creating a greater sense of being 'in' your body.

You do need to be careful not to over-release. Bear in mind that muscular tightness in a hypermobile body may be driven by a nervous-system requirement to create compensatory tension. Rigorously releasing may feel great temporarily, but give it an hour or so and the nervous system tends to respond by clamping down muscles with a vengeance. The aim is to gently coax your body to let go, in a climate of self-talk that is soothing and reassuring to the nervous system. Because of the potential for this kind of reactivity, MFR is, in my experience, often most effective when combined with strengthening activities that increase general resting muscle tone.

Using MFR yourself

As far as I remember, no one really taught me myofascial release. It's something I kind of picked up out of the hypermobility/movement work ether. Subsequently, physios and other movement professionals have suggested different ways and places to release, and kindly given me new myofascial toys. If you have health conditions, make sure you check with an appropriate medical professional before trying myofascial release yourself – this is important: there are contraindications, and these require individual medical clearance. Never release directly into:

- burn sites

- fracture sites

- a site where there is heat, inflammation or a trapped nerve

- the site of herniations

- the site of recent surgery.

Other than that, MFR is generally low risk for hypermobile people, so feel free to gather some tactile objects and roll on them. Different tissues and different degrees of fascial restriction will respond better to different degrees of hardness, so intend to acquire a range from soft to penetrating. You will be able to access some areas better with a pointed, thumb-like surface (hence the Thumbby™), and other areas will prefer something broader and flatter, such as a large firm ball. Be aware that a trigger point can cause pain at a site remote from its actual location, so explore broadly. On the whole, be creative, be intuitive, be playful and follow your own thread. I start most days with MFR, taking at least 20 minutes, and up to an hour. MFR can be a practice in its own right and is also great as a general mobilisation prior to a physically challenging activity.

If you'd like some help and guidance to get started with MFR, Ariele Foster, a yoga teacher and physiotherapist with a specialism in hypermobility, has lots of YouTube resources. Find them at www.youtube.com/user/sacredsourceyoga/videos. Ariele also offers paid-for online MFR courses at https://yogaanatomyacademy.com.

Melissa West also has a series of gentle yoga and myofascial release classes on YouTube at: www.youtube.com/user/drmelissawest.

Trauma awareness

Be aware that working with myofascia can release traumatic memories which have been stored in the safe house of the body. Most of the time, this is helpful: memories are arising because they are ready to be received into conscious mind, and the process of integration will naturally happen. If you are activating emotional material that feels overwhelming, stop. Seek out the help of a Somatic Experiencing therapist, Phoenix Rising yoga therapist or body-based psychotherapist with a specialism in trauma. They will be able to guide you through the process of remembering and embodying in a safe and supported way.

Working with pain

Nowadays, even if I have an acute injury or am in a lot of chronic pain, I still turn up for sessions with my amazing personal trainer. If I can't lift weights, maybe I can do some cardio, or some isometric work, or I can just use my upper body, or just my lower body. There's always some way to work with what I've got. Knowing that makes me feel better, more in control. I know that there are always ways of continuing to move with my EDS, and when I move, the pain is more manageable.

Zara (yoga practitioner with hEDS)

I was 18 when I did my first yoga class – almost unbelievably young (or so it seems from the perspective of 57) and living in a kind of embodiment haze, through which I only dimly apprehended most of my sensate experience. (Actually, although I didn't recognise it at the time, I was propelled into movement practice by an urgent need to find my way into my body.) In early yoga classes I experienced a fair amount of low-level pain, but I normalised it because I heard other students joking about how the postures 'hurt'. I didn't realise that the types of sensation they were describing were (for the most part) the enjoyable good-hurts of muscles stretching and strengthening... whereas I was experiencing (for the most part) the not-so-positive pain of ligaments and tendons being pulled beyond their healthy range of motion, and joints destabilising.

Working physically inevitably entails breadth and intensity of sensation, and the journey into it can feel like walking a maze, full of dead ends, confusing double backs and sudden unexpected openings. Interpreting all of this information with some degree of accuracy is a complex business. While some intense sensations – such as those associated with aggressive passive stretching or working muscles repeatedly beyond the point of fatigue – do signal potential harm, not everything we categorise as painful is a stop signal. When working with pain, it helps a lot to be able to let yourself off the hook: it's unrealistic to expect to be able to divine perfectly the significance of every pain and discomfort you feel in your body. At times overshooting and at other times stopping short is a given. These are not so much mistakes as intricate steps in the ongoing choreography of the dance of edge. However, given time and experience you can become a little more sure-footed in discriminating between sensations you can beneficially stay with and observe, and those that require you to back off and take a different approach.

Experiential work: exploring pain and uncomfortable sensations

This exploration is designed for any time you encounter pain or discomfort in your yoga practice. You may want to introduce it initially into a slower practice, in which you will have lots of time to feel into what's happening. As you develop more facility in the exploration, you will be able to move through it more quickly and easily, and eventually, given time and consistency, it will become a natural and automatic part of every practice you do.

When you feel a painful or uncomfortable sensation, or a sensation you are not sure about, pause...notice what you are experiencing...and ask yourself some of the following questions – whichever feel relevant, interesting or juicy in the moment. Just go with whichever ones call you:

- Is this sensation dull, achy, deep-lying or close to the surface?

- Do any images go with this sensation?

- Do any emotions go with this sensation?

- Does it feel good to press on into this sensation? Does the sensation dissipate if I do this?

- Is this sensation hot, sharp, electric or burning? (If the answer is 'yes', there may be nerve involvement. Take this as a signal to back off. Excessive stretching or compression can cause nerve damage.)

- Am I pulling on ligaments and tendons (at the site of the joint) or do I feel as if I'm stretching into the belly of the muscle? (Generally, we want to be experiencing any stretch in the main body of the muscle, not where it attaches to bone.)

- Does this sensation feel like fatigue? Do I need to rest?

- Can I feel that muscles are engaged or am I passively sitting in joints?

Feel free to improvise, ask your own questions and follow your own thread of enquiry.

Take some time at the end of your practice to reflect quietly on your experiences and mark anything significant you noticed.

Over time, be aware of any correlations between types of sensation, ways of responding and outcomes.

Responding to acute pain

If you have just sprained your ankle or cut your finger, you are experiencing acute pain. 'Acute' refers not to the intensity of the sensation but to the immediacy of the situation. This type of pain is a clear response to injury and disappears as the injury heals. Whereas the standard approach to any tear, sprain or break used to be immobilisation, the opposite is now usually the case. With stable fractures, for example, early mobilisation has been found to be more beneficial than a cast.[24] Similarly, NHS advice for sprained and ruptured knee ligaments is to mobilise as early as possible.[25]

Remember that mobilisation is not the same thing as passive stretching, that it may involve tolerable discomfort but should not cause excruciating pain and that continuing to perform extreme manoeuvres with the affected body part is not advisable – if you just tore a hamstring bending forwards, don't go on trying to touch your toes. The aim of mobilisation is to keep the circulation moving through the injury site, and gently, slowly restore normal range of movement.

Responding to chronic pain

As we saw in Chapter 1, chronic (or ongoing) pain can have anatomical drivers. For hypermobile people these may include:

- micro-tears (often resulting from quite ordinary actions that would be benign for non-hypermobile people)

- muscles in spasm

- inflammation due to osteoarthritic degeneration.

But chronic pain can also be driven (partly or wholly) by a kind of hyperactivity of the nervous system. In this situation, pain is no longer an accurate indicator of tissue damage. Usually, this sort of nervous-system dysregulation comes on slowly, perhaps initiated by an acute injury, and is a learned, or conditioned, mal-response. Neil Pearson explains that the nervous system can change in this way because it is to a large extent plastic. Fortunately, by token of this same plasticity it can also be encouraged back into more even, functional ways of responding.[26] Some scientifically endorsed methods for re-regulating the nervous system in this way are familiar components of yoga practice. For example:

- Knowledge: understanding how the nervous system works, being aware that pain is not always a red light and can sometimes be safely ignored.

- Physical activity.

- Imagination: visualising a body part and imagining it moving without pain.

- Meditation.

- Breathing practices.[27]

In line with what I have learnt more broadly about yoga and hypermobility from working with many hypermobile yoga practitioners over the years, it turns out that, while yoga is widely acknowledged to be helpful in nervous-system regulation and recovery from chronic pain, there is no single unique yoga recipe that works for everyone. Neil Pearson says:

> Modern science does not support a highly prescriptive approach to *asana* or yoga practice for those with chronic pain. To date, there is no evidence that one style of *asana* is best, or that specific *asanas* are required for specific chronic pain problems.[28]

For more on information about pain, see 'Pain' in Chapter 1, and 'Restorative yoga for pain management' in Chapter 5.

Yoga addiction versus cross training and supportive practices

#yogaeverydamnday has a lot to answer for. The blogosphere is replete with articles by yoga practitioners – many of them hypermobile – for whom daily practice, unmediated by other strength-building and stabilising activities, has created serious injury. At the age of 35, hypermobile yoga practitioner and yoga educator, Julie Tran, ended up with two herniated cervical disks, a stage 2 tear in the coracohumeral ligament (of the shoulder) and a necrotic left hip that repeatedly dislocated. She says: 'I fell victim to the idea that *asana* is the only necessary exercise, and I didn't do enough to mitigate the effects of doing the same movements over and over.'[29]

If ancient teachers ever advised their students to practise yoga every day, I'm guessing they were referring to following yogic precepts in a regular and ongoing way, not to maintaining a high-intensity, vinyasa-based exercise programme. In order to be taken seriously as a 'yogi' in more recent times, however, it appears to have become mandatory to perform rigorous sequences of postures on a daily basis – and ideally to be seen to be performing them. Be that as it may, if you are hypermobile, *don't* do *asana* every damn day, whatever your tradition says. It is by now more or less universally agreed by those with expertise in movement for hypermobility that hypermobile people need to do a wide range of different types and intensities of movement. In other words, where hypermobility is concerned, be a generalist. Rosemary Keer and Jane Butler say:

> The emphasis is on maximising tissue health and endurance with a range of exercises and activities. Variety is key, with frequent changes between more active and more sedentary tasks, different postures (flexed, extended), smaller movements and larger movements, more intense and less intense muscle work as well as balancing flexibility with strength and endurance.[30]

Be aware, too, that it is entirely possible to overdo your medicinal strength activities. These also need to be varied, mixed up with other types and intensities of movement, and slow and steady in progression.

Life's short, so cultivate movement forms you can enjoy. If you hate lifting weights, you're very unlikely to stick to a weightlifting programme, no matter how beneficial it may be – whereas if you really like cycling, you'll probably have no problem in doing it regularly. Be curious, and try all sorts of things. Letting go of my hyper-focused seven-day-a-week ballet habit, followed by my six-day-a-week ashtanga routine, freed me up to explore widely. It turns out there's a lot of movement out there to love. My approach to ashtanga has shifted significantly, but I still practise it and still adore it. A couple of years ago I returned to ballet after an 18-year break – similarly, with a very different attitude and intention. I've always swum and walked, and I've been a long-time conscious dancer (I also teach Open Floor dance movement). A game changer was adding floor barre for strength and stability, and ending each day with yoga nidra has been a gift to my nervous system. Breaking a metatarsal a couple of years ago introduced me to chair cardio – great for those with orthostatic issues – and this is now quite often the warm-up for my morning movement practice and for my day.[31]

I generally do everything in smaller chunks than I used to, rarely the same activity two days on the trot, and I'm always looking for the ways I can foster strength and cultivate biomechanical integrity. I've learnt that making small and apparently quite subtle changes can give rise to significant gains in terms of health, energy and physical capacity. Allowing practices to flow in and out of each other and giving myself permission to flow in and out of the practices in an intuitive way has made everything more workable, as has shifting my interest away from goals and outcomes, and towards process and pleasure. The end point now is what I need of the practice or activity rather than what the practice or activity wants of me.

I asked hypermobile yoga practitioners in two online groups what they did as supportive practices. These are some of their responses. It's beyond the scope of this book (and of my knowledge) to go into what each activity entails, but they're all easily google-able if you want to give any of them a try.

- Alexander Technique.

- Barre workout.

- Belly dance.

- Chair cardio.

- Callisthenics.

- Climbing.

- Cycling.

- Elliptical trainer. One autistic person mentioned also loving the rocking motion of this.

- Feldenkrais Method®/Functional Integration. Joanne, a yoga practitioner with HSD, says:

  The Feldenkrais Method® is the core support for everything I do. It helps my body to learn what's comfortable, safe and easy, and it gets all my muscles firing in a more coordinated fashion so I feel stronger and am less likely to hurt myself.

- Functional Range Conditioning®.

- HIIT (High Impact Interval Training).

- Mindful Strength (the work of Kathryn Bruni-Young).

- 'Natural' fitness – climbing trees, balancing on railings, walking barefoot on grass.

- Nordic walking.

- Pilates.

- Pole dancing.

- Running. Alina, a yoga teacher with hEDS, says:

  We often get told not to run, but I find running tremendously useful for strengthening my legs and supporting my knees. In fact, if I have to go through periods of time where I don't run, my knees start to feel more unstable and my connective tissue pain returns.

- Somatics.

- Swimming. I think I was designed to be a fish. For me, water provides external support and a sense of containment. Other hypermobile people also appreciated the lower gravity of water and the resistance it provides.

- Tai chi/qigong.

- Tango.

- Walking. Suzie, a yoga practitioner with hEDS, says:

  Walking gives me space to think about what muscles I'm

activating. I have to remind myself to activate my glutes and use my muscles rather than taking all the impact through my knees.

Don't you love that as hypermobile people we have to think about how to walk?!

- Weights. Arlette, a yoga teacher with HSD, says:

  I really enjoy powerlifting. It's strengthening, and the weights offer feedback in my joints. Although I also teach yoga and I like doing Pilates, it's weight training that has benefited me the most.

  Weightlifting (in a variety of forms) was a very popular activity, which many people found helpful, and not just for strength: all the weightlifters mentioned gains in proprioception.

- Yoga Tune Up and Tune Up Fitness® (the work of Jill Miller).

Self-guidance and intuition

While input from experienced, hypermobility-aware professionals can be very helpful, especially in the beginning stages of a yoga practice, it's also important to stay connected with the thread of our own experience on the mat. Despite the many commonalities, everybody with hypermobility is different and is experiencing a unique interplay of factors on physical, emotional, psychological, social and other levels. These all help to determine whether a particular technique or approach will work for us.

The same applies to theories and approaches supported by scientific research. None of us is a neutral subject in a blind trial, and no research result is going to apply equally to every person. Research is also frequently contested by other experts in the field, subject to the belief systems and cultural norms of its time, and may eventually be superseded. Pragmatism is helpful in working out what to take on and what can be allowed to fall away as irrelevant or unhelpful to you. Trust your own intuition. A sense of open curiosity and a willingness to experiment is key to practising with hypermobility. Diane, a Mysore-style ashtanga teacher with MFS, says:

When my practice started to cause pain and injury, I had good advice from an excellent physiotherapist, but I also had to start investigating myself – because only I really knew what I was experiencing in my practice on a daily basis. My practice was my laboratory – and sometimes it looked nothing like ashtanga. In the early days, I would resolve one issue and then another would happen. It was like solving a Rubik's cube. But gradually, over time, my body as a whole started to work better and hurt less. Ultimately, it's your body and your practice, and you're the only one who's going to work it all out.

On the whole, you should be experiencing gains in strength, structure and control, and a lessening of fatigue and nervous-system stress and lability as a result of any approaches you are using. Enjoyment is important too. If you're flogging through an exercise routine with no sense of pleasure or satisfaction, let it go. There are other ways that will work for you.

Suck it and see

Let me tell you a secret. I'm a poet, not an anatomy geek. I'm dyspraxic and find structural patterns difficult to understand. Many years of practical experience have taught me an enormous amount about biomechanics, but I'm never going to be a native in the land of organisms and parts. When I'm working with my own body, I'm very much of the school of suck it and see. If a movement's hurting one way, I try it another way – engage something different, change the alignment of a foot or a hip, tip or rotate my pelvis in one direction or another. And it's *fine* to approach your hypermobility like this. While knowledge is a good thing, you don't have to have a degree in physiotherapy to work intelligently with your own movement patterns. You just need to be curious and committed, willing to think out of the box and experiment. When you don't have access to a skilled teacher and can't afford a physiotherapist, pragmatism will get you a long way. Read, research, try things on. Be open to professional input, but don't be afraid to trust your own experience of your body.

Finding your flow

In the process of creating stability as a hypermobile mover, it's easy to go from Gumby to Woodentop. While engaging, strengthening and activating is a good – an essential – thing, it isn't *every*thing. I sometimes work with hypermobile yoga practitioners who have made postures so tiny and minimal in order to feel in control of them that they hardly have any room for manoeuvre. It's OK to use your muscles to move your bones. It's OK to be fluid and to feel into the full expression of your body in motion. There's a gain/gain paradox at work here. The harder you work on biomechanical integrity, the greater will be your freedom in movement. Don't forget to move!

Menopause and beyond

As we saw in Chapter 1 ('Hormones, more periods and menopause'), at menopause, when oestrogen levels fall, joint laxity can also increase. At the time of writing, I am about three years post my last bleed, and have experienced many hypermobility-related changes over the perimenopausal and menopausal period. An increase in joint laxity has, indeed, been one of them. While in the early stages of perimenopause, this was very difficult in terms of the joint pain, escalating subluxation and biomechanical dysfunction that ensued, ultimately it hasn't been quite such a bad thing as you might think. Menopause is, of course, highly individual in its effects, and we each have to plot our own course through its sometimes turbulent waters. That said, there are some general guidelines for creating the best possible outcome in a hypermobile body. The following are some things that helped me to navigate the voyage – and make landfall noticeably stronger, healthier and more securely embodied than before.

- Keep on keeping on. As always with hypermobility, whatever your phase of life, the least helpful thing you can do is allow yourself to become deconditioned.

- Be fluid and open to doing differently. Not for nothing is menopause often referred to as 'the change'. Your orientation to practising as well as your repertoire of practices is likely to need to shift somewhat. At the same time…

- Don't throw the baby out with the bath water. What's required may not be as drastic as you might think. Tiny shifts and subtle changes can make a big difference. At many points during perimenopause I agonised over whether to give up my ashtanga vinyasa practice, which no longer seemed to suit my body. What I've actually ended up doing is splitting it into shorter segments (no more two-to-three-hour stints; 90 minutes is usually about my max now), limiting the number of practices I do each week to three and slightly modifying some of the sequences. I actually wish I'd done all of this years ago. It has turned a cycle of attrition and inflammation into one of steady strength building. I'm now re-approaching postures and sequences with a more solid foundation, increased muscular engagement and better proprioception, and I love ashtanga once more (whereas I had started to hate it).

- Focus on working for strength and stability. You may be thinking, 'I'm hypermobile. Heh, what's new?'. Nothing, really, but what you get away with when you're younger sometimes comes back to bite you on the bum. Pilates and body conditioning have been my friends here.

- Move in diverse ways. My weekly movement repertoire now includes ashtanga, swimming, a classical ballet barre, Pilates and conditioning, dance movement, yoga nidra, lots of myofascial release – oh, and sensible stretching. I found that I needed to reintroduce more of that once I'd shifted the emphasis towards strength work.

- Pay attention to how your body is responding to physical activities and adapt what you do on any given day accordingly. If your shoulders are sore, for example, don't do sun salutations. It seems obvious, doesn't it? But some of us do tend to keep hammering away at the same old thing. This also means letting go of rigid schedules. You don't have to lift weights just because it's Tuesday. It may turn out that Tuesday is the day your body wants you to put on some music and dance.

- Take care of emotional work. Our bodies are not just physical entities but are also the guardian of our emotional experiences. When we don't engage in regular embodied practice designed to help us process our feelings, we end up carrying around a lot of excess baggage in the form of pain and muscular tension. Restorative practices, conscious dance, body-centred meditation and so on offer us an opportunity to feel our feelings, express them and then let them dissolve.

Spiralling

The process of being with the totality of our experience is the end point of yoga. All yoga practitioners eventually have to encounter this lesson, but for hypermobile people, it may be stitched into the fabric of our practice from an early stage. It's easy to get frustrated with the two-steps-forward-one-step-back choreography of a hypermobile practice and long for the kind of linear progress CT-typical people seem to make. Transformation happens when we understand – not just theoretically but deep down in our bones – that in yoga there is no 'forwards' and there is no 'back'. If yoga practice has a trajectory, it's a spiral, at every turn of which we are offered an opportunity to revisit old places with new degrees of subtlety and awareness, and to gather up and weave in loose threads. This way, in the long term, we make a stronger and sturdier fabric. When you understand the difficult experiences you meet – injury, pain, fatigue and so on – as essential elements in the process of yoga, rather than annoying hurdles you have to jump in order to get somewhere else, your practice will always feel rich and fulfilling and will be in line with the remit of yoga, one of deepening attention rather than attainment.

Resources

Autism

Autistic Women and Nonbinary Network (AWN): https://awnnetwork.org.

The Autisticats, 'four autistic young adults, figuring out life and sharing our experiences as neurodivergent people': https://theautisticats.weebly.com / @the.autisticats.

Bristol Autism Support's list of autistic bloggers and YouTubers in the UK and around the world: www.bristolautismsupport.com/actuallyautistic-blog-youtube-bloggers.

Samantha Craft, 'Females and Aspergers: A Checklist', currently available on The Art of Autism website: https://the-art-of-autism.com/females-and-aspergers-a-checklist/?fbclid=IwAR1uJs7zGH52bgf37unaIcYfzmWtOsyvtpytsM4PgDe7ZGNP7lqYN1kiPYE.

Nick Walker, Neurocosmopolitanism blog, http://neurocosmopolitanism.com/what-is-autism.

Books about hypermobility

Isobel Knight, *A Guide to Living with Ehlers-Danlos Syndrome (Hypermobility Type): Bending Without Breaking*, Jessica Kingsley Publishers, London, 2015. The first edition (2011) was called, *A Guide to Living with Hypermobility Syndrome*.

Claire Smith, *Understanding Hypermobile Ehlers-Danlos Syndrome and Hypermobility Spectrum Disorder*, Redcliff-House Publications, 2017. Get it here: www.redcliffhousepublications.co.uk/product-page/understanding-hypermobile-ehlers-danlos-syndrome-hypermobility-spectrum-disord.

Children with hypermobility

Excellent and fascinating site of Pam Versfeld, specialist physiotherapist based in Cape Town, about how hypermobility (and neurodifference) affect movement development in infants and children: www.skillsforaction.com.

Chronic Fatigue Syndrome (CFS)

When I had CFS, I wanted positive resources that offered holistic approaches. The two following books were my favourites – oldies but goodies:

- Alexandra Barton (ed.), *Recovery from CFS: 50 Personal Stories*, AuthorHouse UK, Milton Keynes, 2008.
- William Collinge, *Recovering from ME: A Guide to Self-Empowerment*, Souvenir Press, London, 1993.

A more recent addition is:

- Donna Owens, *Yoga, my Bed and ME*, CreateSpace Independent Publishing Platform, 2016.

Diagnosis and services

The Ehlers-Danlos Syndromes Toolkit, a diagnostic tool devised for GPs by the Royal College of General Practitioners: www.rcgp.org.uk/clinical-and-research/resources/toolkits/ehlers-danlos-syndromes-toolkit.aspx.

The Hypermobility Clinic, Department of Rheumatology, University College London Hospitals, NW1 (referral by rheumatologist): www.uclh.nhs.uk/OurServices/ServiceA-Z/MEDSPEC/RHEUM/HMC/Pages/Home.aspx. **Please note**: At the time of writing the Hypermobility Clinic is closed to new referrals due to increased demand and is redesigning services to increase capacity. Please check the link above for updates

The London Hypermobility Unit, Platinum Medical Centre (The Wellington Hospital), 15–17 Lodge Road London NW8 7JA, (private service): www.thelondonhypermobilityunit.co.uk.

The Ehlers-Danlos Society has an international list of EDS-friendly medical professionals: www.ehlers-danlos.com/medical-professionals-directory/#uk.

Dyspraxia

Dyspraxia Foundation: www.dyspraxiafoundation.org.uk.
Dyspraxia Foundation USA: https://dyspraxiausa.org

Facebook group

For new resources, questions, experiences, announcements, etc., the Hypermobility on the Yoga Mat Facebook group is at: www.facebook.com/groups/hypermobilityontheyogamat.

Marfan Syndrome exercise guidelines

Downloadable from: http://info.marfan.org/physical-activities-guidelines.

Myofascial release

YouTube resources by Ariele Foster, yoga teacher and physiotherapist with a specialism in hypermobility: www.youtube.com/user/sacredsourceyoga/videos. Paid-for online MFR courses with Ariele: https://yogaanatomyacademy.com.

Gentle yoga and myofascial release classes with Melissa West: www.youtube.com/user/drmelissawest.

Pain management

Neil Pearson, Shelly Prosko, Marlysa Sullivan (eds), *Yoga and Science in Pain Care: Treating the Person in Pain*, Singing Dragon, London, 2019.

Neil Pearson's article, 'Yoga Therapy in Practice: Yoga for People in Pain', is a great resource for teaching people in chronic pain: https://paincareu.com/wp-content/uploads/2019/02/IJYT-Yoga_Chronic_2008.pdf.

Pelvic floor health

'Yoga for the Pelvic Floor: Keys to Lifelong Health': online course on hyper- and hypotonic pelvic floor with Lesley Howard: https://yogauonline.com/yogau-product/6661.

Dr Uchenna Ossai's introduction to the pelvic floor and sexual function at the O.School: www.o.school/originals/pelvic-floor-health.

Postural orthostatic tachycardia syndrome (POTS)

POTS UK: www.potsuk.org.

Standing Up to POTS: http://standinguptopots.org.

I was diagnosed with POTS at King's College Hospital London, where Dr Nicholas Gall, consultant cardiologist, and team have a special interest in POTS: www.kch.nhs.uk. There is a listing of other doctors with a POTS specialism (in the UK and internationally) at: www.potsuk.org/doctors.

Resistance bands

Laurel Beversdorf's 'Yoga with Resistance' online course: https://laurelbeversdorf.com.

SI joint health

'Yoga For Lower Back Pain: Keys to Sacroiliac Stability and Ease of Movement': online course on SI joint integrity with Donna Farhi: https://yogauonline.com/yogau-product/7746.

Support organisations for hypermobility

The Ehlers-Danlos Society: www.ehlers-danlos.com.

Ehlers-Danlos Support UK: www.ehlers-danlos.org.

The Hypermobility Syndromes Association: http://hypermobility.org.

The Marfan Foundation: www.marfan.org.

Endnotes

Introduction

1   @bonniebainbridgecohen, Instagram, 4 February 2020.

Chapter 1

1   C. Smith, *Understanding Hypermobile Ehlers-Danlos Syndrome and Hypermobility Spectrum Disorder*, Redcliff-House Publications, 2017.

2   US National Library of Medicine, Genetics Home Reference: Your Guide to Understanding Genetic Conditions, 'Ehlers-Danlos Syndrome': https://ghr.nlm.nih.gov/condition/ehlers-danlos-syndrome#genes (accessed on 6/4/20).

3   So far, so simple; however, the FBN1 gene can mutate in more than 3,000 different ways! NHS, 'Marfan Syndrome', 2019: www.nhs.uk/conditions/marfan-syndrome (accessed on 6/4/20).

4   US National Library of Medicine, Genetics Home Reference: Your Guide to Understanding Genetic Conditions, 'Marfan Syndrome': https://ghr.nlm.nih.gov/condition/marfan-syndrome#genes (accessed on 6/4/20).

5   The Ehlers-Danlos Society, 'HEDGE Study: Hypermobile Ehlers-Danlos Genetic Evaluation': www. ehlers-danlos.com/heds-genetic-research-study (accessed on 6/4/20).

6   The Ehlers-Danlos Society, 'Hypermobile Ehlers-Danlos Syndrome (hEDS) vs. Hypermobility Spectrum Disorders (HSD): What's the Difference?': https://ehlers-danlos.com/wp-content/uploads/ hEDSvHSD.pdf (accessed on 6/4/20).

7   Fight vEDS, 'What is Vascular Ehlers-Danlos Syndrome?', 2019: www.fightveds.org/what-is-vascular-eds (accessed on 6/4/20).

8   P. Byers, J. Belmont, J. Black, J. De Backer, *et al.*, 'Diagnosis, Natural History and Management in Vascular Ehlers-Danlos Syndrome', *American Journal of Medical Genetics* Part C (Seminars in Medical Genetics), 175C, 40–47, 2017: https://onlinelibrary.wiley.com/doi/full/10.1002/ajmg.c.31553 (accessed on 6/4/20).

9   Fight vEDS, 'Diet and Exercise', 2017: www.fightveds.org/diet-exercise (accessed on 6/4/20).

10   The Ehlers-Danlos Society, 'The 2017 EDS International Classification: Your Questions Answered': https://ehlers-danlos.com/wp-content/uploads/QandA-2.pdf (accessed on 6/4/20).

11   The Marfan Foundation, 'What is Marfan Syndrome?': www.marfan.org/about/marfan (accessed on 6/4/20).

12   The Marfan Foundation, 'Physical Activity Guidelines': https://info.marfan.org/physical-activities-guidelines (accessed on 6/4/20).

13   The Marfan Foundation, 'What is Marfan Syndrome?': www.marfan.org/about/marfan (accessed on 6/4/20).

14   The Ehlers-Danlos Society, 'The Ehlers-Danlos Society Responds to the Recent Paper on the Prevalence of EDS and HSD', 2019: www.ehlers-danlos.com/society-responds-to-bmj-paper-on-prevalence (accessed on 6/4/20).

15   A.J. Hakim, L.F. Cherkas, R. Grahame, T.D. Spector, A.J. MacGregor, 'The Genetic Epidemiology of Joint Hypermobility: A Population Study of Female Twins', *Arthritis & Rheumatism*, 50, 8, 2004: https://onlinelibrary.wiley.com/doi/pdf/10.1002/art.20376 (accessed on 6/4/20).

16   The Ehlers-Danlos Society, 'How Bias and a Lack of Access to Healthcare Impacts EDS Patients of African Descent', 2020: www.ehlers-danlos.com/breaking-down-barriers-nia/?fbclid=IwAR3SCtrH JeiAKSBoCZT4RM4RScaFxeKN6uZQel8wCbNAyPsrzj0OGcmwt4k (accessed on 6/4/20).

17   C. Smith, *Understanding Hypermobile Ehlers-Danlos Syndrome and Hypermobility Spectrum Disorder*, Redcliff-House Publications, 2017.

18   C. Smith, *Understanding Hypermobile Ehlers-Danlos Syndrome and Hypermobility Spectrum Disorder*, Redcliff-House Publications, 2017.

19   K. Malterud, 'The (Gendered) Construction of Diagnosis: Interpretation of Medical Signs in Women Patients', *Theoretical Medicine and Bioethics*, 20, 275–286, 1999: https://link.springer.com/article/10.1023/A:1009905523228 (accessed on 6/4/20).

20   The Ehlers-Danlos Society, 'Yes, Men Have Ehlers-Danlos: For Men's Health Month the Ehlers-Danlos Society Raises Awareness for Men with EDS/HSD': www.ehlers-danlos.com/menhaveeds (accessed on 6/4/20).

21   NHS, 'Marfan Syndrome', 2019: www.nhs.uk/conditions/marfan-syndrome (accessed on 6/4/20).

22   C. Chan, L. Hopper, F. Zhang, V. Pacey, L. Nicholson, 'The prevalence of Generalised and Syndromic Hypermobility in Elite Australian Dancers', *Physical Therapy in Sport*, 32, 15–21, 2018: www.ncbi.nlm.nih.gov/pubmed/29655088 (accessed on 6/4/20).

23   M. McCormack, J. Briggs, A. Hakim, R. Grahame, 'Joint Laxity and the Benign Joint Hypermobility Syndrome in Student and Professional Ballet Dancers', *Journal of Rheumatology*, 1, 173–178, 2004: www.ncbi.nlm.nih.gov/pubmed/14705238 (accessed on 6/4/20).

24   Hypermobility MD, Bendy Bodies podcast, 'Episode 1: Reducing injury and Increasing Education with Moira McCormack', 2020: www.hypermobilitymd.com/podcast/episode/c3a267d5/episode-1-reducing-injury-and-increasing-education-with-moira-mccormack-part-1 (accessed on 6/4/20). (If you're interested in hypermobility in dance, this is a fascinating episode of a promising new podcast.)

25   L-G. Larsson, J. Baum, G.S. Mudholkar, G.D. Kollia, 'Benefits and Advantages of Joint Hypermobility Among Musicians', *The New England Journal of Medicine*, 329, 1079–1082, 1993: www.nejm.org/doi/full/10.1056/NEJM199310073291504#article_citing_articles (accessed on 6/4/20).

26   J. Simmonds, 'Webinar: Managing EDS and Muscle Conditioning', Ehlers-Danlos Support UK: www.ehlers-danlos.org/information/webinar-managing-eds-and-muscle-conditioning (accessed on 6/4/20).

27   C. Baeza-Velasco, M-C. Gély-Nargeot, G. Pailhez, A. Vilarrasa, A. Bulbena, 'Joint Hypermobility and Sport: A Review of Advantages and Disadvantages', *Current Sports Medicine Reports*, 12, 5, 291–295, 2013: https://journals.lww.com/acsm-csmr/Fulltext/2013/09000/Joint_Hypermobility_and_Sport___A_Review_of.7.aspx (accessed on 6/4/20).

28   M. Scheper, J. de Vries, J. Verbunt, R. Engelbert, 'Chronic Pain in Hypermobility Syndrome and Ehlers–Danlos Syndrome (Hypermobility Type): It Is a Challenge', *Journal of Pain Research*, 8, 591–601, 2015: www.ncbi.nlm.nih.gov/pmc/articles/PMC4548768 (accessed on 6/4/20).

29   L. Winship, *Evening Standard*, 'Sylvie Guillem on Her Retirement From Ballet: "It's a Big Goodbye!"', 28 July 2015: www.standard.co.uk/go/london/theatre/sylvie-guillem-on-her-retirement-from-ballet-its-a-big-goodbye-10420577.html (accessed on 6/4/20).

30   The Ehlers-Danlos Society, 'Born This Way? When Hypermobility Has its Privileges – and Problems': www.ehlers-danlos.com/edsgad (accessed on 6/4/20).

31   A. Behrmann, *The Daily Mail*, 'Hypermobility: When Being Flexible May Not Be Such a Good Thing After All', 2019: www.dailymail.co.uk/health/article-7025227/Hypermobility-flexible-not-good-thing-all.html?fbclid=IwAR1ZbzsFEp32odmPP1r2UDTrtHe_qIgPWWMv8T8eAYI4T03EcOtJsGAJiiI (accessed on 6/4/20).

32   T. Leckie, Independent Living guest blog: 'Managing Hypermobility: A Musician's View': www.independentliving.co.uk/guest-blog/managing-hypermobility-musicians-view (accessed on 6/4/20).

33   British Association for Performing Arts Medicine, 'Arts Health Practitioners in Focus: Massage Therapy', 2018: https://bapam.org.uk/news/tag/hypermobility (accessed on 6/4/20).

34   D. Tilley, Shift: Movement Science and Gymnastics Education, 'How Much Flexibility Is Too Much for a Gymnast?': https://shiftmovementscience.com/how-much-flexibility-is-too-much-for-a-gymnast (accessed on 6/4/20).

35 The best definition of autism for my money is by Nick Walker, on his Neurocosmopolitanism blog: Nick Walker, 'What Is Autism?', 2014: http://neurocosmopolitanism.com/what-is-autism (accessed on 6/4/20).

36 C. Baeza-Velasco, D. Cohen, C. Hamonet, E. Vlamynck, *et al.*, 'Autism, Joint-Hypermobility Disorders and Pain', *Frontiers in Psychiatry*, 2018: www.frontiersin.org/articles/10.3389/fpsyt.2018.00656/full (accessed on 6/4/20).

37 J. Eccles, V. Iodice, N.G. Dowell, A. Owens *et al.*, 'Joint Hypermobility and Autonomic Hyperactivity: Relevance to Neurodevelopmental Disorders', *Journal of Neurology, Neurosurgery & Psychiatry*, 85, e3, 2014: https://jnnp.bmj.com/content/85/8/e3.40 (accessed on 6/4/20).

38 B. Clark, *The Complete Guide to Yin Yoga: The Philosophy and Practice of Yin Yoga*, White Cloud Press, Ashland, OR, 2012.

39 Fascia Research Society: https://fasciaresearchsociety.org/about (accessed on 6/4/20).

40 N. Blair, *Brightening Our Inner Skies: Yin and Yoga*, MicMac Margins, London, 2017.

41 B. Clark, *The Complete Guide to Yin Yoga: The Philosophy and Practice of Yin Yoga*, White Cloud Press, Ashland, OR, 2012.

42 I. Knight, *A Guide to Living with Ehlers-Danlos Syndrome (Hypermobility Type): Bending Without Breaking*, Singing Dragon, London, 2014.

43 J. Meyersohn, K. Launier, A. Valiente, ABC News, 'Rare Medical Condition is the Secret to Contortionist's Ability', 2015: https://abcnews.go.com/health/rare-medical-condition-secret-contortionists-ability/story?id=29054612 (accessed on 6/4/20).

44 C. Smith, *Understanding Hypermobile Ehlers-Danlos Syndrome and Hypermobility Spectrum Disorder*, Redcliff-House Publications, 2017.

45 C. Smith, *Understanding Hypermobile Ehlers-Danlos Syndrome and Hypermobility Spectrum Disorder*, Redcliff-House Publications, 2017.

46 Cited in C. Smith, *Understanding Hypermobile Ehlers-Danlos Syndrome and Hypermobility Spectrum Disorder*, Redcliff-House Publications, 2017.

47 T. Gullo, Y. Golightly, P. Flowers, J. Jordan, *et al.* 'Joint Hypermobility Is Not Positively Associated with Prevalent Multiple Joint Osteoarthritis: a Cross-sectional Study of Older Adults. *BMC Musculoskeletal Disorders*, 20, 165, 2019: https://bmcmusculoskeletdisord.biomedcentral.com/articles/10.1186/s12891-019-2550-z (accessed on 6/4/20).

48 D. Goldenberg 'Osteoarthritis and central pain', *Practical Pain Management*, 16, 6, 2017: www.practicalpainmanagement.com/pain/myofascial/osteoarthritis/osteoarthritis-central-pain (accessed on 6/4/20).

49 C. Smith, *Understanding Hypermobile Ehlers-Danlos Syndrome and Hypermobility Spectrum Disorder*, Redcliff-House Publications, 2017.

50 PhysioWorks, 'Why do your Joints Click? Are You Tired of Your Joints Clicking? Can You Be Click Free?': https://physioworks.com.au/FAQRetrieve.aspx?ID=30987 (accessed on 6/4/20).

51 P. Grilley, 'The truth about clicking + popping joints', *Yoga Journal*, 2007 updated 2017: www.yogajournal.com/poses/cracking-and-popping-joints (accessed on 6/4/20).

52 P. Grilley, 'The truth about clicking + popping joints', *Yoga Journal*, 2007 updated 2017: www.yogajournal.com/poses/cracking-and-popping-joints (accessed on 6/4/20).

53 PhysioWorks, 'Why do your Joints Click? Are You Tired of Your Joints Clicking? Can You Be Click Free?': https://physioworks.com.au/FAQRetrieve.aspx?ID=30987 (accessed on 6/4/20).

54 Scoliosis Association UK, 'Syndromic Scoliosis': www.sauk.org.uk/types-of-scoliosis/syndromic-scoliosis (accessed on 6/4/20).

55 Scoliosis Research Society, 'Congenital Scoliosis': www.srs.org/professionals/online-education-and-resources/conditions-and-treatments/congenital-scoliosis (accessed on 6/4/20).

56 Scoliosis Research Society, 'Congenital Scoliosis': www.srs.org/professionals/online-education-and-resources/conditions-and-treatments/congenital-scoliosis (accessed on 6/4/20).

57 H. Bird, C. Eastmond, A. Hudson, V. Wright, 'Is Generalized Hypermobility a Factor in Spondylolisthesis?', *Scandinavian Journal of Rheumatology*, 9, 4: www.ncbi.nlm.nih.gov/pubmed/7455631 (accessed on 6/4/20).

58 J. Highsmith, Spine Universe, 'Causes of Spondylolisthesis', 2019: www.spineuniverse.com/conditions/spondylolisthesis/causes-spondylolisthesis (accessed on 6/4/20).

59 D. Keil, 3D Muscle Lab, 'Is Yoga Tearing Labrums?', 2015: www.yoganatomy.com/yoga-tearing-labrums (accessed on 6/4/20).

60   S. Porter, Ehlers-Danlos Support UK, 'Oral and Dental Implications of the Ehlers-Danlos Syndromes', 2016: www.ehlers-danlos.org/information/aaoral-and-dental-implications-of-the-ehlers-danlos-syndromes (accessed on 6/4/20).

61   C. Smith, *Understanding Hypermobile Ehlers-Danlos Syndrome and Hypermobility Spectrum Disorder*, Redcliff-House Publications, 2017.

62   A. Erickson Gabbey, medically reviewed by G. Minnis, Healthline, 'Hypermobile Joints', 2017: www.healthline.com/health/hypermobile-joints#outlook (accessed on 6/4/20).

63   A. Pocinki, The Zebra Network, 'Joint Hypermobility and Joint Hypermobility Syndrome': http://thezebranetwork.org/pagef (accessed on 6/4/20).

64   Previously cited on Claire Smith's EDS-H & JHS website, now archived.

65   NHS, 'Overview: Hypotonia', 2018: www.nhs.uk/conditions/hypotonia (accessed on 6/4/20).

66   C. Smith, *Understanding Hypermobile Ehlers-Danlos Syndrome and Hypermobility Spectrum Disorder*, Redcliff-House Publications, 2017.

67   Cited by R. Schierling, 'Fascia, Proprioception and Chronic Pain', 2017: www.doctorschierling.com/blog/fascia-as-a-proprioceptive-organ-and-its-relationship-to-chronic-pain (accessed on 6/4/20).

68   T. Myers, *Anatomy Trains: Myofascial Meridians for Manual and Movement Therapists*, Churchill Livingstone, London, 2013.

69   T. Myers, IDEA Health & Fitness Association, 'Fascial Fitness: Training in the Neuromyofascial Web', 2011: www.ideafit.com/fitness-library/fascial-fitness (accessed on 6/4/20).

70   T.R. Mukhopadhyay, *The Mind Tree: A Miraculous Child Breaks the Silence of Autism*, Arcade Publishing, New York, 2000.

71   E. Beater, 'Studying with Dyspraxia: "I Never Truly Understood an Academic Text"', *The Guardian*, 5 March 2019: www.theguardian.com/education/2019/mar/05/studying-with-dyspraxia-i-never-truly-understood-an-academic-text (accessed on 6/4/20).

72   E. Beater, 'Studying with Dyspraxia: "I Never Truly Understood an Academic Text"', *The Guardian*, 5 March 2019: www.theguardian.com/education/2019/mar/05/studying-with-dyspraxia-i-never-truly-understood-an-academic-text (accessed on 6/4/20).

73   C. Smith, *Understanding Hypermobile Ehlers-Danlos Syndrome and Hypermobility Spectrum Disorder*, Redcliff-House Publications, 2017.

74   Restless Legs Syndrome Foundation, 'Symptoms and Diagnosis: How Do I Know If I Have RLS?': www.rls.org/understanding-rls/symptoms-diagnosis (accessed on 6/4/20).

75   C&S Patient Education Foundation, 'What Is Chiari Malformation?', 2012: www.conquerchiari.org/documents/presentations/OVERVIEW%20Presentation.pdf (accessed on 6/4/20).

76   F. Henderson, C. Austin, E. Benzel, P. Bolognese, *et al.*, adapted by B. Guscott, 'Neurological and Spinal Manifestations of the Ehlers-Danlos Syndromes (for Non-experts)', 2017: www.ehlers-danlos.com/2017-eds-classification-non-experts/neurological-spinal-manifestations-ehlers-danlos-syndromes (accessed on 6/4/20).

77   Children's Hospital of Georgia, Augusta University Health, 'The Relationship between Chiari Malformations and Connective Tissue Disorders: Is It Casual or Causal?', 2018: https://advances.augusta.edu/689 (accessed on 6/4/20).

78   F. Henderson, C. Austin, E. Benzel, P. Bolognese, *et al.*, adapted by B. Guscott, 'Neurological and Spinal Manifestations of the Ehlers-Danlos Syndromes (for Non-experts)', 2017: www.ehlers-danlos.com/2017-eds-classification-non-experts/neurological-spinal-manifestations-ehlers-danlos-syndromes (accessed on 6/4/20).

79   Brain and Spine Foundation, *Chiari Malformation: A Guide for Patients and Carers*, 2018: www.brainandspine.org.uk/wp-content/uploads/2018/04/Chiari-malformations-booklet.pdf (accessed on 6/4/20).

80   F. Henderson, C. Austin, E. Benzel, P. Bolognese, et al., adapted by B. Guscott, 'Neurological and Spinal Manifestations of the Ehlers-Danlos Syndromes (for Non-experts)', 2017: www.ehlers-danlos.com/2017-eds-classification-non-experts/neurological-spinal-manifestations-ehlers-danlos-syndromes (accessed on 6/4/20).

81   Children's Hospital of Georgia, Augusta University Health, 'The Relationship between Chiari Malformations and Connective Tissue Disorders: Is It Casual or Causal?', 2018: https://advances.augusta.edu/689 (accessed on 6/4/20).

82   myheart.net, 'POTS: Explained by Doctors and Patients': https://myheart.net/pots-syndrome (accessed on 6/4/20).

83   POTS UK, 'Symptoms', 2015 reviewed 2018: www.potsuk.org/symptoms (accessed on 6/4/20).

84   C. Smith, *Understanding Hypermobile Ehlers-Danlos Syndrome and Hypermobility Spectrum Disorder*, Redcliff-House Publications, 2017.

85   J. Stewart, P. Pianosi, M. Shaban, C. Terilli, *et al.*, 'Postural Hyperventilation as a Cause of Postural Tachycardia Syndrome: Increased Systemic Vascular Resistance and Decreased Cardiac Output When Upright in All Postural Tachycardia Syndrome', *Journal of the American Heart Association*, 7, 13, 2018: www.ahajournals.org/doi/pdf/10.1161/JAHA.118.008854 (accessed on 6/4/20).

86   myheart.net, 'POTS: Explained by Doctors and Patients': https://myheart.net/pots-syndrome (accessed on 6/4/20).

87   American College of Rheumatology, 'Raynaud's Phenomenon?', 2019: www.rheumatology.org/I-Am-A/Patient-Caregiver/Diseases-Conditions/Raynauds-Phenomenon (accessed on 6/4/20).

88   Scleroderma and Raynaud's UK, 'What Causes Raynaud's': www.sruk.co.uk/raynauds/what-causes-raynauds (accessed on 6/4/20).

89   C. Smith, *Understanding Hypermobile Ehlers-Danlos Syndrome and Hypermobility Spectrum Disorder*, Redcliff-House Publications, 2017.

90   E. Soyucen and F. Esen, 'Benign Joint Hypermobility Syndrome: A Cause of Childhood Asthma?', *Medical Hypotheses*, 74, 5, 2010: www.sciencedirect.com/science/article/pii/S0306987709008056?via%3Dihub (accessed on 6/4/20).

91   A. Hunter, Ehlers-Danlos Support UK, 'Speech, Language, Voice and Swallowing in the Ehlers-Danlos Syndromes', 2017: www.ehlers-danlos.org/information/speech-language-voice-and-swallowing-in-the-ehlers-danlos-syndromes (accessed on 6/4/20).

92   A. Hunter, Ehlers-Danlos Support UK, 'Speech, Language, Voice and Swallowing in the Ehlers-Danlos Syndromes', 2017: www.ehlers-danlos.org/information/speech-language-voice-and-swallowing-in-the-ehlers-danlos-syndromes (accessed on 6/4/20).

93   B. Peters, Verywell Health, 'The Link Between Ehlers Danlos Syndrome and Sleep Apnoea: Breathing Difficulties in Sleep Due to Cartilage Defects in the Airway', 2019: www.verywellhealth.com/ehlers-danlos-syndrome-and-sleep-apnea-4129568 (accessed on 6/4/20).

94   C. Guilleminault, M. Primeau, H. Chiu, K. Yuen, D. Leger, A. Metlaine, 'Sleep-Disordered Breathing in Ehlers-Danlos Syndrome (a Genetic Model of Sleep Apnoea)', *Sleep Medicine*, 14, S1, e145, 2013: www.sciencedirect.com/science/article/pii/S138994571301544X (accessed on 6/4/20).

95   The Marfan Foundation, 'Lungs': www.marfan.org/about/body-systems/lungs (accessed on 6/4/20).

96   The Marfan Foundation, 'Lungs': www.marfan.org/about/body-systems/lungs (accessed on 6/4/20).

97   The Marfan Foundation, 'Lungs': www.marfan.org/about/body-systems/lungs (accessed on 6/4/20).

98   E. McGeorge, The Pelvic Hub, 'Pelvic Floor Basics Part Two: Pelvic Floor Dysfunction', 2018: www.thepelvichub.com/post/pelvic-floor-basics-part-two-pelvic-floor-dysfunction (accessed on 6/4/20).

99   E. McGeorge, The Pelvic Hub, 'Pelvic Floor Basics Part Two: Pelvic Floor Dysfunction', 2018: www.thepelvichub.com/post/pelvic-floor-basics-part-two-pelvic-floor-dysfunction (accessed on 6/4/20).

100 N. Veit-Rubin, R. Cartwright, G. Digesu, R. Fernando, V. Khullar, 'Association Between Joint Hypermobility and Pelvic Organ Prolapse in Women: A Systematic Review and Meta-analysis', *International Urogynecology Journal*, 2015: www.ncbi.nlm.nih.gov/pubmed/26658756 (accessed on 6/4/20).

101 H. Mastoroudes, I. Giarenis, L. Cardozo, S. Srikrishna, *et al.*, 'Prolapse and Sexual Function in Women with Benign Joint Hypermobility Syndrome', *British Journal of Obstetrics and Gynaecology*, 120, 2, 2013: https://obgyn.onlinelibrary.wiley.com/doi/full/10.1111/1471-0528.12082 (accessed on 6/4/20).

102 M. Castori, S. Morlino, C. Dordoni, C. Celletti, *et al.*, 'Gynecologic and Obstetric Implications of the Joint Hypermobility Syndrome (a.k.a. Ehlers-Danlos Syndrome Hypermobility Type) in 82 Italian Patients', *American Journal of Medical Genetics*, 158A, 9, 2012: https://onlinelibrary.wiley.com/doi/abs/10.1002/ajmg.a.35506 (accessed on 6/4/20).

103 J. Hugon-Rodin, G. Lebègue, S. Becourt, C. Hamonet, A. Gompel, 'Gynecologic Symptoms and the Influence on Reproductive Life in 386 Women with Hypermobility Type Ehlers-Danlos Syndrome: a Cohort Study', *Orphanet Journal of Rare Diseases*, 11, 2016: https://ojrd.biomedcentral.com/articles/10.1186/s13023-016-0511-2 (accessed on 6/4/20).

104 C. Smith, *Understanding Hypermobile Ehlers-Danlos Syndrome and Hypermobility Spectrum Disorder*, Redcliff-House Publications, 2017.

105 Source unknown.

106 H. Bird, Hypermobility Syndromes Association, 'Hormones and Hypermobility', 2017: www.hypermobility.org/hormones-and-hypermobility (accessed on 6/4/20).

107 H. Bird, Hypermobility Syndromes Association, 'Hormones and Hypermobility', 2017: www.hypermobility.org/hormones-and-hypermobility (accessed on 6/4/20).

108 H. Bird, Hypermobility Syndromes Association, 'Hormones and Hypermobility', 2017: www.hypermobility.org/hormones-and-hypermobility (accessed on 6/4/20).

109 I. Knight, *A Guide to Living with Ehlers-Danlos Syndrome (Hypermobility Type): Bending Without Breaking*, Singing Dragon, London, 2014.

110 H. MacIver, 'Joints, Hypermobility and Hormones', *Women's Health Journal*, Sherborne Gibbs Ltd, 2013: www.womenshealthj.com/browse/editorial/item/5687-disease-focus-joints-hypermobility-and-hormones.html (accessed on 6/4/20).

111 In a paper by P. Beighton, J. Murdoch, T. Votteler, 'Gastrointestinal Complications of the Ehlers-Danlos Syndrome', *Gut*, 10, 12, 1969: www.ncbi.nlm.nih.gov/pubmed/5308459 (accessed on 6/4/20).

112 H. Collins, 'Gastrointestinal Complications of Ehlers-Danlos Syndrome', EDNF Physicians Conference, 15 September 2014: www.ehlers-danlos.com/2014-physicians-conference/Collins.pdf (accessed on 6/4/20).

113 Quoted in C. Smith, *Understanding Hypermobile Ehlers-Danlos Syndrome and Hypermobility Spectrum Disorder*, Redcliff-House Publications, 2017.

114 NHS, 'Symptoms: Irritable Bowel Syndrome (IBS)': www.nhs.uk/conditions/irritable-bowel-syndrome-ibs/symptoms (accessed on 6/4/20).

115 Hypermobility Syndromes Association, 'Bowel Problems': www.hypermobility.org/keeping-bowels-healthy (accessed on 6/4/20).

116 Z. Al-Rawi, K. Al-Dubaikel, H. Al-Sikafi, 'Joint Mobility in People with Hiatus Hernia', *Rheumatology*, 43, 574–576, May 2004: https://academic.oup.com/rheumatology/article/43/5/574/1788299 (accessed on 6/4/20).

117 L. Brockway, Ehlers-Danlos Support UK, 'Gastro-Intestinal Problems in Hypermobile Ehlers-Danlos Syndrome and Hypermobility Spectrum Disorders', 2016: www.ehlers-danlos.org/information/gastrointestinal-problems-in-hypermobile-ehlers-danlos-syndrome-and-hypermobility-spectrum-disorders (accessed on 6/4/20).

118 M. Castori, S. Morlino, G. Pascolini, C. Blundo, P. Grammatico, 'Gastrointestinal and Nutritional Issues in Joint Hypermobility Syndrome/Ehlers-Danlos Syndrome, Hypermobility Type', *American Journal of Medical Genetics*, 169, 1, 2015: https://onlinelibrary.wiley.com/doi/full/10.1002/ajmg.c.31431 (accessed on 6/4/20).

119 Ehlers-Danlos Support UK, 'Diet and EDS Research Fund': www.ehlers-danlos.org/studies/diet-and-eds-research-fund (accessed on 6/4/20).

120 J. Di Bon, 'Small Steps: the Role of Diet and Nutrition in Hypermobility', 2018: https://jeanniedibon.com/wellness/small-steps-role-diet-nutrition-hypermobility (accessed on 6/4/20).

121 A. Hunter, Ehlers-Danlos Support UK, 'Speech, Language, Voice and Swallowing in the Ehlers-Danlos Syndromes', 2017: www.ehlers-danlos.org/information/speech-language-voice-and-swallowing-in-the-ehlers-danlos-syndromes (accessed on 6/4/20).

122 C. Smith, *Understanding Hypermobile Ehlers-Danlos Syndrome and Hypermobility Spectrum Disorder*, Redcliff-House Publications, 2017.

123 M. Castori, F. Camerota, C. Celletti, C. Denese, *et al.*, 'Natural History and Manifestations of the Hypermobility Type Ehlers-Danlos Syndrome: a Pilot Study on 21 Patients', *American Journal of Medical Genetics*, 152A, 3, 556–564, 2010: www.ncbi.nlm.nih.gov/pubmed/20140961 (accessed on 6/4/20).

124 Urology Care Foundation, 'What is a Bladder Diverticulum?': www.urologyhealth.org/urologic-conditions/bladder-diverticulum (accessed on 6/4/20).

125 J. Rawston, Real Life Unlimited Blog, 'Infections and Ehlers-Danlos Syndrome', 2015: https://reallifeunlimited.wordpress.com/2015/05/25/infections-and-ehlers-danlos-syndrome (accessed on 6/4/20).

126 M. Castori, S. Morlino, G. Pascolini, C. Blundo, P. Grammatico, 'Gastrointestinal and Nutritional Issues in Joint Hypermobility Syndrome/Ehlers-Danlos Syndrome, Hypermobility Type', *American Journal of Medical Genetics*, 169, 1, 2015: https://onlinelibrary.wiley.com/doi/full/10.1002/ajmg.c.31431 (accessed on 6/4/20).

127 K. Rodgers, J. Gui, M. Dinulos, R. Cou, 'Ehlers-Danlos Syndrome Hypermobility Type Is Associated with Rheumatic Diseases', *Scientific Reports*, 7, 39636, 2017: www.ncbi.nlm.nih.gov/pmc/articles/PMC5209734 (accessed on 6/4/20).

128 D. Driscoll, 'Ocular Manifestations of Ehlers-Danlos Syndrome': https://totaleyecare.com/ocular-complications-ehlers-danlos-syndrome (accessed on 6/4/20).

129 D. Driscoll, 'Ocular Manifestations of Ehlers-Danlos Syndrome': https://totaleyecare.com/ocular-complications-ehlers-danlos-syndrome (accessed on 6/4/20).

130 D. Driscoll, 'Ocular Manifestations of Ehlers-Danlos Syndrome': https://totaleyecare.com/ocular-complications-ehlers-danlos-syndrome (accessed on 6/4/20).

131 The Marfan Foundation, 'Eyes': www.marfan.org/about/body-systems/eyes (accessed on 6/4/20).

132 D. Driscoll, 'Ocular Manifestations of Ehlers-Danlos Syndrome': https://totaleyecare.com/ocular-complications-ehlers-danlos-syndrome (accessed on 6/4/20).

133 C. Smith, *Understanding Hypermobile Ehlers-Danlos Syndrome and Hypermobility Spectrum Disorder*, Redcliff-House Publications, 2017.

134 M.C. Stöppler, MedicineNet, 'Medical Definition of Blue Sclera': www.medicinenet.com/script/main/art.asp?articlekey=201242 (accessed on 6/4/20).

135 D. Driscoll, 'Ocular Manifestations of Ehlers-Danlos Syndrome': https://totaleyecare.com/ocular-complications-ehlers-danlos-syndrome (accessed on 6/4/20).

136 The Marfan Foundation, 'Eyes': www.marfan.org/about/body-systems/eyes (accessed on 6/4/20).

137 D. Driscoll, 'Ocular Manifestations of Ehlers-Danlos Syndrome': https://totaleyecare.com/ocular-complications-ehlers-danlos-syndrome (accessed on 6/4/20).

138 Ehlers-Danlos Support UK, 'Fibromyalgia and Chronic Fatigue', 2016: www.ehlers-danlos.org/information/fibromyalgia-and-chronic-fatigue (accessed on 6/4/20).

139 C. Akin, P. Valent, D. Metcalfe, 'Mast Cell Activation Syndrome: Proposed Diagnostic Criteria', *The Journal of Allergy and Clinical Immunology*, 126, 6, 1099–1104, 2010: www.jacionline.org/article/S0091-6749(10)01333-3/abstract (accessed on 6/4/20).

140 Wikipedia, 'Mast Cell': https://en.wikipedia.org/wiki/mast_cell (accessed on 6/4/20).

141 C. Smith, *Understanding Hypermobile Ehlers-Danlos Syndrome and Hypermobility Spectrum Disorder*, Redcliff-House Publications, 2017.

142 Mast Cell Action, 'About MCAS': www.mastcellaction.org/about-mcas (accessed on 6/4/20).

143 I. Cheung, P. Vadas, 'A New Disease Cluster: Mast Cell Activation Syndrome, Postural Orthostatic Tachycardia Syndrome, and Ehlers-Danlos Syndrome', *The Journal of Allergy and Clinical Immunology*, 135, 2, Supplement, AB65, 2015: www.researchgate.net/publication/276340960_a_new_disease_cluster_mast_cell_activation_syndrome_postural_orthostatic_tachycardia_syndrome_and_ehlers-danlos_syndrome (accessed on 7/4/20).

144 Mast Cell Action, 'About MCAS': www.mastcellaction.org/about-mcas (accessed on 7/4/20).

145 C. Smith, *Understanding Hypermobile Ehlers-Danlos Syndrome and Hypermobility Spectrum Disorder*, Redcliff-House Publications, 2017.

146 M. Castori, S. Morlino, C. Celletti, G. Ghibellini, *et al.*, 'Rewriting the Natural History of Pain and Related Symptoms in the Joint Hypermobility Syndrome/Ehlers-Danlos Syndrome, Hypermobility Type', *American Journal of Medical Genetics*, 161, 12, 2013: www.ncbi.nlm.nih.gov/pubmed/24254847 (accessed on 7/4/20).

147 M. Castori, S. Morlino, C. Celletti, G. Ghibellini, *et al.*, 'Rewriting the Natural History of Pain and Related Symptoms in the Joint Hypermobility Syndrome/Ehlers-Danlos Syndrome, Hypermobility Type', *American Journal of Medical Genetics*, 161, 12, 2013: www.ncbi.nlm.nih.gov/pubmed/24254847 (accessed on 7/4/20).

148 C. Smith, *Understanding Hypermobile Ehlers-Danlos Syndrome and Hypermobility Spectrum Disorder*, Redcliff-House Publications, 2017.

149 M. Castori, S. Morlino, C. Celletti, G. Ghibellini, *et al.*, 'Rewriting the Natural History of Pain and Related Symptoms in the Joint Hypermobility Syndrome/Ehlers-Danlos Syndrome, Hypermobility Type', *American Journal of Medical Genetics*, 161, 12, 2013: www.ncbi.nlm.nih.gov/pubmed/24254847 (accessed on 7/4/20).

150 Brain and Spine Foundation, 'Neuropathic Pain', 2016: www.brainandspine.org.uk/information-and-support/living-with-a-neurological-problem/neuropathic-pain (accessed on 7/4/20).

151 F. Camerota, C. Celletti, M. Castori, P. Grammatico, L. Padua, 'Neuropathic Pain Is a Common Feature in Ehlers-Danlos Syndrome', *Journal of Pain and Symptom Management*, 41, 1, e2–e4, 2011: www.jpsmjournal.com/article/S0885-3924(10)00668-8/fulltext (accessed on 7/4/20).

152 C. Smith, *Understanding Hypermobile Ehlers-Danlos Syndrome and Hypermobility Spectrum Disorder*, Redcliff-House Publications, 2017.

153 S. DeWeerdt, Spectrum, 'Unseen Agony: Dismantling Autism's House of Pain', 2015: www.spectrumnews.org/features/deep-dive/unseen-agony-dismantling-autisms-house-of-pain (accessed on 7/4/20).

154 S. DeWeerdt, Spectrum, 'Unseen Agony: Dismantling Autism's House of Pain', 2015: www.spectrumnews.org/features/deep-dive/unseen-agony-dismantling-autisms-house-of-pain (accessed on 7/4/20).

155 C. Baeza-Velasco, D. Cohen, C. Hamonet, E. Vlamynck, *et al.*, 'Autism, Joint-Hypermobility Disorders and Pain', *Frontiers in Psychiatry*, 2018: www.frontiersin.org/articles/10.3389/fpsyt.2018.00656/full (accessed on 6/4/20).

156 P. Roth, Medical Xpress, 'Study Suggests Link Between Autism, Pain Sensitivity', 2017: https://medicalxpress.com/news/2017-07-link-autism-pain-sensitivity.html (accessed on 7/4/20).

157 S. DeWeerdt, Spectrum, 'Unseen Agony: Dismantling Autism's House of Pain', 2015: www.spectrumnews.org/features/deep-dive/unseen-agony-dismantling-autisms-house-of-pain (accessed on 7/4/20).

158 J. Di Bon, 'Small Steps – Hypermobility and Sleep', 2018: https://jeanniedibon.com/wellness/small-steps-hypermobility-sleep (accessed on 7/4/20).

159 EDHS.info, 'Fatigue and EDS-H/JHS', now archived.

160 J. Southall, The Mighty, 'Inside the Mind of Someone with Hypermobile EDS at Night', 2019: https://themighty.com/2017/03/hypermobile-ehlers-danlos-syndrome-pain-at-night (accessed on 7/4/20).

161 J. Di Bon, 'Small Steps – Hypermobility and Sleep', 2018: https://jeanniedibon.com/wellness/small-steps-hypermobility-sleep (accessed on 7/4/20).

162 J. Southall, The Mighty, 'Inside the Mind of Someone with Hypermobile EDS at Night', 2019: https://themighty.com/2017/03/hypermobile-ehlers-danlos-syndrome-pain-at-night (accessed on 7/4/20).

163 J. Morrison, Ehlers-Danlos Support UK, 'Managing Fatigue, Sleeping Problems and Brain Fog', 2017: www.ehlers-danlos.org/information/managing-fatigue-sleeping-problems-and-brain-fog (accessed on 7/4/20).

164 The Mighty, '28 People With Chronic Illness Explain What Brain Fog Feels Like to Them', 2016: https://themighty.com/2016/02/what-brain-fog-feels-like (accessed on 3/3/19).

165 EDHS.info, 'Anxiety and EDS-H/JHS', now archived.

166 A. Bulbena-Cabré and A. Bulbena, 'Anxiety and Joint Hypermobility: An Unexpected Association', 17, 4, 15–21, 2018: www.mdedge.com/psychiatry/article/161887/anxiety-disorders/anxiety-and-joint-hypermobility-unexpected-association (accessed on 7/4/20).

167 I. Knight, *A Guide to Living with Ehlers-Danlos Syndrome (Hypermobility Type): Bending Without Breaking*, Singing Dragon, London, 2014.

168 Quoted in I. Knight, *A Guide to Living with Ehlers-Danlos Syndrome (Hypermobility Type): Bending Without Breaking*, Singing Dragon, London, 2014.

169 N. Mallorquí-Bagué, S. Garfinkel, M. Engles, J. Eccles, *et al.*, 'Neuroimaging and Psychophysiological Investigation of the Link Between Anxiety, Enhanced Affective Reactivity and Interoception in People with Joint Hypermobility', *Frontiers in Psychology*, 5, 1162, 2014: www.frontiersin.org/articles/10.3389/fpsyg.2014.01162/full (accessed on 7/4/20).

170 J. Eccles, F. Beacher, M. Gray, C. Jones, *et al.*, 'Brain Structure and Joint Hypermobility: Relevance to the Expression of Psychiatric Symptoms', *The British Journal of Psychiatry*, 200, 6, 508–509, 2012: www.ncbi.nlm.nih.gov/pmc/articles/PMC3365276 (accessed on 7/4/20).

171 J. Eccles, F. Beacher, M. Gray, C. Jones, *et al.*, 'Brain Structure and Joint Hypermobility: Relevance to the Expression of Psychiatric Symptoms', *The British Journal of Psychiatry*, 200, 6, 508–509, 2012: www.ncbi.nlm.nih.gov/pmc/articles/PMC3365276 (accessed on 7/4/20).

172 I. Knight, *A Guide to Living with Ehlers-Danlos Syndrome (Hypermobility Type): Bending Without Breaking*, Singing Dragon, London, 2014.

173 I. Knight, *A Guide to Living with Ehlers-Danlos Syndrome (Hypermobility Type): Bending Without Breaking*, Singing Dragon, London, 2014.

174 I. Knight, *A Guide to Living with Ehlers-Danlos Syndrome (Hypermobility Type): Bending Without Breaking*, Singing Dragon, London, 2014.

175 H. Westwood, K. Tchanturia, 'Autism Spectrum Disorder in Anorexia Nervosa: An Updated Literature Review', *Current Psychiatry Reports*, 19, 7, 2017: www.ncbi.nlm.nih.gov/pmc/articles/PMC5443871 (accessed on 7/4/20).

176 A word coined by Gordon Gates, in *Trauma, Stigma, and Autism: Developing Resilience and Loosening the Grip of Shame*, Jessica Kingsley Publishers, London, 2019.

177 Move Daily, 'Top 5 Ehlers-Danlos Hypermobility Considerations: Stress and Anxiety', 2018: www.movewelldaily.com/ehlers-danlos-hypermobility-stress-anxiety (accessed on 7/4/20).

178 A. Pocinki, 'Joint Hypermobility and Joint Hypermobility Syndrome', 2010: www.dynainc.org/docs/hypermobility.pdf (accessed on 7/4/20).

179 M. Castori, S. Morlino, C. Celletti, G. Ghibellini, *et al.*, 'Rewriting the Natural History of Pain and Related Symptoms in the Joint Hypermobility Syndrome/Ehlers-Danlos Syndrome, Hypermobility Type', *American Journal of Medical Genetics*, 161, 12, 2013: www.ncbi.nlm.nih.gov/pubmed/24254847 (accessed on 7/4/20).

180 Instagram, 21 May 2019.

181 M. Castori, S. Morlino, C. Celletti, G. Ghibellini, *et al.*, 'Rewriting the Natural History of Pain and Related Symptoms in the Joint Hypermobility Syndrome/Ehlers-Danlos Syndrome, Hypermobility Type', *American Journal of Medical Genetics*, 161, 12, 2013: www.ncbi.nlm.nih.gov/pubmed/24254847 (accessed on 7/4/20).

182 A. Ebba, 'So Much More than Tired: Three Ways to Explain What Chronic Fatigue is Really Like', Healthline, 2018: www.healthline.com/health/how-i-explain-chronic-fatigue-syndrome (accessed on 7/4/20).

183 J. Nijs, A. Aerts, K. De Meirleir, 'Generalised Joint Hypermobility Is More Common in Chronic Fatigue Syndrome than in Healthy Control Subjects', *Journal of Manipulative and Physiogical Therapeutics*, 29, 1, 32–39, 2006: https://www.ncbi.nlm.nih.gov/pubmed/16396727 (accessed on 7/4/20).

184 A. Hakim, I. De Wandele, C. O'Callaghan, A. Pocinki, P. Rowe, adapted by B. Guscott, 'Chronic Fatigue in Ehlers-Danlos-Syndrome Hypermobile-Type (For Non-experts)', *The Ehlers-Danlos Society, 2019*: www.ehlers-danlos.com/2017-eds-classification-non-experts/chronic-fatigue-ehlers-danlos-syndrome-hypermobile-type (accessed on 7/4/20).

185 A. Hakim 'Hypermobility Syndromes and Local Anaesthetic', June 2013: www.hypermobility.org/local-anaesthetic (accessed on 7/4/20).

186 J. Schubart, E. Schaefer, P. Janicki, S. Adhikary, *et al.* 'Resistance to Local Anaesthesia in People with the Ehlers-Danlos Syndromes Presenting for Dental Surgery', *Journal of Dental Anesthesia and Pain Medicine*, 19, 5, 261–270, 2019: www.ncbi.nlm.nih.gov/pmc/articles/PMC6834718 (accessed on 7/4/20).

187 C. Baraniuk, BBC Future, 'Some of Her Patients Have Told Her That Their Doctor or Dentist Simply Won't Believe Them When They Say, "Local Anaesthetic Doesn't Work On Me"', 2017: www.bbc.com/future/story/20170106-the-people-who-cant-go-numb-at-the-dentists (accessed on 7/4/20).

188 C. Smith, *Understanding Hypermobile Ehlers-Danlos Syndrome and Hypermobility Spectrum Disorder*, Redcliff-House Publications, 2017.

189 T. Wiesmann, M. Castori, F. Malfait, H. Wulf, 'Recommendations for Anesthesia and Perioperative Management in Patients with Ehlers-Danlos Syndrome(s)', *Orphanet Journal of Rare Diseases*, 9, 109, 2014: www.ncbi.nlm.nih.gov/pmc/articles/PMC4223622/?fbclid=IwAR0LTrz7TF4EOciIDsU-Yjd_wbg8uT5u0SOVo0ALfpINKurW8kgQO2Yfgn4 (accessed on 7/4/20).

190 R. Grahame, 'Joint Hypermobility: Emerging Disease or Illness Behaviour', *Clinical Medicine*, 13, S6, s50–s52, 2013: www.researchgate.net/publication/272872930_Joint_hypermobility_Emerging_disease_or_illness_behaviour (accessed on 7/4/20).

191 Instagram, 31 May 2019.

192 Instagram, 2 May 2019.

193 R. Keer, K. Butler, 'Physiotherapy and Occupational Therapy in the Hypermobile Adult', in A. Hakim, R. Keer, R. Grahame (eds), *Hypermobility, Fibromyalgia and Chronic Pain*, Churchill Livingstone Elsevier, 2010. Free download at: https://epdf.pub/hypermobility-fibromyalgia-and-chronic-pain.html (accessed on 7/4/20).

194 @ehlers.danlos, Instagram, 2 January 2020.

195 @ehlers.danlos, Instagram, 2 January 2020.
196 @ehlers.danlos, Instagram, 2 January 2020.

Chapter 2

1   A. Wilds, 'Hypermobility in Yoga', 2018: www.learntoloveyoga.co.uk/yoga-anatomy/hypermobility-in-yoga (accessed on 11/4/20).

2   B. Birney, Yoga International, 'Joint Hypermobility Syndrome: Yoga's Enigmatic Epidemic': https://yogainternational.com/article/view/joint-hypermobility-syndrome-yogas-enigmatic-epidemic (accessed on 11/4/20).

3   R. Keer, K. Butler, 'Physiotherapy and Occupational Therapy in the Hypermobile Adult', in A. Hakim, R. Keer, R. Grahame (eds), *Hypermobility, Fibromyalgia and Chronic Pain*, Churchill Livingstone Elsevier, 2010. Free download at: https://epdf.pub/hypermobility-fibromyalgia-and-chronic-pain.html (accessed on 7/4/20).

4   J. Glenny, *The Yoga Teacher Mentor: A Reflective Guide to Holding Spaces, Maintaining Boundaries, and Creating Inclusive Classes*, Singing Dragon, London, 2020.

5   R. Keer, K. Butler, 'Physiotherapy and Occupational Therapy in the Hypermobile Adult', in A. Hakim, R. Keer, R. Grahame (eds), *Hypermobility, Fibromyalgia and Chronic Pain*, Churchill Livingstone Elsevier, 2010. Free download at: https://epdf.pub/hypermobility-fibromyalgia-and-chronic-pain.html (accessed on 7/4/20).

6   J. Glenny, *The Yoga Teacher Mentor: A Reflective Guide to Holding Spaces, Maintaining Boundaries, and Creating Inclusive Classes*, Singing Dragon, London, 2020.

7   R. Keer, J. Simmonds, Ehlers-Danlos Support UK, 'Physical Therapy for Hypermobility': www.ehlers-danlos.org/information/physical-therapy-for-hypermobility (accessed on 11/4/20).

8   For more on the ethics of touch, see J. Glenny, *The Yoga Teacher Mentor: A Reflective Guide to Holding Spaces, Maintaining Boundaries, and Creating Inclusive Classes*, Singing Dragon, London, 2020.

9   K. Bruni Young, Mindful Strength: Whole Body Immersion Online, week 1, 'Tissue Adaptation': https://kathrynbruniyoung.com (accessed on 11/4/20).

10 K. Bruni Young, Mindful Strength: Whole Body Immersion Online, week 1, 'Tissue Adaptation': https://kathrynbruniyoung.com (accessed on 11/4/20).

11 R. Keer, J. Simmonds, Ehlers-Danlos Support UK, 'Physical Therapy for Hypermobility': www.ehlers-danlos.org/information/physical-therapy-for-hypermobility (accessed on 11/4/20).

12 T. Ghose, LiveScience, 'Does Stretching Increase Flexibility?', 2014: www.livescience.com/48744-how-does-stretching-work.html (accessed on 11/4/20).

13 See: www.julesmitchell.com. Jules Mitchell's recent book on this subject is *Yoga Biomechanics: Stretching Redefined*, Handspring Publishing Ltd, Pencaitland, UK, 2019.

14 R. Long, Daily Bandha, 'Stretching, Ageing and Your Down Dog', 2015, : www.dailybandha.com/2015/03/stretching-growing-older-and-your-down.html (accessed on 11/4/20).

15 R. Mulready, The Australian Ballet Blog, 'Strength Beats Stretch', 2018: https://australianballet.com.au/behind-ballet/strength-beats-stretch (accessed on 11/4/20).

16 J. Ringer, *Dancing Through It: My Journey in the Ballet*, Viking Penguin, 2014.

17 J. Parry, 'Dislocation/Subluxation Management, Or "I'm Just Popping Out for a While"', webinar for The Ehlers-Danlos Society, 21 August 2019.

18 J. Parry, 'Dislocation/Subluxation Management, Or "I'm Just Popping Out for a While"', webinar for The Ehlers-Danlos Society, 21 August 2019.

19 J. Glenny, *The Yoga Teacher Mentor: A Reflective Guide to Holding Spaces, Maintaining Boundaries, and Creating Inclusive Classes*, Singing Dragon, London, 2020.

20 R. Keer, K. Butler, 'Physiotherapy and Occupational Therapy in the Hypermobile Adult', in A. Hakim, R. Keer, R. Grahame (eds), *Hypermobility, Fibromyalgia and Chronic Pain*, Churchill Livingstone Elsevier, 2010. Free download at: https://epdf.pub/hypermobility-fibromyalgia-and-chronic-pain.html (accessed on 7/4/20).

21 J. Glenny, *The Yoga Teacher Mentor: A Reflective Guide to Holding Spaces, Maintaining Boundaries, and Creating Inclusive Classes*, Singing Dragon, London, 2020.

Chapter 3

1   The Yoga Sutras of Patanjali, II.46.

2   J. Rawlings, T. Pollen, 'Seven Prominent Yogis Weigh In On Yoga Injuries and What to Do About Them', 2019: www.jennirawlings.com/blog/7-prominent-yogis-weigh-in-on-yoga-injuries-and-what-to-do-about-them?fbclid=IwAR0uJMWFdaED-8HGQr2pn6DCFI0GZTUJS1kb5nKpfXDn6Mfp4Pl0FzqHlUE (accessed on 11/4/20).

3   R. Cole, 'Protect Your Knees: Learn to Avoid Hyperextension', *Yoga Journal*, 2009, updated 2017: www.yogajournal.com/practice/please-your-knees (accessed on 11/4/20).

4   R. Cole, 'Protect Your Knees: Learn to Avoid Hyperextension', *Yoga Journal*, 2009, updated 2017: www.yogajournal.com/practice/please-your-knees (accessed on 11/4/20).

5   R. Keer, J. Butler, 'Physiotherapy and Occupational Therapy in the Hypermobile Adult', in A. Hakim, R. Keer, R. Grahame (eds), *Hypermobility, Fibromyalgia and Chronic Pain*, Churchill Livingstone Elsevier, London, 2010. Free download at: https://epdf.pub/hypermobility-fibromyalgia-and-chronic-pain.html (accessed on 7/4/20).

6   R. Strong, Daily Bandha, 'A Tip for Helping to Correct Alignment in Hyperextended Elbows and Knees in Yoga', 2011: www.dailybandha.com/2011/03/tip-for-helping-hyperextended-elbows.html (accessed on 11/4/20).

7   R. Keer, J. Butler, 'Physiotherapy and Occupational Therapy in the Hypermobile Adult', in A. Hakim, R. Keer, R. Grahame (eds), *Hypermobility, Fibromyalgia and Chronic Pain*, Churchill Livingstone Elsevier, London, 2010. Free download at: https://epdf.pub/hypermobility-fibromyalgia-and-chronic-pain.html (accessed on 7/4/20).

8   J. Gudmestad, 'The Danger of a Hyperextended Knee and How to Fix It', *Yoga Journal*, 2007, updated 2017: www.yogajournal.com/practice-section/the-hyperextended-knee (accessed on 11/4/20).

9   R. Long, Bandha Yoga, 'A Tip for Helping Hyperextended Knees in Yoga': www.bandhayoga.com/keys_knee_hype.html (accessed on 14/4/20).

10   R. Long, Daily Bandha, 'A Tip for Helping to Correct Alignment in Hyperextended Elbows and Knees in Yoga', 2011: www.dailybandha.com/2011/03/tip-for-helping-hyperextended-elbows.html (accessed on 14/4/20).

11   S. Lucett, National Academy of Sports Medicine (NASM), 'The Effects of Pronation Distortion Syndrome and Solutions for Injury Prevention', 2013: https://blog.nasm.org/fitness/the-effects-of-pronation-distortion-syndrome-and-solutions-for-injury-prevention (accessed on 14/4/20).

12   Physiopedia, 'Supraspinatus': www.physio-pedia.com/supraspinatus (accessed on 14/4/20).

13   M. McCrary, 'A Yogi's Guide to the Shoulder Girdle and its Actions', *Yoga Journal*, 2015, updated 2017: www.yogajournal.com/teach/tiffany-cruikshanks-guide-shoulder-girdle-stability (accessed on 14/4/20).

14   L.-J. Lee, 'Thoracic Ring Approach™': https://ljlee.ca/teaching-models/the-thoracic-ring-approach (accessed on 14/4/20).

15   J. Gudmestad, 'Spread Your Wings', *Yoga Journal*, 2007, updated 2017: www.yogajournal.com/practice-section/spread-your-wings (accessed on 14/4/20).

16   D. Keil, *Functional Anatomy of Yoga: A Guide for Practitioners and Teachers*, Lotus Publishing, Chichester, 2014.

17   Bone shapes in the ankle also play a role here.

18   @bonniebainbridgecohen, Instagram, 2 October 2019.

19   D. Keil, *Functional Anatomy of Yoga: A Guide for Practitioners and Teachers*, Lotus Publishing, Chichester, 2014.

20   D. Keller, YogaUOnine, 'The Origins of Misalignment In Yoga: Focus on Forward Bends': https://yogauonline.com/yogau-product/7871 (accessed on 14/4/20).

21   D. Keller, YogaUOnine, 'The Origins of Misalignment In Yoga: Focus on Forward Bends': https://yogauonline.com/yogau-product/7871 (accessed on 14/4/20).

22   S. Bailey, 'Do You Have "Yoga Butt"? Here's How You Fix It': www.bodyandsoul.com.au/fitness/workouts/do-you-have-yoga-butt-heres-how-you-fix-it/news-story/0aa26d85cf4cdb70aea2452822305e12 (accessed on 14/4/20).

23   D. Keller, YogaUOnline, 'The Origins of Misalignment In Yoga: Focus on Forward Bends': https://yogauonline.com/yogau-product/7871 (accessed on 14/4/20).

24 D. Keller, YogaUOnline, 'The Origins of Misalignment In Yoga: Focus on Forward Bends': https://yogauonline.com/yogau-product/7871 (accessed on 14/4/20).

25 C. Jordan, Caroline Jordan Fitness, 'How I Got My Butt Back. A Surprising Yoga Injury Experience', 2014: https://carolinejordanfitness.com/butt-back-surprising-yoga-injury (accessed on 14/4/20).

26 C. Jordan, Caroline Jordan Fitness, 'How I Got My Butt Back. A Surprising Yoga Injury Experience', 2014: https://carolinejordanfitness.com/butt-back-surprising-yoga-injury (accessed on 14/4/20).

27 D. Keil, *Functional Anatomy of Yoga: A Guide for Practitioners and Teachers*, Lotus Publishing, Chichester, 2014.

28 J. Heafner, The Student Physical Therapist, 'The Ups and Downs of the Clamshell Exercise', 2017: www.thestudentphysicaltherapist.com/featured-articles/the-ups-and-downs-of-the-clamshell-exercise#.

29 D. Keller, 'Recruit the Glutes', *Yoga Plus*, September–October 2008: www.doyoga.com/articles_all/14_sept_08_gluteals.pdf (accessed on 14/4/20).

30 I was not able to find any research in this area.

31 R. Cole, 'Glute-Free Backbends?', *Yoga Journal*, 2009, updated 2017: www.yogajournal.com/practice/the-max-factor (accessed on 14/4/20).

32 R. Cole, 'Glute-Free Backbends?', *Yoga Journal*, 2009, updated 2017: www.yogajournal.com/practice/the-max-factor (accessed on 14/4/20).

33 D. Keil, YogAnatomy, 'A Reality Check on the SI Joint in Yoga', website: www.yoganatomy.com/si-joint-in-yoga/#ref (accessed on 14/4/20).

34 J. Lasater, 'The Best Yoga Poses for Sacroiliac Joint Pain', *Yoga Journal*, 2014, updated 2018: www.yogajournal.com/lifestyle/out-of-joint (accessed on 14/4/20).

35 D. Farhi, YogaUOnline, 'Yoga for Lower Back Pain: Keys to Sacroiliac Stability and Ease of Movement': https://yogauonline.com/yogau-product/7746 (accessed on 14/4/20).

36 D. Farhi, YogaUOnline, 'Yoga for Lower Back Pain: Keys to Sacroiliac Stability and Ease of Movement': https://yogauonline.com/yogau-product/7746 (accessed on 14/4/20).

37 For a helpful explanation of the two types of *uddiyana bandha*, see G. Maehle, Chintamani Yoga 'Uddiyana Bandha Elusive No More', 2019: https://chintamaniyoga.com/uddiyana-bandha-elusive-no-more (accessed on 14/4/20).

38 According to Dr Timothy McCall, 'One of yoga's secrets, documented in research from the Swami Vivekananda Yoga Research Foundation near Bangalore, is that more active practices followed by relaxing ones lead to deeper relaxation than relaxing practices alone' ('The Scientific Basis of Yoga Therapy', *Yoga Journal*, 2007, updated 2017: www.yogajournal.com/teach/the-scientific-basis-of-yoga-therapy (accessed on 14/4/20)).

39 J. Glenny, *The Yoga Teacher Mentor: A Reflective Guide to Holding Spaces, Maintaining Boundaries, and Creating Inclusive Classes*, Singing Dragon, London, 2020.

40 S. Hepner, in a private group.

41 J. Rawlings, T. Pollen, Jenni Rawlings Blog, 'Physical Touch in Yoga: Do Teachers and Students Agree?': https://jennirawlingsblog.com/blog/physical-touch-in-yoga-do-teachers-and-students-agree (accessed on 14/4/20).

42 J. Glenny, *The Yoga Teacher Mentor: A Reflective Guide to Holding Spaces, Maintaining Boundaries, and Creating Inclusive Classes*, Singing Dragon, London, 2020.

43 R. Keer, J. Simmonds, Ehlers-Danlos Support UK, 'Physical Therapy for Hypermobility': www.ehlers-danlos.org/information/physical-therapy-for-hypermobility (accessed on 11/4/20).

44 R. Keer, J. Butler, 'Physiotherapy and Occupational Therapy in the Hypermobile Adult', in A. Hakim, R. Keer, R. Grahame (eds), *Hypermobility, Fibromyalgia and Chronic Pain*, Churchill Livingstone Elsevier, London, 2010. Free download at: https://epdf.pub/hypermobility-fibromyalgia-and-chronic-pain.html (accessed on 7/4/20).

45 R. Keer, J. Butler, 'Physiotherapy and Occupational Therapy in the Hypermobile Adult', in A. Hakim, R. Keer, R. Grahame (eds), *Hypermobility, Fibromyalgia and Chronic Pain*, Churchill Livingstone Elsevier, London, 2010. Free download at: https://epdf.pub/hypermobility-fibromyalgia-and-chronic-pain.html (accessed on 7/4/20).

Chapter 4

1   For example, 11 years for @edsunplugged, 51 years for @elhedberg61 and 20 years for @lady-command, who says: '…but [I] wasn't given the name for another 10 years! Why? Between visits my specialist changed practices and [the] old practice destroyed patient records. Worse than that is how few doctors know, really know, what #ehlersdanlossyndrome is and that it affects the whole body, not just "loose joints" as most are taught in a book.' Shared by @ehlersdanlosuk, Instagram, 3 July 2019: www.instagram.com/p/Bzc5sEdAgkJ (accessed on 22/4/20).

2   Mitchell LaBerge, Speaking About Autism, LLC, 'Help For My Ears', 2017: www.speakingaboutautism.com/blog/ait-auditory-integration-training-journey-by-mitchell-laberge (accessed on 22/4/20). Research shows that Mitchell's experience is generalisable among the autistic population: UCL News, 'Greater Capacity to Detect Sound Gives Autistic People an Advantage', 2017: www.ucl.ac.uk/news/2017/may/greater-capacity-detect-sound-gives-autistic-people-advantage (accessed on 22/4/20).

3   The autistic self-advocacy network within the blogosphere is vast, and examples are legion, but include:
Ryan Boren, Boren blog, 'Autistic Empathy', 2017: https://boren.blog/2017/09/04/autistic-empathy (accessed on 22/4/20); Holly Wilkinson, StimSensory blog, 'Autism Stereotypes: "Autistic People Have No Empathy"', 2019: www.stimsensory.co.uk/blog/autism-stereotypes-autistic-people-have-no-empathy (accessed on 22/4/20); Ann Memmott, Ann's Autism Blog, 'Autism, Morality, Love, Empathy', 2017: http://annsautism.blogspot.com/2017/10/autism-morality-love-empathy.html (accessed on 22/4/20).

4   Helen Wallace-Iles, The Art of Autism blog, 'Autistic People and Empathy: What's the Real Story', 6 August 2018: https://the-art-of-autism.com/autistic-people-empathy-whats-the-real-story (accessed on 22/4/20).

5   Helen Wallace-Iles, The Art of Autism blog, 'Autistic People and Empathy: What's the Real Story', 6 August 2018: https://the-art-of-autism.com/autistic-people-empathy-whats-the-real-story (accessed on 22/4/20).

6   J. Glenny, *The Yoga Teacher Mentor: A Reflective Guide to Holding Spaces, Maintaining Boundaries, and Creating Inclusive Classes*, Singing Dragon, London, 2020.

7   Doug Keller, Yoga International, '9 Poses to Prevent Bunions and Relieve Bunion Pain': https://yogainternational.com/article/view/9-poses-to-prevent-bunions-relieve-bunion-pain (accessed on 22/4/20).

8   Foundation Podiatry, 'Bunions': www.foundationpodiatry.com.au/bunions/ (accessed on 22/4/20).

9   Doug Keller, Yoga International, '9 Poses to Prevent Bunions and Relieve Bunion Pain': https://yogainternational.com/article/view/9-poses-to-prevent-bunions-relieve-bunion-pain (accessed on 22/4/20).

10 Doug Keller, Yoga International, '9 Poses to Prevent Bunions and Relieve Bunion Pain': https://yogainternational.com/article/view/9-poses-to-prevent-bunions-relieve-bunion-pain (accessed on 22/4/20).

11 Doug Keller, Yoga International, '9 Poses to Prevent Bunions and Relieve Bunion Pain': https://yogainternational.com/article/view/9-poses-to-prevent-bunions-relieve-bunion-pain (accessed on 22/4/20).

12 Mayfield Chiari Center, 'Treatments': www.mayfieldchiaricenter.com/chiari_Treatments.php.

13 Conquer Chiari, 'Chiari FAQ's': www.conquerchiari.org/education/chiari-faqs.html.

14 Conquer Chiari, 'Chiari FAQ's': www.conquerchiari.org/education/chiari-faqs.html.

15 Personal communication.

16 Personal communication.

17 Donna Owens, *Yoga, my Bed and M.E.*, CreateSpace Independent Publishing Platform, 2016.

18 Donna Owens, The Health Sessions blog, 'How to Start Doing Yoga in Bed When You Have M.E./C.F.S.': https://thehealthsessions.com/how-to-start-doing-yoga-in-bed.

19 In a private group.

20 D. A. Parker MD, Sports-health, 'Hip Labral Tear Risk Factors and Causes', 2018: www.sports-health.com/sports-injuries/hip-injuries/hip-labral-tear-risk-factors-and-causes (accessed on 22/4/20).

21 D. A. Parker MD, Sports-health, 'Hip Labral Tear Risk Factors and Causes', 2018: www.sports-health.com/sports-injuries/hip-injuries/hip-labral-tear-risk-factors-and-causes (accessed on 22/4/20).

22　L. Howell, YouTube, 'Is Over Stretching Bad?', 2019: https://youtu.be/-fwxTGWlp0g (accessed on 22/4/20).

23　W. Ericson, R. Wolman, 'Orthopaedic Management of the Ehlers-Danlos Syndromes', *American Journal of Medical Genetics*, 2017: https://onlinelibrary.wiley.com/doi/full/10.1002/ajmg.c.31551 (accessed on 22/4/20).

24　YogAnatomy, 'Is Yoga Tearing Labrums?': www.yoganatomy.com/yoga-tearing-labrums (accessed on 22/4/20).

25　D. A. Parker MD, Sports-health, 'Hip Labral Tear Risk Factors and Causes', 2018: www.sports-health.com/sports-injuries/hip-injuries/hip-labral-tear-risk-factors-and-causes (accessed on 22/4/20).

26　YogAnatomy, 'Is Yoga Tearing Labrums?': www.yoganatomy.com/yoga-tearing-labrums (accessed on 22/4/20).

27　YogAnatomy, 'Is Yoga Tearing Labrums?': www.yoganatomy.com/yoga-tearing-labrums (accessed on 22/4/20).

28　L. Burkhart, '10 Ways to Get Real About Your Body's Limitations and Avoid Yoga Injuries', *Yoga Journal*, 2018: www.yogajournal.com/practice/10-ways-to-get-real-about-your-bodys-limitations-avoid-yoga-injuries (accessed on 22/4/20).

29　L. Burkhart, '10 Ways to Get Real About Your Body's Limitations and Avoid Yoga Injuries', *Yoga Journal*, 2018: www.yogajournal.com/practice/10-ways-to-get-real-about-your-bodys-limitations-avoid-yoga-injuries (accessed on 22/4/20).

30　L. Burkhart, '10 Ways to Get Real About Your Body's Limitations and Avoid Yoga Injuries', *Yoga Journal*, 2018: www.yogajournal.com/practice/10-ways-to-get-real-about-your-bodys-limitations-avoid-yoga-injuries (accessed on 22/4/20).

31　A. Foster, 'Yoga and Your Hips: Deciphering Femoroacetabular Impingement and Hip Labral Tears': https://sacredsourceyoga.com/physicaltherapy/yoga-and-your-hips-deciphering-femoroacetabular-impingement-and-labral-tears (accessed on 22/4/20).

32　R. Long, Daily Bandha, 'Preventing Yoga Injury vs. Preventing Yoga, Part II: Joint Hypermobility', 2013: www.dailybandha.com/2013/11/preventing-yoga-injuries-vs-preventing_19.html (accessed on 22/4/20).

33　A. Foster, 'Yoga and Your Hips: Deciphering Femoroacetabular Impingement and Hip Labral Tears': https://sacredsourceyoga.com/physicaltherapy/yoga-and-your-hips-deciphering-femoroacetabular-impingement-and-labral-tears (accessed on 22/4/20).

34　In a private group.

35　In a private group.

36　In a private group.

37　In a private group.

38　L. Howard, YogaUOnline course, 'Yoga for the Pelvic Floor: Keys to Lifelong Health': https://yogauonline.com/yogau-product/6661 (accessed on 22/4/20).

39　M. Rabbitt, 'Core Concept: Soften Your Middle for a Stronger Core', *Yoga Journal*, 2016, updated 2017: www.yogajournal.com/practice/core-concept-soften-middle-for-stronger-core (accessed on 22/4/20).

40　H. Shaheed, Continence Foundation of Australia, 'The Hypertonic Pelvic Floor', 2019: https://continence.org.au/news.php/577/the-hypertonic-pelvic-floor (accessed on 22/4/20).

41　L. Howard, YogaUOnline course, 'Yoga for the Pelvic Floor: Keys to Lifelong Health': https://yogauonline.com/yogau-product/6661 (accessed on 22/4/20).

42　S. Prosko, Yoga For Healthy Aging blog, 'The Treatment of Incontinence: The Physio-Yoga Therapy Approach', 2014: http://yogaforhealthyaging.blogspot.com/2014/02/treatment-of-incontinence-physio-yoga.html (accessed on 22/4/20).

43　J. Steward, P. Pianosi, M. Shaban, C. Terilli, *et al.* 'Postural Hyperventilation as a Cause of Postural Tachycardia Syndrome: Increased Systemic Vascular Resistance and Decreased Cardiac Output When Upright in All Postural Tachycardia Syndrome Variants', *Journal of the American Heart Association*, 2018: www.ncbi.nlm.nih.gov/pmc/articles/PMC6064900 (accessed on 22/4/20).

44　Personal communication.

45　D. Keil, YogAnatomy, 'A Reality Check on the SI Joint in Yoga': www.yoganatomy.com/si-joint-in-yoga/#ref (accessed on 22/4/20).

46　R. Cole, 'Practice Tips for the SI Joints', *Yoga Journal*, 2007, updated 2017: www.yogajournal.com/teach/practice-tips-for-the-si-joints (accessed on 22/4/20).

47   R. Cole, 'Practice Tips for the SI Joints', *Yoga Journal*, 2007, updated 2017: www.yogajournal.com/teach/practice-tips-for-the-si-joints (accessed on 22/4/20).

48   R. Cole, 'Practice Tips for the SI Joints', *Yoga Journal*, 2007, updated 2017: www.yogajournal.com/teach/practice-tips-for-the-si-joints (accessed on 22/4/20).

49   B. Bell, Yoga for Healthy Aging, 'Friday Q&A: Yoga for Spondylolisthesis', 2018: http://yogaforhealthyaging.blogspot.com/2018/03/friday-q-yoga-for-spondylolisthesis.html (accessed on 22/4/20).

50   K. Ellis, 'Spondylolisthesis She Wrote': https://pilatesnerd.com/spondylolistesis-she-wrote (accessed on 22/4/20).

51   B. Bell, Yoga for Healthy Aging, 'Friday Q&A: Yoga for Spondylolisthesis', 2018: http://yogaforhealthyaging.blogspot.com/2018/03/friday-q-yoga-for-spondylolisthesis.html (accessed on 22/4/20).

52   W. Ericson, R. Wolman, 'Orthopaedic Management of the Ehlers-Danlos Syndromes', *American Journal of Medical Genetics*, 175, 1 (Special Issue: The Ehlers-Danlos Syndromes: Reports from the International Consortium on the Ehlers-Danlos Syndromes), 188–194, 2017: https://onlinelibrary.wiley.com/doi/full/10.1002/ajmg.c.31551 (accessed on 22/4/20).

53   R. Cole, 'Have You Gone Numb?', *Yoga Journal*, 2010, updated 2017: www.yogajournal.com/practice/numbness-hand-and-arm-pain-yoga-tension (accessed on 22/4/20).

54   R. Cole, 'Have You Gone Numb?', *Yoga Journal*, 2010, updated 2017: www.yogajournal.com/practice/numbness-hand-and-arm-pain-yoga-tension (accessed on 22/4/20).

Chapter 5

1   www.pauliezink.com.

2   https://paulgrilley.com.

3   https://sarahpowers.com/sp.

4   B. Clark, Yinsights, 'Original Yin': https://yinyoga.com/yinsights/original-yin (accessed on 22/4/20).

5   B. Clark, *The Complete Guide to Yin Yoga: The Philosophy and Practice of Yin Yoga*, White Cloud Press, 2012.

6   B. Clark, 'In Defence of Yin Yoga': https://yinyoga.com/in-defense-of-yin-yoga/?fbclid=IwAR3Qx-Dxx8qQiCA23ScAsuqxWpev99xz7C3qlqdyQmOWjsJtQ4nJG-i2V_o (accessed on 22/4/20).

7   B. Clark, 'In Defence of Yin Yoga': https://yinyoga.com/in-defense-of-yin-yoga/?fbclid=IwAR3Qx-Dxx8qQiCA23ScAsuqxWpev99xz7C3qlqdyQmOWjsJtQ4nJG-i2V_o (accessed on 22/4/20).

8   N. Blair, *Brightening Our Inner Skies: Yin and Yoga*, MicMac Margins, London, 2017.

9   P. Grilley, *Yin Yoga: A Quiet Practice*, White Cloud Press, Ashland, OR, 2002.

10   Quoted in P. Grilley, *Yin Yoga: A Quiet Practice*, White Cloud Press, Ashland, OR, 2002.

11   S. Powers, 'Yin/Yang Yoga: Sarah Powers Finds Power in Stillness', (first published in *Yoga Chicago*, 2001): https://sarahpowers.com/sp/media/articles/yinyang-yoga (accessed on 22/4/20).

12   'Yin Yoga': https://moveyourframe.com/class/yin-yoga (accessed on 22/4/20).

13   Yoga with Kassandra, YouTube, 'One-Hour Yin Yoga Class Without Props – Full Body Yin Yoga Class': https://youtu.be/mzf2kFNf8Yw (accessed on 22/4/20).

14   'Yin Yoga': https://yogasoulmcr.co.uk/classes/yin-yoga (accessed on 22/4/20).

15   'Yin Yoga: All Levels': https://yogahome.com/apps/mindbody/classes/343 (accessed on 22/4/20).

16   B. Clarke, 'What Stops Me?', *Your Body Your Yoga: Learn Alignment Cues that are Skillful, Safe and Best Suited to You*, Wild Strawberry Productions, Vancouver, 2016.

17   R. Cole, 'Which Poses Treat Adrenal Exhaustion?' *Yoga Journal*, 2007, updated 2017: www.yogajournal.com/practice/treating-adrenal-exhaustion (accessed on 22/4/20).

18   Reported by Karen Macklin in 'When Restorative Yoga Doesn't Feel Relaxing…', *Yoga Journal*, 2009, updated 2017: www.yogajournal.com/practice/on-solid-ground (accessed on 22/4/20).

19   M. West, 'Yoga Nidra for Mental Overwhelm, Attention Economy Series, Yoga With Melissa 496': https://melissawest.com/496 (accessed on 22/4/20).

20   N. Pearson, 'Yoga Therapy in Practice: Yoga for People in Pain', *International Journal of Yoga Therapy*, 18, 2008: https://paincareu.com/wp-content/uploads/2019/02/IJYT-Yoga_Chronic_2008.pdf (accessed on 22/4/20).

21 N. Pearson, 'Yoga Therapy in Practice: Yoga for People in Pain', *International Journal of Yoga Therapy*, 18, 2008: https://paincareu.com/wp-content/uploads/2019/02/IJYT-Yoga_Chronic_2008.pdf (accessed on 22/4/20).

22 N. Pearson, 'Yoga Therapy in Practice: Yoga for People in Pain', *International Journal of Yoga Therapy*, 18, 2008: https://paincareu.com/wp-content/uploads/2019/02/IJYT-Yoga_Chronic_2008.pdf (accessed on 22/4/20).

23 N. Pearson, 'Yoga Therapy in Practice: Yoga for People in Pain', *International Journal of Yoga Therapy*, 18, 2008: https://paincareu.com/wp-content/uploads/2019/02/IJYT-Yoga_Chronic_2008.pdf (accessed on 22/4/20).

Chapter 6

1   Ehlers-Danlos Support UK, 'Children': www.ehlers-danlos.org/what-is-eds/information-on-eds/children (accessed on 22/4/20).

2   @ehlersdanlosuk, Instagram, 7 June 2019.

3   B. Smith, Complex Child, 'Living with Ehlers-Danlos Syndrome': https://complexchild.org/articles/2015-articles/september/living-eds (accessed on 22/4/20).

4   The Ehlers-Danlos Society, 19 January 2020: www.facebook.com/ehlers.danlos (accessed on 22/4/20).

5   B. Smith, Complex Child, 'Living with Ehlers-Danlos Syndrome': https://complexchild.org/articles/2015-articles/september/living-eds (accessed on 22/4/20).

6   A further reason for obtaining diagnosis may be that the frequent bruising and dislocation that often accompany hypermobility can – rarely – lead to accusations of child abuse. Beth says: 'The frightening part of the lack of awareness in the medical community is that EDS is known to look like child abuse – bruises, frequent injuries, new wounds and old scars, even fractures in various stages of healing thanks to Vitamin D deficiency. An innocent parent who is unaware of the genetic fault that causes all of those red flags will have no explanation for his or her child's injuries.' B. Smith, Complex Child, 'Living with Ehlers-Danlos Syndrome': https://complexchild.org/articles/2015-articles/september/living-eds (accessed on 22/4/20).

7   A. D. Klein MD, The Ehlers-Danlos Society, 'Hypermobile Ehlers-Danlos Syndrome in Children': www.ehlers-danlos.com/wp-content/uploads/Kline-hEDS-in-Children-S.pdf (accessed on 22/4/20).

8   @ehlersdanlosuk, Instagram, 30 November 2019.

9   L. Howell, The Ballet Blog, 'My Daughter Is Hypermobile': www.theballetblog.com/portfolio/my-daughter-is-hypermobile (accessed on 22/4/20).

10 C. Cook, Quora, 'Is Gymnastics a Safe Sport for a Child with Hypermobility of the Joints', 2019: www.quora.com/Is-gymnastics-a-safe-sport-for-a-child-with-hypermobility-of-the-joints (accessed on 22/4/20).

11 P. Versfeld, Skills for Action, 'How Hypermobility and Low Muscle Tone Affect Your Baby's Development': www.skillsforaction.com/infant-joint-hypermobility (accessed on 22/4/20).

12 P. Versfeld, Skills for Action, 'How Hypermobility and Low Muscle Tone Affect Your Baby's Development': www.skillsforaction.com/infant-joint-hypermobility (accessed on 22/4/20).

13 P. Versfeld, Skills for Action, 'How Hypermobility and Low Muscle Tone Affect Your Baby's Development': www.skillsforaction.com/infant-joint-hypermobility (accessed on 18/5/20).

14 P. Versfeld, Skills for Action, 'How Hypermobility and Low Muscle Tone Affect Your Baby's Development': www.skillsforaction.com/infant-joint-hypermobility (accessed on 18/5/20).

15 P. Versfeld, Skills for Action, 'How Hypermobility and Low Muscle Tone Affect Your Baby's Development': www.skillsforaction.com/infant-joint-hypermobility (accessed on 18/5/20).

16 P. Versfeld, Skills for Action, 'How Hypermobility and Low Muscle Tone Affect Your Baby's Development': www.skillsforaction.com/infant-joint-hypermobility (accessed on 18/5/20).

17 J. Campbell, 700 Children's Blog, 'Why Crawling Is Important for Your Baby', 2016: www.nationwidechildrens.org/family-resources-education/700childrens/2016/11/why-crawling-is-important-for-your-baby (accessed on 18/5/20).

18 P. Versfeld, Skills for Action, 'How Hypermobility and Low Muscle Tone Affect Your Baby's Development': www.skillsforaction.com/infant-joint-hypermobility (accessed on 18/5/20).

19 P. Versfeld, Skills for Action, 'How Hypermobility and Low Muscle Tone Affect Your Baby's Development': www.skillsforaction.com/infant-joint-hypermobility (accessed on 18/5/20).

20 P. Versfeld, Skills for Action, 'How Hypermobility and Low Muscle Tone Affect Your Baby's Development': www.skillsforaction.com/infant-joint-hypermobility (accessed on 18/5/20).

21 A. Green Gilbert, Creative Dance Center, 'BrainDance': www.creativedance.org/about__trashed/braindance (accessed on 18/5/20).

22 A. Pawlowski, 'Why W Sitting Is Really Not So Bad for Kids, After All', Today, 2016: www.today.com/parents/why-w-sitting-really-not-so-bad-kids-after-all-t69806 (accessed on 22/4/20).

23 The Movement Team, 'W-Sitting? Don't Stress, Read This…', 2016: http://themovementteam.com.au/blog/2016/5/16/w-sitting-dont-stress-read-this (accessed on 22/4/20).

24 Z. Mulroy, 'Why the "W" Sitting Position IS Bad for Kids – and How to Stop Your Child Adopting it', Mirror, 2017: www.mirror.co.uk/lifestyle/family/w-sitting-position-bad-prevent-7081066 (accessed on 22/4/20).

25 C. Shortsleeve, 'Why It's Totally Fine to Let Your Kid Sit in the "W" Position': www.parents.com/baby/health/kids-sitting-in-the-w-position (accessed on 22/4/20).

26 P. Versfeld, 'The Trouble with W-sitting': https://skillsforaction.com/w-sitting (accessed on 22/4/20).

27 P. Versfeld, 'The Trouble with W-sitting': https://skillsforaction.com/w-sitting (accessed on 22/4/20).

28 K. Askins, Child's Play Therapy Center blog, 'W-sitting: What Is It and Why Should I Correct it?', 2014: www.childsplaytherapycenter.com/w-sitting-correct (accessed on 22/4/20).

29 K. Askins, Child's Play Therapy Center blog, 'W-sitting: What Is It and Why Should I Correct it?', 2014: www.childsplaytherapycenter.com/w-sitting-correct (accessed on 22/4/20).

30 K. Askins, Child's Play Therapy Center blog, 'W-sitting: What Is It and Why Should I Correct it?', 2014: www.childsplaytherapycenter.com/w-sitting-correct (accessed on 22/4/20).

31 G. Forrester, The Conversation blog, 'How Children's Brains Develop to Make them Right- or Left-Handed', 2016: http://theconversation.com/how-childrens-brains-develop-to-make-them-right-or-left-handed-55272 (accessed on 22/4/20).

32 G. Forrester, The Conversation blog, 'How Children's Brains Develop to Make them Right- or Left-Handed', 2016: http://theconversation.com/how-childrens-brains-develop-to-make-them-right-or-left-handed-55272 (accessed on 22/4/20).

33 P. Versfeld, 'The Trouble with W-sitting': https://skillsforaction.com/w-sitting (accessed on 22/4/20).

34 P. Versfeld, 'The Trouble with W-sitting': https://skillsforaction.com/w-sitting (accessed on 22/4/20).

35 I was recently reassessed for hEDS in order to take part in the HEDGE study; the question is still there.

36 @ehlersdanlosuk, Instagram, 7 June 2019.

37 L. Russek, The Ehlers-Danlos Society, 'Self-care for Kids & Teens with Hypermobility Spectrum Disorder', 2017: www.ehlers-danlos.com/wp-content/uploads/Russek-Self-Care-for-Kids-Teens-with-Hypermobility-Spectrum-Disorder-S.pdf (accessed on 25/6/20).

38 L. Russek, The Ehlers-Danlos Society, 'Self-care for Kids & Teens with Hypermobility Spectrum Disorder', 2017: www.ehlers-danlos.com/wp-content/uploads/Russek-Self-Care-for-Kids-Teens-with-Hypermobility-Spectrum-Disorder-S.pdf (accessed on 25/6/20).

39 L. Russek, The Ehlers-Danlos Society, 'Self-care for Kids & Teens with Hypermobility Spectrum Disorder', 2017: www.ehlers-danlos.com/wp-content/uploads/Russek-Self-Care-for-Kids-Teens-with-Hypermobility-Spectrum-Disorder-S.pdf (accessed on 25/6/20).

40 In a straw poll of children's yoga teachers, only one had received any input on working with hypermobility in children.

41 For more information about Iris's work, go to www.mrswallerstribe.earth.

42 For more information about Melissa's work, go to www.facebook.com/intercalm.

43 J. Smith, '10 Myths about Yoga for Children', Mosaic Kids Yoga: https://mosaickidsyoga.com/myths-about-kids-yoga (accessed on 22/4/20).

44 J. Smith, '10 Myths about Yoga for Children', Mosaic Kids Yoga: https://mosaickidsyoga.com/myths-about-kids-yoga (accessed on 22/4/20).

45 L. Howell, YouTube, 'Is Over Stretching Bad?', 2019: https://youtu.be/-fwxTGWlp0g (accessed on 22/4/20).

Chapter 7

1 J. Simmonds, A. Herbland, A. Hakim, N. Ninis, et al. 'Exercise Beliefs and Behaviours of Individuals with Joint Hypermobility Syndrome/Ehlers-Danlos Syndrome – Hypermobility Type', Disability Rehabilitation, 41, 4, 445–455, 2019: www.ncbi.nlm.nih.gov/pubmed/29125009 (accessed on 22/4/20).

2   M. Scheper, J. de Vries, J. Verbunt, R. Engelbert, 'Chronic Pain in Hypermobility Syndrome and Ehlers–Danlos Syndrome (Hypermobility Type): It Is a Challenge', *Journal of Pain Research*, 8, 591–601, 2015: www.ncbi.nlm.nih.gov/pmc/articles/PMC4548768 (accessed on 6/4/20).

3   @anoushehusain, Instagram, 15 May 2019.

4   Posted by Ehlers-Danlos Support UK, Facebook, 23 June 2019.

5   L. Maple, POTS UK, 'How Exercise Has Helped Me': www.potsuk.org/stories/54 (accessed on 22/4/20).

6   N. Pearson, 'Know Pain? A Brief Guide to Understanding Pain for Yoga Therapists', *Yoga Therapy Today*, Summer 2012: https://paincareu.com/wp-content/uploads/2015/10/KnowPain_Yoga_Therapy_Today_2012.pdf (accessed on 22/4/20).

7   The Ehlers-Danlos Society, 'Living in the Grey': www.ehlers-danlos.com/amyac (accessed on 22/4/20).

8   L. Greaves, 'What Is Scaravelli Yoga?': https://welldoing.org/article/yoga-pt-10-what-is-scaravelli-yoga (accessed on 22/4/20).

9   L. Greaves, 'What Is Scaravelli Yoga?': https://welldoing.org/article/yoga-pt-10-what-is-scaravelli-yoga (accessed on 22/4/20).

10 Healthline, 'Hot Yoga: Is It Super-Heated Exercise or a Health Danger?', 2018: www.healthline.com/health-news/hot-yoga-booming-but-it-may-be-bad-for-you-051515#1 (accessed on 22/4/20).

11 It's Yoga International, 'Overview': https://itsyoga.com/the-rocket (accessed on 22/4/20).

12 American Viniyoga Institute, 'What Is Viniyoga?': www.viniyoga.com/about/what-is-viniyoga (accessed on 22/4/20).

13 B. Delaney, 'The Yoga Industry Is Booming – But Does It Make You a Better Person?', *The Guardian*, 17 September 2017: www.theguardian.com/lifeandstyle/2017/sep/17/yoga-better-person-lifestyle-exercise (accessed on 22/4/20).

14 Causely, 'Double Revenue at Your Yoga Studio with a Teacher Training Program': www.causely.com/blog/double-revenue-at-your-yoga-studio-with-a-teacher-training-program (accessed on 22/4/20).

15 C. Jones, Quora, 'How Much Experience is Necessary Before You Get into Yoga Teacher Training', 2018: www.quora.com/how-much-experience-is-necessary-before-you-get-into-yoga-teacher-training (accessed on 22/4/20).

16 For a more detailed discussion of regulation of yoga in the UK see The Independent Yoga Network's 'Regulation: The Facts: www.namaskaram.co.uk/regulation-the-facts (accessed on 22/4/20). For more information on the US situation, see 'Yoga Alliance's Official Stance on Government Regulation': www.yogaalliance.org/about_yoga/article_archive/our_official_stance_on_government_regulation (accessed on 22/4/20).

17 J. Gudmestad, 'The Danger of a Hyperextended Knee and How to Fix It', *Yoga Journal*, 2007: www.yogajournal.com/practice-section/the-hyperextended-knee (accessed on 22/4/20).

18 E. Schiffmann, *Yoga: The Spirit and Practice of Moving into Stillness*, Pocket Books, New York, 1996.

19 R. Keer, J. Butler, 'Physiotherapy and Occupational Therapy in the Hypermobile Adult', in A. Hakim, R. Keer, R. Grahame (eds), *Hypermobility, Fibromyalgia and Chronic Pain*, Churchill Livingstone Elsevier, London, 2010. Free download at: https://epdf.pub/hypermobility-fibromyalgia-and-chronic-pain.html (accessed on 7/4/20).

20 R. Keer, J. Butler, 'Physiotherapy and Occupational Therapy in the Hypermobile Adult', in A. Hakim, R. Keer, R. Grahame (eds), *Hypermobility, Fibromyalgia and Chronic Pain*, Churchill Livingstone Elsevier, London, 2010. Free download at: https://epdf.pub/hypermobility-fibromyalgia-and-chronic-pain.html (accessed on 7/4/20).

21 R. Keer, J. Butler, 'Physiotherapy and Occupational Therapy in the Hypermobile Adult', in A. Hakim, R. Keer, R. Grahame (eds), *Hypermobility, Fibromyalgia and Chronic Pain*, Churchill Livingstone Elsevier, London, 2010. Free download at: https://epdf.pub/hypermobility-fibromyalgia-and-chronic-pain.html (accessed on 7/4/20).

22 A conical massage ball made out of silicon which is designed to mimic the shape of the thumb. I was given a Thumbby™ ten years ago, and it is my absolutely favourite myofascial tool. I use it every day: www.thumbby.com.

23 J. Barnes, 'What Is Myofascial Release': www.myofascialrelease.com/about/definition.aspx (accessed on 22/4/20).

24   H. Kreder, 'Review: Early Mobilisation Is Better Than Cast Immobilisation for Injured Limbs', *British Medical Journal Evidence-Based Medicine*, 10, 118, 2005: https://ebm.bmj.com/content/10/4/118.info (accessed on 22/4/20).

25   Oxford University Hospitals NHS Foundation Trust, Trauma Physiotherapy Department, *Helping Your Knee to Recover After a Ligament Sprain or Rupture: Information for Patients*, 2016, reviewed 2019: www.ouh.nhs.uk/patient-guide/leaflets/files/14217pkneesprain.pdf (accessed on 22/4/20).

26   N. Pearson, 'Yoga Therapy in Practice: Yoga for People in Pain', *International Journal of Yoga Therapy*, 18, 2008: https://paincareu.com/wp-content/uploads/2019/02/IJYT-Yoga_Chronic_2008.pdf (accessed on 22/4/20).

27   N. Pearson, 'Yoga Therapy in Practice: Yoga for People in Pain', *International Journal of Yoga Therapy*, 18, 2008: https://paincareu.com/wp-content/uploads/2019/02/IJYT-Yoga_Chronic_2008.pdf (accessed on 22/4/20).

28   N. Pearson, 'Yoga Therapy in Practice: Yoga for People in Pain', *International Journal of Yoga Therapy*, 18, 2008: https://paincareu.com/wp-content/uploads/2019/02/IJYT-Yoga_Chronic_2008.pdf (accessed on 22/4/20).

29   J. Tran, ShutUpAndYoga, 'Recovering From Yoga: A Sobering Tale of Injuries, Dogma and Waking the F*ck up', website: https://shutupandyoga.com/recovering-from-yoga-a-sobering-tale-of-injuries-dogma-and-waking-the-fck-up/?fbclid=IwAR3mW0qxgWTnZDhA393n9ZtOTnVhF9WHgBdEAG6weVKMu5cXkQdZg7U06M0 (accessed on 22/4/20).

30   R. Keer, J. Butler, 'Physiotherapy and Occupational Therapy in the Hypermobile Adult', in A. Hakim, R. Keer, R. Grahame (eds), *Hypermobility, Fibromyalgia and Chronic Pain*, Churchill Livingstone Elsevier, London, 2010. Free download at: https://epdf.pub/hypermobility-fibromyalgia-and-chronic-pain.html (accessed on 7/4/20).

31   Fitness coach Caroline Jordan has a number of challenging chair cardio workouts. Find them on YouTube.

Index